Artificial Neural Networks for IoT-Enabled Smart Applications

Artificial Neural Networks for IoT-Enabled Smart Applications

Editors

Andrei Velichko
Dmitry Korzun
Alexander Meigal

MDPI • Basel • Beijing • Wuhan • Barcelona • Belgrade • Manchester • Tokyo • Cluj • Tianjin

Editors
Andrei Velichko
Petrozavodsk State University
Petrozavodsk, Russia

Dmitry Korzun
Petrozavodsk State University
Petrozavodsk, Russia

Alexander Meigal
Petrozavodsk State University
Petrozavodsk, Russia

Editorial Office
MDPI
St. Alban-Anlage 66
4052 Basel, Switzerland

This is a reprint of articles from the Special Issue published online in the open access journal *Sensors* (ISSN 1424-8220) (available at: https://www.mdpi.com/journal/sensors/special_issues/IoT_SmartApp).

For citation purposes, cite each article independently as indicated on the article page online and as indicated below:

LastName, A.A.; LastName, B.B.; LastName, C.C. Article Title. *Journal Name* **Year**, *Volume Number*, Page Range.

ISBN 978-3-0365-8428-7 (Hbk)
ISBN 978-3-0365-8429-4 (PDF)

Contents

About the Editors . . . . **vii**

Andrei Velichko, Dmitry Korzun and Alexander Meigal
Artificial Neural Networks for IoT-Enabled Smart Applications: Recent Trends
Reprinted from: *Sensors* **2023**, *23*, 4853, doi:10.3390/10.3390/s23104853 . . . . **1**

Panagiotis Kasnesis, Vasileios Doulgerakis, Dimitris Uzunidis, Dimitris G. Kogias, Susana I. Funcia, Marta B. González, et al.
Deep Learning Empowered Wearable-Based Behavior Recognition for Search and Rescue Dogs
Reprinted from: *Sensors* **2022**, *22*, 993, doi:10.3390/10.3390/s22030993 . . . . **5**

Mustafa Aljasim and Rasha Kashef
E2DR: A Deep Learning Ensemble-Based Driver Distraction Detection with Recommendations Model
Reprinted from: *Sensors* **2022**, *22*, 1858, doi:10.3390/10.3390/s22051858 . . . . **31**

Ana-Luiza Rusnac and Ovidiu Grigore
CNN Architectures and Feature Extraction Methods for EEG Imaginary Speech Recognition
Reprinted from: *Sensors* **2022**, *22*, 4679, doi:10.3390/10.3390/s22134679 . . . . **55**

Mehmet Tahir Huyut and Andrei Velichko
Diagnosis and Prognosis of COVID-19 Disease Using Routine Blood Values and LogNNet Neural Network
Reprinted from: *Sensors* **2022**, *22*, 4820, doi:10.3390/10.3390/s22134820 . . . . **75**

Juan Carlos Cepeda-Pacheco and Mari Carmen Domingo
Deep Learning and 5G and Beyond for Child Drowning Prevention in Swimming Pools
Reprinted from: *Sensors* **2022**, *22*, 7684, doi:10.3390/10.3390/s22197684 . . . . **101**

Andrei Velichko, Mehmet Tahir Huyut, Maksim Belyaev, Yuriy Izotov and Dmitry Korzun
Machine Learning Sensors for Diagnosis of COVID-19 Disease Using Routine Blood Values for Internet of Things Application
Reprinted from: *Sensors* **2022**, *22*, 7886, doi:10.3390/10.3390/s22207886 . . . . **125**

Alexander Y. Meigal, Liudmila I. Gerasimova-Meigal, Sergey A. Reginya, Alexey V. Soloviev and Alex P. Moschevikin
Gait Characteristics Analyzed with Smartphone IMU Sensors in Subjects with Parkinsonism under the Conditions of "Dry" Immersion
Reprinted from: *Sensors* **2022**, *22*, 7915, doi:10.3390/10.3390/s22207915 . . . . **155**

Sarita Limbu and Sivanesan Dakshanamurthy
Predicting Chemical Carcinogens Using a Hybrid Neural Network Deep Learning Method
Reprinted from: *Sensors* **2022**, *22*, 8185, doi:10.3390/10.3390/s22218185 . . . . **173**

Cheng-Han Liu, Tsun-Hua Yang and Obaja Triputera Wijaya
Development of an Artificial Neural Network Algorithm Embedded in an On-Site Sensor for Water Level Forecasting
Reprinted from: *Sensors* **2022**, *22*, 8532, doi:10.3390/10.3390/s22218532 . . . . **189**

Umara Umar, Sanam Nayab, Rabia Irfan, Muazzam A. Khan, Amna Umer
E-Cardiac Care: A Comprehensive Systematic Literature Review
Reprinted from: *Sensors* **2022**, *22*, 8073, doi:10.3390/10.3390/s22208073 . . . . **211**

About the Editors

Andrei Velichko

Dr. Andrei Velichko received a Ph.D. degree in physics and mathematics with the specialization "Physical Electronics" from Petrozavodsk State University, Petrozavodsk, Russia, in 2002. From 2001 to 2015, he worked as a senior lecturer in the Department of Electronic and Ion Devices, and since 2016, he has worked as a leading research scientist at PetrSU. Dr. Velichko's research mainly focuses on artificial neural networks, oxide ReRAM, and metal–insulator transitions. He is the author of the LogNNet neural network configuration for IoT devices as well as the time series entropy estimation algorithm called Neural Network Entropy (NNetEn).

Dmitry Korzun

Dr. Dmitry Korzun received his B.Sc. (1997) and M.Sc (1999) degrees in Applied Mathematics and Computer Science from Petrozavodsk State University (PetrSU, Russia). He received a Ph.D. degree in Physics and Mathematics from St. Petersburg State University (Russia) in 2002. He is an Associate Professor in the Department of Computer Science of PetrSU (since 2003 and ongoing). He was a Visiting Research Scientist at the Helsinki Institute for Information Technology HIIT, Aalto University, Finland (2005-2014). In 2014–2016, he performed the duties of Vice Dean for Research in the Faculty of Mathematics and Information Technology of PetrSU. Since 2014, he has acted as a Leading Research Scientist at PetrSU, originating research and development activity within fundamental and applied research projects on emerging topics in ubiquitous computing, smart spaces, and Internet technology. Dmitry Korzun serves on technical program committees and editorial boards of a number of international conferences and journals. His research interests include the modeling and evaluation of distributed systems, mathematical modeling and concept engineering of cyber–physical systems, ubiquitous computing and smart spaces, Internet of Things and its applications, software engineering and programming methods, algorithm design and complexity, linear Diophantine analysis and its applications, theory of formal languages and parsing. His educational activity started in 1997 in the Faculty of Mathematics of PetrSU.

Alexander Meigal

Prof. Alexander Meigal received a Candidate of Sciences degree in Biology in the field of "Physiology" from the Institute of Experimental Physiology, St. Petersburg, Russia (1991), and a Doctor of Science degree in Medicine from Archangelsk State Medical University, Russia (1997). He has been a Head of the Department of Human and Animal Physiology and Pathophysiology at the Medical Institute of PetrSU since 20018, and Head of the laboratory of novel methods in physiology, PetrSU, since 2014. He was also a Visiting Research Scientist at the University of Eastern Finland (Kuopio, Finland, 2006–2014). His research interests are in the field of signal processing and evaluation of electromyogram (EMG), accelerogram, heart rate variability (HRV), kinematics, nonlinear dynamics of EMG and HRV, diagnostics of Parkinsonism and multiple sclerosis, muscle tone disorders, tremor, gravitational and space physiology, thermoregulation, wearable and textile sensors, and the instrumentalization of tools and gadgets, including smartphones.

sensors

MDPI

Editorial

Artificial Neural Networks for IoT-Enabled Smart Applications: Recent Trends

Andrei Velichko [1,*], Dmitry Korzun [2] and Alexander Meigal [3]

1 Institute of Physics and Technology, Petrozavodsk State University, 33 Lenin Ave., 185910 Petrozavodsk, Russia
2 Department of Computer Science, Institute of Mathematics and Information Technology, Petrozavodsk State University, 33 Lenin Ave., 185910 Petrozavodsk, Russia; dkorzun@cs.karelia.ru
3 Medical Institute, Petrozavodsk State University, 33 Lenin Ave., 185910 Petrozavodsk, Russia; meigal@petrsu.ru
* Correspondence: velichko@petrsu.ru

In the age of neural networks and the Internet of Things (IoT), the search for new neural network architectures capable of operating on devices with limited computing power and small memory size is becoming an urgent agenda. Trends in the development of artificial intelligence (AI) applications in the field of the Internet of Things include smart healthcare services [1–5], smart object-recognition [6–8], smart environment monitoring [9,10], and smart disaster rescue [11]. Traditionally, such applications operate in real time. For example, security camera-based object-recognition tasks operate with detection intervals of 500 ms to capture and respond to target events. The data processing of human health and physiological parameters from different sensors (heart rate monitoring, glucose monitoring, oxygen saturation, etc.) generally requires immediate processing. Often, commercial smart IoT devices transfer information to the cloud for subsequent intelligent processing. However, stable network connections are not available everywhere, and it is a limitation for meeting real-time requirements. The solution to this problem can be the execution of information processing using neural networks installed directly on IoT devices. In this case, the quality of the Internet connection would not have a significant impact. Enabling artificial intelligence directly on the device is a challenge because of the limited computing power and small memory size of IoT devices. Frequently, smart applications need to run on a lightweight OS with a minimal set of libraries that imposes limitations on the operation of resource-intensive neural networks.

AI technologies for IoT devices and edge computing are demanded in mobile healthcare (m-Health), as well as in close application domains. Ambient intelligence (AmI) environments are constructed in IoT domains to provide smart services based on real-time analysis of human cognitive and motion functions. This Special Issue focuses on recent developments in the constantly growing application field of computing technologies and artificial intelligence algorithms. It includes new approaches to the organization of artificial intelligence on edge devices, as well as the organization of modular, feed forward, distributed, reservoir, recurrent, convolutional, and deep neural networks for various IoT-enabled smart applications. The guest editors are Andrei Velichko (Institute of Physics and Technology), Dmitry Korzun (Institute of Mathematics and Information Technology), and и Alexander Meigal (Medical Institute); they are all from Petrozavodsk State University, Russia.

The Special Issue collects eleven papers to provide a multi-domain overview of the trends and developments in the edge computing and starts with the illustration of achievements in smart healthcare services. The digitalization of healthcare driven by the IoT and AmI leads to the effective use of sensors, when various parameters of the human body are instantly tracked and processed in daily life [1,2]. The concept of machine learning sensors is applied to the diagnosis of COVID-19 as IoT application in healthcare and ambient

Citation: Velichko, A.; Korzun, D.; Meigal, A. Artificial Neural Networks for IoT-Enabled Smart Applications: Recent Trends. *Sensors* **2023**, *23*, 4853. https://doi.org/10.3390/s23104853

Received: 10 May 2023
Accepted: 15 May 2023
Published: 18 May 2023

assisted living. An important task is to determine the status of infection with COVID-19 using various diagnostic tests. This study provides a fast, reliable, and cost-effective alternative tool for diagnosing COVID-19 based on routine blood values measured at clinic admission. Popular machine learning classifiers were studied and their important features were identified to ensure the high accuracy of disease diagnostics. The study [2] continues the topic of COVID-19 diagnostic and reviews the routine blood values using a backward feature elimination algorithm and the LogNNet reservoir neural network. The proposed method reduces the negative pressures on the health sector and helps doctors to understand the pathogenesis of COVID-19 using the key blood values. The method demonstrates high opportunity of the LogNNet network to be applied in IoT smart applications.

An IoT-enabled system to monitor gait in subjects with Parkinson's disease is presented in study [3]. Parkinson's disease is one of the most studied pathologies in the field of neurology and is suitable for application of science-intensive study methods, virtual reality technologies and even robotics. Wearable sensors and IoT-enabled technologies look promising for monitoring motor activity and gait in Parkinson's disease patients. The gait was measured and characterized with help of the accelerometer signal acquired from inertial measurement unit of a smartphone attached to the head during the timed up and go test. Smartphones as a measuring device are well suited for the creation of IoT-enabled systems. The use of accelerometer signals received from a smartphone inertial measurement unit creates high potential for AI-supported systems and makes the proposed method applicable not only in healthcare laboratories but in the daily life settings.

Smart healthcare applications, the Internet of Things (IoT), and artificial intelligence are arguably the most appropriate customized solutions for such shortcomings of traditional healthcare systems, such as long waiting times, unnecessary long trips to health centers, high costs, and mandatory periodic doctor visits. The comprehensive literature review [4] determines the impact of IoT, AI, various communication technologies, sensor networks, and disease detection in Cardiac healthcare. The results of the review show that deep learning is emerging as a promising technology along with the combination of IoT in the field of cardiac care with increased accuracy and real-time clinical monitoring. In addition, this study points out the main advantages and major challenges of e-cardiology in the areas of IoT and AI.

Another illustration of the effective application of neural networks in healthcare is presented in study [5]. Speech is a complex mechanism that allows us to communicate our needs, desires, and thoughts. In some cases of nervous dysfunction, this ability is severely affected, making daily activities that require communication difficult. This study explores various options for an intelligent imaginary speech recognition system that can be installed on low-cost devices with limited resources. The authors used a method based on covariance in the frequency domain, which performed better than other methods in the time domain. Several architectures of convolutional neural networks have been studied and it has been demonstrated that a more complex architecture does not necessarily lead to better results. The results prove that cheap IoT devices can be effectively used in speech recognition and contribute to the development of IoT-enabled smart applications.

The realm of smart object-recognition applications of AI systems is presented in the subsequent articles [6–8]. Driver assistants have become a more and more popular class of smart IoT-enabled smart applications, as illustrated in study [6] that detects distracting actions in driver activities. According to the World Health Organization, the increase in car accidents is a major problem in today's transportation systems, and is the eighth leading cause of death worldwide. More than 80% of traffic accidents are caused by distraction while driving. A practical approach to solving this problem is to introduce quantitative indicators of driver activity and develop a classification system that identifies distracting activities. Authors implemented a portfolio of different ensemble deep learning models that have been proven to effectively classify driver distractions and provide in-vehicle recommendations to minimize distraction levels and improve safety. Another lifesaving application based on deep learning is a child drowning prevention system [7]. The proposed deep convolutional neural networks-based models can be used to automatically detect the possible distractions of a caregiver who is supervising a child and generate alerts to warn them. The system was tested in a swimming pool, and we think it could be implemented in natural water reservoirs to avoid possible child drowning. Such smart applications for the rapid detection of dangerous situations are of critical importance, as they are able to observe persons and their activity more effectively than humans.

For the IoT-enabled smart applications, point clouds are one of the most widely used data formats created by depth sensors. Research on feature extraction from disordered and irregular point cloud data has advanced recently. The overview [8] of the different types of models is presented, and studies of point clouds and remote sensing problems have been carried out using deep learning methods. It is concluded that convolutional neural networks achieve the best performance in various remote sensing applications that operate directly with raw cloud data. The lightweight models are especially important for IoT edge computing.

The research direction of smart environment monitoring is presented by the study [9], in which a model of artificial neural network was integrated into a Raspberry Pi-based sensor to implement edge computing for hourly river level prediction. The model that consists of a three-layer perceptron is able to predict river levels with a high degree of accuracy using only previously observed water levels, precipitation, and runoff information as input, without the need for other hydrological and meteorological parameters. This study is a first attempt to combine real-time customized sensors and artificial neural network algorithms in practice. The model was built into a low-cost, open-source, and low-energy-consumption custom sensor to forecast the water level. A high level of model performance applied to real events, and the low-cost system is of interest for environmental monitoring. Another potential reference case for the development of smart IoT-enabled systems for environmental monitoring is presented in the study of determining the carcinogenicity of thousands of wide-variety classes of real-life exposure chemicals [10]. Authors have developed carcinogen prediction models based on the hybrid neural network deep learning method. The proposed model has a high potential for use in various IoT environmental projects.

Smart disaster rescue is presented by an interesting development of a wearable device for search dogs that recognizes the behavior of a dog when a victim is found, using deep learning models [11]. With their exceptional sense of smell and hearing, search and rescue dogs are important in first aid because they are able to locate a victim in conditions that are difficult for humans to reach. The authors propose an implementation of a wearable device that supports deep learning, including a base station, a mobile application, and a cloud infrastructure. The device can, firstly, track the activity, sounds and location of the search and rescue dog in real time, and, secondly, recognize and alert the rescue team whenever the dog spots a victim. For activity recognition, deep convolutional neural networks were used for classifying dog sounds, as well as inertial sensors. The developed deep learning models operated on a wearable IoT device. The functioning of the system was tested in two separate search and rescue scenarios, which allowed to successfully locate the victim and inform the rescue team in real time based on IoT technology.

In conclusion, this Special Issue illustrates advanced cases of using the AI technology for IoT-enabled smart applications. Each case demonstrates a promising trend for applying AI in IoT environments, making a step towards the effective use of modern technologies in our everyday life.

Author Contributions: All authors contributed equally to this editorial. All authors have read and agreed to the published version of the manuscript.

Funding: The first part of this research is implemented with financial support by Russian Science Foundation, project no. 22-11-20040 (https://rscf.ru/en/project/22-11-20040/, accessed on 1 May 2023) jointly with Republic of Karelia and funding from Venture Investment Fund of Republic of Karelia (VIF RK). The concept of machine learning sensor is studied using practical examples of COVID-19 infectious disease and IoT-enabled monitoring of human gait. Additionally, edge-oriented sensorics are studied for implementing smart object-recognition. The second part of the research was supported by the Russian Science Foundation (grant no. 22-11-00055, https://rscf.ru/en/project/22-11-00055/, accessed on 30 March 2023). Diagnosis and prognosis of COVID-19 disease using the LogNNet Neural Network and an overview of the directions of smart environment monitoring and smart disaster rescue were made.

Acknowledgments: The authors express their gratitude to Andrei Rikkiev for valuable comments made in the course of the article translation and revision.

Conflicts of Interest: The authors declare no conflict of interest.

References

1. Velichko, A.; Huyut, M.T.; Belyaev, M.; Izotov, Y.; Korzun, D. Machine Learning Sensors for Diagnosis of COVID-19 Disease Using Routine Blood Values for Internet of Things Application. *Sensors* **2022**, *22*, 7886. [CrossRef] [PubMed]
2. Huyut, M.T.; Velichko, A. Diagnosis and Prognosis of COVID-19 Disease Using Routine Blood Values and LogNNet Neural Network. *Sensors* **2022**, *22*, 4820. [CrossRef] [PubMed]
3. Meigal, A.Y.; Gerasimova-Meigal, L.I.; Reginya, S.A.; Soloviev, A.V.; Moschevikin, A.P. Gait Characteristics Analyzed with Smartphone IMU Sensors in Subjects with Parkinsonism under the Conditions of "Dry" Immersion. *Sensors* **2022**, *22*, 7915. [CrossRef] [PubMed]
4. Umar, U.; Nayab, S.; Irfan, R.; Khan, M.A.; Umer, A. E-Cardiac Care: A Comprehensive Systematic Literature Review. *Sensors* **2022**, *22*, 8073. [CrossRef] [PubMed]
5. Rusnac, A.-L.; Grigore, O. CNN Architectures and Feature Extraction Methods for EEG Imaginary Speech Recognition. *Sensors* **2022**, *22*, 4679. [CrossRef] [PubMed]
6. Aljasim, M.; Kashef, R. E2DR: A Deep Learning Ensemble-Based Driver Distraction Detection with Recommendations Model. *Sensors* **2022**, *22*, 1858. [CrossRef] [PubMed]
7. Cepeda-Pacheco, J.C.; Domingo, M.C. Deep Learning and 5G and Beyond for Child Drowning Prevention in Swimming Pools. *Sensors* **2022**, *22*, 7684. [CrossRef] [PubMed]
8. Diab, A.; Kashef, R.; Shaker, A. Deep Learning for LiDAR Point Cloud Classification in Remote Sensing. *Sensors* **2022**, *22*, 7868. [CrossRef] [PubMed]
9. Liu, C.-H.; Yang, T.-H.; Wijaya, O.T. Development of an Artificial Neural Network Algorithm Embedded in an On-Site Sensor for Water Level Forecasting. *Sensors* **2022**, *22*, 8532. [CrossRef] [PubMed]
10. Limbu, S.; Dakshanamurthy, S. Predicting Chemical Carcinogens Using a Hybrid Neural Network Deep Learning Method. *Sensors* **2022**, *22*, 8185. [CrossRef] [PubMed]
11. Kasnesis, P.; Doulgerakis, V.; Uzunidis, D.; Kogias, D.G.; Funcia, S.I.; González, M.B.; Giannousis, C.; Patrikakis, C.Z. Deep Learning Empowered Wearable-Based Behavior Recognition for Search and Rescue Dogs. *Sensors* **2022**, *22*, 933. [CrossRef] [PubMed]

sensors MDPI

Article

Deep Learning Empowered Wearable-Based Behavior Recognition for Search and Rescue Dogs

Panagiotis Kasnesis [1,*], Vasileios Doulgerakis [1], Dimitris Uzunidis [1], Dimitris G. Kogias [1], Susana I. Funcia [2], Marta B. González [2], Christos Giannousis [1] and Charalampos Z. Patrikakis [1]

1 Department of Electrical and Electronic Engineering, University of West Attica, 12244 Athens, Greece; v.doulger@uniwa.gr (V.D.); duzunidis@uniwa.gr (D.U.); dimikog@uniwa.gr (D.G.K.); giannousis@uniwa.gr (C.G.); bpatr@uniwa.gr (C.Z.P.)
2 Spanish School of Rescue and Detection with Dogs (ESDP), 28524 Madrid, Spain; s.izquierdo@escuelasalvamento.org (S.I.F.); esdp.eu@escuelasalvamento.org (M.B.G.)
* Correspondence: pkasnesis@uniwa.gr; Tel.: +30-210-5381549

Abstract: Search and Rescue (SaR) dogs are important assets in the hands of first responders, as they have the ability to locate the victim even in cases where the vision and or the sound is limited, due to their inherent talents in olfactory and auditory senses. In this work, we propose a deep-learning-assisted implementation incorporating a wearable device, a base station, a mobile application, and a cloud-based infrastructure that can first monitor in real-time the activity, the audio signals, and the location of a SaR dog, and second, recognize and alert the rescuing team whenever the SaR dog spots a victim. For this purpose, we employed deep Convolutional Neural Networks (CNN) both for the activity recognition and the sound classification, which are trained using data from inertial sensors, such as 3-axial accelerometer and gyroscope and from the wearable's microphone, respectively. The developed deep learning models were deployed on the wearable device, while the overall proposed implementation was validated in two discrete search and rescue scenarios, managing to successfully spot the victim (i.e., obtained F1-score more than 99%) and inform the rescue team in real-time for both scenarios.

Keywords: deep learning; canine activity recognition; bark detection; wearable computing; search and rescue system

Citation: Kasnesis, P.; Doulgerakis, V.; Uzunidis, D.; Kogias, D.G.; Funcia, S.I.; González, M.B.; Giannousis, C.; Patrikakis, C.Z. Deep Learning Empowered Wearable-Based Behavior Recognition for Search and Rescue Dogs. *Sensors* **2022**, *22*, 993. https://doi.org/10.3390/s22030993

Academic Editors: Andrei Velichko, Dmitry Korzun and Alexander Meigal

Received: 20 December 2021
Accepted: 25 January 2022
Published: 27 January 2022

1. Introduction

Animal Activity Recognition (AAR) and monitoring is an emerging research area enhanced mainly by the recent advances in computing, Deep Learning (DL) algorithms, and motion sensors. AAR attracted significant attention as it can provide significant insights about the behavior, health condition, and location of the observing animal [1]. In addition, if a proper network implementation is considered (e.g., with the proper devices, software, and communication protocol) the monitoring of the animal can be performed in real-time to allow exploitation of AAR for various purposes, e.g., study of the interaction between different animals, search and rescue missions [2], protection of animals from poaching and theft, etc. [3]. To perform this, the use of inertial sensors is mandated, such as accelerometers, gyroscopes, and magnetometers as well as a Machine Learning (ML) method, which after the proper training can accurately classify the animal activity [4].

Acknowledging the fact that AAR is a rich source of information that not only provides insights into animals life and well-being but also about their environment, over the past years, several works reporting on the use of animal activity recognition were published, increasingly focusing on the use of ML [5], while several open access datasets [6] were available, assisting the development of models and tools for accurate activity recognition of different animals.

In this work, we focus on the Dog Activity Recognition (DAR) for search and rescue (SaR) missions. SaR dogs are important assets in the hands of first responders due to their inherent talents with olfactory and auditory senses. However, in some cases the dog handler is impossible to be present in the same spot with the SaR dog, and thus, a life-critical amount of time is spent as the dog must return to the trainer and guide him to the victim [7]. To solve this problem, we introduce a novel implementation comprised of a wearable device, a base station, a cloud server, a mobile application, and Deep Convolutional Neural Networks (CNN), which were shown in [8–10] to be more accurate compared with that of other ML algorithms due to their ability to extract features automatically. More specifically, we developed a back-mounted wearable device for the SaR dogs that can:

1. collect audio and motion signals, exploiting its inertial sensors (e.g., 3-axial accelerometer and 3-axial gyroscope) and the embedded microphone;
2. process the produced sensor signals using DL algorithms (e.g., Deep CNNs);
3. communicate the critical message via the candidate network architecture; and
4. display in real-time the dog activity and location to its handler via a mobile application.

The proposed implementation is validated in two SaR scenarios managing to successfully locating the victim and communicating this message to the first responders in real-time with more than 99% F1-score.

In the rest of the paper, we analyze the related work in the field to provide a wider view in the problem we address (Section 2). In Section 3, we propose the core modules of our implementation along with their details and specifications, and we illustrate the overall network architecture developed to communicate the messages between the first responder and the SaR dog. Section 4 elaborates the data collection/annotation steps as well as the employed CNN architectures, while in Section 5 we evaluate the algorithmic results in terms of efficiency and efficacy. Next, in Section 6 the validation of the proposed solution is discussed, proving that our prototype satisfies all the desired functional and nonfunctional requirements. Finally, Section 7 discusses the obtained results, the limitations of the approach, and the future steps, while Section 8 concludes the paper.

2. Related Work

In the current section, we present the related works presenting results on canine behavior recognition, audio classification, and existing SaR systems based on animal wearables.

2.1. Activity Recognition

In prior research, animal activity recognition and monitoring was exploited to study various types of animals, spanning from livestock animals [10–15] to wild animals [16–18]. In the former case, the animal monitoring can (a) optimize the asset management, as the animals can be maintained always within preset "virtual fences", (b) provide insights about the animals' health through tracking the fluctuation on their activity levels, and (c) designate the optimal pastures. In wild animals, the animal activity monitoring can (a) minimize the poaching illegal activity and stock theft, (b) extract the state of health of the observed populations, and (c) assist the observations about the behavior of the wild animals and the interactions between them and other species.

In the category of pet animals, a literature review which analyzes the different technologies used to monitor various target features, such as location, health, behavior, etc. can be found in [19]. In the domain of DAR, these results can aid us towards a better interpretation of the everyday routine of the animals and their needs, which in turn can directly benefit the interaction with their handlers or can be exploited to perceive the behavior SaR units, providing valuable information to their trainers (e.g., victim discovery). The field of DAR emerged over the last decade due to the availability of low-cost sensors and smart devices that can acquire data and perform the ML algorithmic procedure in real-time [6,20–28]. Usually, the sensors are located in the back, collar, withers, and tail of the dog, while the employed sensors are mainly 3-axial accelerometers, 3-axial gyroscopes and sensors which monitor biometric data (e.g., heart rate). After completing the data collection process from the various sensors and performing their proper preprocessing, the data are then fed into an ML algorithm for training to classify any forthcoming activity.

For the purposes of DAR, various ML algorithms were utilized to attain sufficient accuracy. A k-NN classifier was employed in [21] to classify 17 different activities by studying the naturalistic behavior of 18 dogs attaining an accuracy of about 70%. In [25], the SVM (Support Vector Machines) classifier was applied into a dataset that comprised 24 dogs performing seven discrete activities and attained an accuracy of above 90%. Further, in [28], the accuracy of various ML classification algorithms was evaluated in a dataset comprising 10 dogs of different breeds, ages, sizes and gender performing seven different activities. The employed algorithms were Random Forest, SVM, k-NN, Naïve Bayes, and Artificial Neural Network (ANN). ANN outperformed the other four algorithms in activity detection, whilst Random Forest outperformed the other four in emotion detection. The attainable accuracy exceeded 96% in all cases. A recent study [6] in dog behavior recognition examined the optimal sensor placement in the dog, through a comparison of various algorithms (e.g., SVM). In particular, the authors attached two sensor devices to each dog, one on the back of the dog in a harness and one on the neck collar. The movement sensor at the back yielded up to 91% accuracy in classifying the dog activities and the sensor placed at the collar yielded 75% accuracy at best. These results helped the current work to decide the optimal sensor placement, which was mounting a harness on the back of the SaR dog with the developed device in it. Finally, the authors in [29] created a huge dataset exploiting a 3-axial accelerometer and collecting data from more than 2500 dogs of multiple breeds. Then they trained a deep learning classifier which was then validated for a real-world detection of eating and drinking behavior. The validated results attained a true positive rate of 95.3% and 94.9%for eating and drinking activities, respectively. The details of the related work on DAR are shown in Table 1.

Table 1. Summary of related work on Dog Activity Recognition (DAR).

Ref.	Location	Sensors	No. of Activities	Subjects	Algorithms
[20]	back	3-axial accelerometer and gyroscope	-	2 dogs of 2 breeds	only measurements from the sensors were performed
[21]	collar	3-axial accelerometer	17	18 dogs of 13 breeds	k-NN
[22]	collar	3-axial accelerometer	8	51 dogs of mainly 8 breeds	analytical algorithms created by the developers
[23]	collar	Heart rate, galvanic skin resistance, and body temperature	-	various dogs	only measurements from the sensors were performed
[24]	collar	3-axial accelerometer	-	6 dogs	generalized linear mixed effect models fit to the activity
[25]	withers	3-axial accelerometer and gyroscope	7	24 dogs of 2 breeds	SVM
[26]	back	ECG, PPG, Inertial Measurement Unit (IMU)	various	5 dogs of 4 breeds	only measurements from the sensors were performed

Table 1. *Cont.*

Ref.	Location	Sensors	No. of Activities	Subjects	Algorithms
[27]	collar, vest, and forelimb	3-axial accelerometer	various	4 dogs of 4 breeds	only measurements from the sensors were performed
[28]	collar, tail	3-axial accelerometer and gyroscope	7	10 dogs of 9 breeds	Random Forest, SVM, KNN, Naïve Bayes, ANN
[6]	back, collar	3-axial accelerometer and gyroscope	7	45 dogs of 26 breeds	Decision Tree, SVM
[29]	collar	3-axial accelerometer	15	more than 2500 dogs of multiple breeds	Deep learning classifier

2.2. Audio Classification

Similar to wearable-based activity recognition, over the last years, there were proposed several audio signal processing techniques relying on DL algorithms and were proved to achieve better results than baseline ML algorithms [30]. DL algorithms, such as Deep CNNs, possess the ability to increase their performance as the training dataset grows; thus, the authors in [31] applied well-known CNN architectures, which were employed successfully in computer vision tasks, to test their effectiveness on classifying large-scale audio data. The networks architectures they used were a fully connected ANN, an AlexNet [32], a VGG [33], an Inception V3 [34], and a ResNet-50 [35]; these networks were trained and evaluated using AudioSet, which consists of 2,084,320 human-labeled 10-second audio clips drawn from YouTube videos. The audio classes are based on an audio ontology [36], which is specified as a hierarchical graph of event categories, covering a wide range of human and animal sounds, musical instruments and genres, and common everyday environmental sounds. Their experiments showed that the ResNet-50 model, which had the most layers (i.e., it was deeper than the others), achieved the best results.

In addition to this, CNNs are also state-of-the-art models, even for relative smaller audio datasets consisting of a few thousand samples. Salamon and Bello [37] compare a baseline system (i.e., using MFCCs features) with unsupervised feature learning performed on patches of PCA-whitened log-scaled mel-spectrograms using the UrbanSound8K dataset. In particular, they utilized the spherical k-means algorithm [38] followed by the Random Forests algorithm and managed an average classification accuracy 5% higher than the baseline system. Furthermore, Karol J. Piczak [30] obtained state-of-the-art results for the UrbanSound8K dataset, training a relatively shallow CNN (two convolutional layers), which had as input the log-scaled mel-spectograms of the audio clips. The proposed CNN model had an average accuracy of about 73.1% against the 68% average accuracy of the baseline model, despite the fact that it seemed to overfit the training data. A deeper, VGG-like CNN model (five convolutional layers) was implemented by A. Kumar [39] and used on the UltraSound8K dataset, reaching a 73.7% average accuracy.

Finally, data augmentation techniques were adopted by the researchers to increase the number of the audio samples. To this end, Salamon and Bello [40] explored the influence of different augmentation techniques ((a) Time Stretching; (b) Dynamic Range Compression; (c) Pitch Shifting; and (d) Adding Background Noise) on the performance of a proposed CNN architecture, and they obtained an average accuracy close to 79% using recordings of the ESC-50 (2000 clips) and ESC-10 (400 clips) datasets [41]. Moreover, Karol J Piczak [41] utilized random time delays to the original recordings of the ESC-50 and ESC-10 datasets. The CNN architecture achieved better accuracy results from the baseline model for both datasets, while in the case of the ESC-50, the difference between the average accuracies was over 20% (baseline accuracy: 44%, best CNN: 64.5%).

2.3. Existing SaR Solutions Based on Animal Wearables

SaR systems are vital components when it comes to disaster recovery due to the fact that every second might be life-critical. Trained animals, such as dogs (i.e., K9s), are exploited by SaR teams due to their augmented senses (e.g., smell), and their small size is ideal for searching under the debris for survivors.

The authors in [2] developed a two-part system consisting of a wearable computer interface for working SaR dogs communicating with their handler via a mobile application. The wearable comprised a bite sensor and a GPS to display the K9s location in the mobile application. The SaR dog bites the bringsel, which is equipped with the bite sensor to notify its handler. In addition to this, the work in [42] demonstrates several interfaces developed for animal–computer interaction purposes, which could be used in SaR missions for notifying the canine handler, such as bite sensors, proximity sensor, and tug sensor. Furthermore, in [7,43] the use of head gestures is examined to establish communication between the SaR dogs and the handlers. The developed wearable is added in a collar and is comprised by motion sensors (3-axial accelerometer, gyroscope and magnetometer), while the systems analyzes motion signals produced by the canine wearable using dynamic time warping. Each detected head gesture is paired with a predetermined message that is voiced to the humans by a smart phone. To this end, the participating K9s were specifically trained to perform the appropriate gesture.

Existing patented canine wearables, such as [44,45], could also be used for SaR purposes. A wirelessly interactive dog collar is presented in [45]; it allows voice commands and tracking over long distances, along with features that facilitate tracking and visualization, exploiting its embedded sensors (GPS, microphone, speaker, light). Moreover, in [44] an enhanced animal collar is presented. This device consists of extra sensors, such as camera, thermographic camera, and infrared camera to enable the transmission of the captured images, in addition to audio signals.

Finally, the animal-machine collaboration was also explored. The authors in [46] introduce a new approach to overcome the mobility problem of canines through narrow paths in the debris utilizing a robot snake. The SaR dog carries this small robot, and when it is close to the victim it barks to release the robot that locates the trapped person. The robot snake is equipped with a microphone and a camera. Rat cyborg is another option for SaR missions [47]. The system is implanted with microelectrodes in the brain of a rat, through which the outer electrical stimuli can be delivered into the brain in vivo to control its behaviors. The authors state that the cyborg system could be useful in search and rescue missions where the rat handler can navigate through the debris by exploiting a camera mounted on the rats.

Table 2 summarizes the aforementioned works including our solution, in terms of equipped sensors/actuators and their capabilities (i.e., communication with handler and victim, edge data processing, delivery package, search through debris, extra animal training, no welfare concerns, no rescuer guidance needed).

Table 2. Summary of the existing SaR solutions based on animal wearables.

Ref.	Animal	Sensors/Actuators	Communic. with Rescuer	Edge Data Processing	Delivery Package	Communication with Victim	Search through Debris	Extra Animal Training	No Welfare Concerns	No Rescuer Guidance Needed
[2]	dog	GPS, Bite sensor	Yes	No	No	No	No	Yes	Yes	Yes
[42]	dog	GPS, Bite sensor, Proximity Sensor, Tug sensor	Yes	No	No	No	No	Yes	Yes	Yes
[7,43]	dog	Accelerometer, Gyroscope, Magnetometer	Yes	Yes	No	No	No	Yes	Yes	Yes
[44]	dog	GPS, Camera, Thermographic camera, Infrared camera, Microphone, Speaker, Light.	Yes	No	No	Yes	No	No	Yes	Yes
[45]	dog	GPS, Microphone, Speaker, Light.	Yes	No	No	Yes	No	No	Yes	Yes
[46]	dog and robot snake	Bark detector (RobotSnake: Microphone, Camera)	No	No	Yes	Nos	Yes	Yes	Yes	Yes
[47]	rat	Microstimulating electrodes, Pressure sensors	No	No	No	Nos	Yes	Yes	No	No
this work	dog	Accelerometer, Gyroscope, Microphone, Camera, Vibrator, Speaker	Yes	Yes	Yes	Yes	Yes	No	Yes	Yes

3. Network Architecture

The overall system architecture for the SaR dog real-time monitoring is illustrated in Figure 1. The architecture is divided into two levels (i.e., layers):

1. the EDGE-level, which contains the architectural modules that have low computational power and are located at the edge of the network (i.e., wearable device, base station and the smartphone application), and
2. the FOG-level, which contains the modules having higher computational power and enhanced communication capabilities (publish-subscribe middleware and the local Portable Command Center (PCOP), used during a SaR mission).

The communication from the EDGE layer to the FOG takes place mainly between the wearable device and the Secure IoT Middleware (SIM), which contains an encrypted KAFKA (https://kafka.apache.org/, accessed on 22 September 2021) Publish-Subscribe broker using Wi-Fi connectivity. When such connectivity is not available at the area of operation, a secondary communication path is deployed. This path represents communication at the EDGE layer and includes an RF (Radio Frequency) connection between the wearable and the Base Station (BS). Once the data are collected by the BS, it uses a Wi-Fi/3G/4G connection to publish them at the FOG layer's KAFKA pub-sub broker through the SIM.

Finally, the smartphone of the first responder, which is the handler of the animal, is notified in real-time about the SaR dog's behavior by the KAFKA broker via his/her mobile application. All these data flows can be seen in Figure 1, while the developed EDGE-level modules are explained in detail in the following subsections.

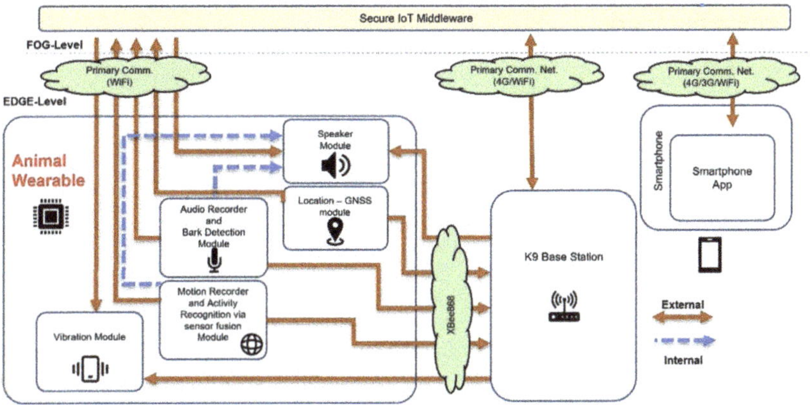

Figure 1. Wearable for animals—system architecture and communication flows.

3.1. Wearable Device

The wearable device is the most important module as it collects various types of data, such as 3-axial accelerometer and 3-axial gyroscope data, audio recordings, and localization data, while it can also provide feedback to the dog via vibration and audio signals. The wearable was developed from our team with the guidance of K9-SaR experts solely for the purposes of the SaR task; however, it can be exploited for various other tasks comprising animal activity monitoring and recognition, e.g., in dogs or even in livestock animals for the purposes of behavioral analysis.

The designed harness is back-mounted vest instead of neck-mounted (i.e., collar) to further improve the animal's comfort by moving the center of mass to a more suitable place, as well as to achieve higher accuracy for the activity recognition task [6]. The new design is completely modular since all the components are attached with Velcro to the wearable. A strip with Velcro is also included at the belly of the animal to provide for further grip. In general, the detachability requirement is related to the dog's safety, as it ensures that the dog will break free from the wearable if tangled.

In Figure 2 the sketch for the designs of the animal wearable is displayed including the strips with velcro attachments (points A and Γ), the pouch for electronics (point B) and the mini-camera position at the animal's front. In particular, point B (back of the animal) contains the main computational platform, the custom board and the battery, while the camera is placed on the animal's chest, always facing in front.

Additionally, except from the pouch for the electronics, another, optional, smaller pouch/pocket was introduced, able to fit a small device (e.g., a mobile phone), or any small item considered useful to be carried by the animal (Figure 3a). This design pertains to rescue scenarios where the delivery of a small item to an unreachable trapped person could be of great importance and contribute to the efficient rescue.

The main features of the wearable device, which is pictorially described in Figure 3b, are the:

- Hardware (processing unit): Raspberry Pi 4 Compute Module (https://www.raspberrypi.com/products/compute-module-4/, accessed on 16 December 2022) (CM4), which features the Broadcom BCM2711, a quad-core ARM Cortex-A72 processor chosen as a processor for the SaR wearable, with dimensions of about 55 × 40 mm. The CM4 offers the processing power required for the complete list of features of the device, including the inference of the DL models as well as the hardware peripherals needed to drive the sensors and modules of the custom board.
- Power Supply Unit: Texas Instruments TPS63002, a Single Inductor Buck-Boost Converter. Since the Raspberry Pi requires a 5 V power supply, a Buck-Boost Converter offers the ability to use a single cell 3.6 V battery and still provide the desired 5 V to the device. The specific model was selected due to its QFN package, measuring 3 mm × 3 mm and due to the small number of additional components needed for the power supply, keeping the overall size on the board minimal.
- Battery Charger Module: Texas Instruments BQ24075 standalone 1-Cell Li-Ion 1.5-A Linear Battery Charger. This battery charger, being in a QFN package offers a small footprint on the device of only 3 mm × 3 mm, and the simplicity of the application circuit assists to the minimalization of the device dimensions. The maximum battery charging current was set to 1.0 A offering a balance between a quick charge for most commercially available batteries and a battery health preservation by keeping the charging rate under 0.5C.
- Battery: 18650 Li-Ion battery cell. The device was designed to operate with a single 18650 type cell, due to the wide adoption of this specific rechargeable battery format, which helps lower the cost of the device and allows for easier maintenance, while offering a balanced solution between energy capacity, size and weight. The operation duration after which the battery was selected is 1 h, which was met with a cell of 3000 mAh. Longer operations can still be covered by carrying multiple spare batteries, since it is a battery type that can be easily replaced in the field.
- RF module: XBee SX 868 modules manufactured by Digi, offering a maximum transmission current of 55 mA. The communication data rate between two modules is set to 10 Kbps to maximize the range and the module is connected to the main processor through the UART interface. These radio modules claim a theoretical maximum range of 14.5 km in line-of-sight with a 2.1 dBi antenna and a maximum transmission current of 55 mA. A maximum range of 750 m was achieved in a line-of-site urban environment. They were chosen over the competition with similar performance, for their setup simplicity and the ability to form a network with as low as two identical modules without the need of third-party involvement and/or subscription fees.
- Audio recording module: SPH0645LM4H-B MEMS digital microphone by Knowles. A very small low-power omnidirectional digital microphone was needed, which uses the I^2S audio bus and requires very few additional components, keeping the device's dimensions to a minimum.
- Audio playback module: the audio signal is constructed from the PWM output of the processor and then it is amplified through Texas Instruments' TPA711DGNR19

low-voltage audio power amplifier, a mono amplifier capable of conducting up to 750 mW of RMS power to an 8Ω speaker continuously. The amplifier's footprint measures 5 mm × 3.1 mm, although the complete audio circuitry also includes an electrolytic capacitor measuring 4.3 mm × 4.3 mm × 5.5 mm.

- Inertia Measurement Unit: BMI160 from Bosch Sensortec featuring a 16-bit triaxial accelerometer and a 16-bit triaxial gyroscope. The module is selected for its very low power consumption of 925 μA and its very small footprint of 2.5 mm × 3 mm. Both the accelerometer and the gyroscope can be operated at high sampling rates of 3200 Hz and 800 Hz respectively, well above the 100 Hz needed for this project.
- GNSS module: Sierra Wireless XA1110 offering a mix of GPS, GLONASS and Galileo satellite system tracking with a maximum update rate of 10 Hz with an integrated patch antenna. This module was selected for its small size of 12.5 × 12.5 × 6.8 mm, which was preferable than a possibly smaller module combined with a larger separate antenna requiring additional space.
- Vibrator module: Texas Instruments' DRV2603 Haptic Drive. The haptic drive comes in a QFN package measuring only 2 mm × 2 mm contributing to the small size needs of the device.
- Camera module: The Raspberry Pi Camera Module v1 was initially selected, but was later dropped in favor of a standalone mini actioncam like the SQ12. This change allowed for a modular design, where the camera can be used when needed or removed when not.

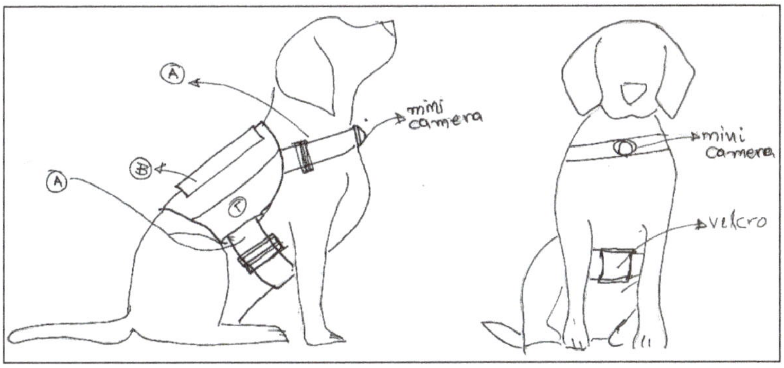

Figure 2. Drawing displaying placement of animal wearable.

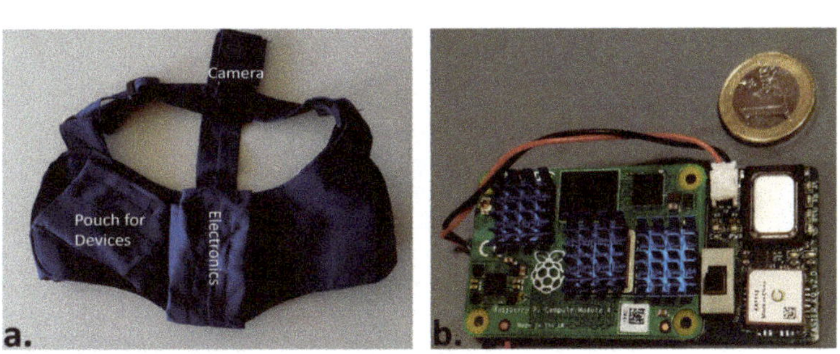

Figure 3. Designed animal harness (**a**) and electronic device (**b**).

The custom board was designed to meet or exceed the predefined specifications covering device functionality and achieve a balance between battery life, weight, and physical dimensions. Therefore, in most cases, the chosen modules are the smallest that would satisfy the consumption and functional requirements. The total weight of the device is 121 g including the battery (47 g), while the total cost for ordering the components and assembling them was equal to 260€. Table 3 provides details on the electrical characteristics, maximum ratings and recommended operating conditions of the device.

Table 3. Electrical characteristics of device.

Parameter	Minimum	Typical	Maximum	Unit
Absolute Maximum Ratings				
Vin—Input Voltage	0.3	-	28	V
Iin—Input Current	-	-	1.6	A
Ichg—Battery Fast Charge Current	0.895	1	1.105	A
Vbat—Battery Charge Voltage	4.16	4.2	4.23	V
Operating Temperature	−40	-	100	°C
Storage Temperature	−65	-	150	°C
Recommended Operating Conditions				
Vin—Input Voltage	4.35	5	6.4	V
Operating Temperature	−40	-	85	°C

3.2. *SaR Base Station*

The BS device is a portable wireless device, based on the Raspberry Pi Zero W (https://www.raspberrypi.com/products/raspberry-pi-zero-w/, accessed on 19 January 2022) and powered by an internal power-bank. It is equipped with an XBee SX 868 RF module (https://www.digi.com/xbee, accessed on 19 January 2022) similar to the wearable devices and creates an XBee network to which all animal wearable devices in range can connect. This results in an extended range of coverage for the animal wearables. The BS device, includes a pocket Wi-Fi module, granting 4G connectivity. Any messages sent from the wearables are received by the BS through the Xbee network and delegated to the SIM over either the Wi-Fi connection to the Pocket Wi-Fi device and then transmitted over 4G network, or to any other known Wi-Fi hot spot. Likewise, any commands issued by the rest of the modules to the wearables (e.g., initiate data collection), are either received directly by the devices through Wi-Fi, or received by the BS and relayed to the devices via the XBee network. The existence of a BS is extremely critical in a disaster scenario, as public telecommunications networks cannot be taken for granted. For this purpose, the animal wearable device cannot rely solely on mobile network coverage.

3.3. *Smartphone Application*

The application of the animal wearable is one feature of a wider application developed for FASTER (First responder Advanced technologies for Safe and efficienT Emergency Response) EU Horizon 2020 project (https://cordis.europa.eu/project/id/833507, accessed on 16 December 2021). As a result, the application contains four tabs for displaying: (a) biometrics of first responders, (b) environmental data, (c) the behavior and location of SaR dogs, and (d) upcoming notifications (e.g., a victim was found). In general, it is an Android application (supporting android version 8.0 and above) that makes use of Google Maps (https://www.google.com/maps, accessed on 16 December 2021) for the depiction of information about the location of the dog. The application receives the information from a KAFKA broker with the aid of a Quarkus Reactive Streams (https://quarkus.io/, accessed on 16 December 2021) service. The information flows continuously from KAFKA to the screen of the user. Reactive streams work by publishing messages whenever they receive new information from a source. This makes the information flow "seamless" and most importantly it does not spam the server with http requests every some seconds. The android system can absorb these streams with the use of a library called okSse (https:

//github.com/biowink/oksse, accessed on 16 December 2021) which helps to establish a connection with a reactive streams service.

Once we get the information, we feed it to our system with the use of LiveData (https://developer.android.com/topic/libraries/architecture/livedata, accessed on 16 December 2021). LiveData is an observable data holder class. Unlike a regular observable, LiveData is lifecycle-aware, meaning it respects the lifecycle of other application components, such as activities, fragments, or services. This awareness ensures LiveData only updates the application component observers that are in an active lifecycle state. With the use of an observer, we "observe" any changes to the state of the information, and when we find something new we draw on the map the new location or behavior of the dog. The dog actions describe the state in which the animal is at a particular time in space (Figure 4). For example, whether the dog is walking/running or standing still.

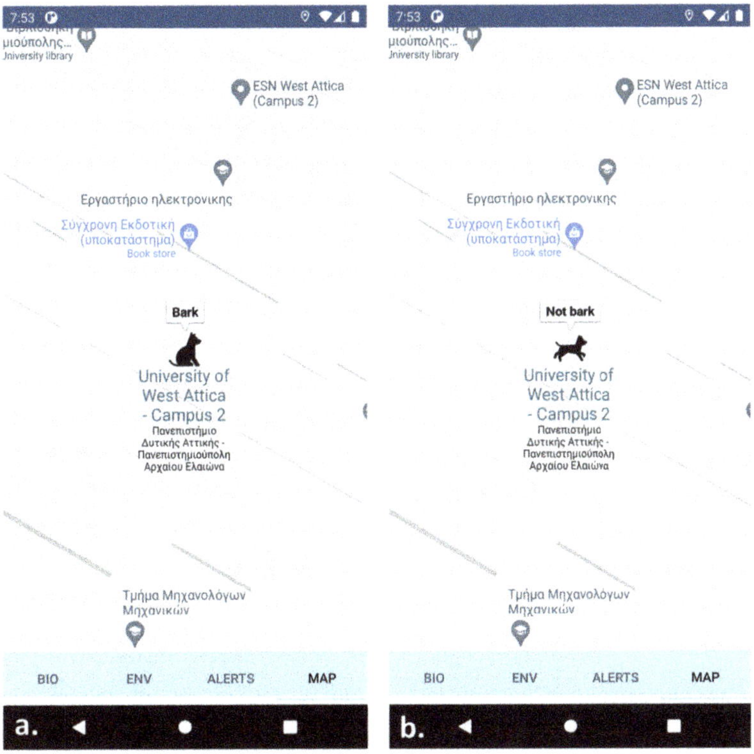

Figure 4. Developed smartphone application displaying SaR dog behavior: (**a**) canine is not moving and barks; (**b**) canine is moving and does not bark.

4. Data Collection, Processing, and Deployment of Deep Learning Algorithms

4.1. Data Collection Process

The tests were performed in an arena covered with ruins to mimic a real search and rescue operation as best as possible (Figure 5). The tests included search and rescue missions both during the day and night. In the former case, adequate vision is considered, while in the latter, only limited vision can be attained. The resulting AI algorithms are trained in both cases, as in a real operation both cases can be encountered.

Next, the testing procedure is as follows. First, a member of the rescuing team, the "victim", hides somewhere in the arena among the ruins, in one of the various spots which are designed for this purpose. Then, after the wearable on the SaR dog is activated by his trainer, the dog is allowed to search for the victim. The test is successfully completed when the SaR dog is able to found the "victim". In this successful case, the SaR dog makes a characteristic bark sound, which lasts for some seconds, while it is in a standing position and stares at the "victim". Depending on the location of the "victim" in the arena, the search and rescue test may last from half a minute up to a few minutes.

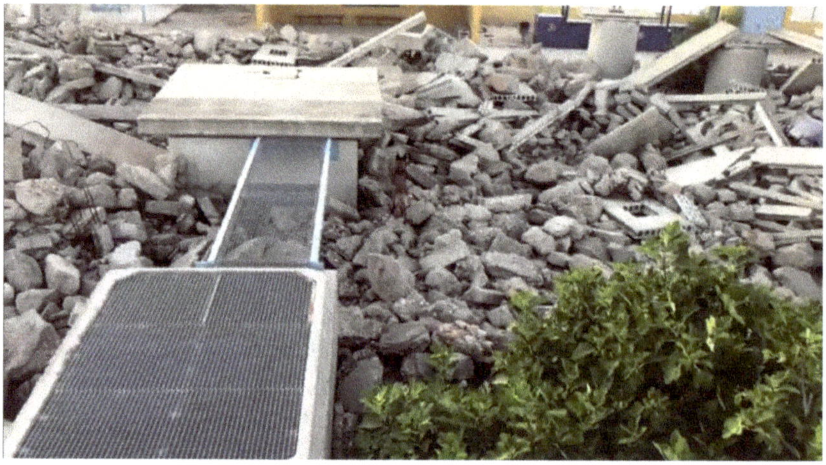

Figure 5. Arena used to conduct search and rescue tests.

4.2. Labeling Process

The labeling process was performed offline using video and audio recordings. The videos were recorded using a smartphone camera which was positioned on a high place on one side of the arena to capture almost the entire search and rescue field. The audio recordings were performed using the wearable device's microphone. Only segments longer than 2 s were considered during the labeling process, which means that a single activity needs to last more than two consecutive seconds to be labeled. The recorded videos were synchronized with sensor data using metadata (e.g., timestamp) and via exploiting the plotted time series of the sensors (e.g., accelerometer). Four activities were considered:

(a) standing—the dog is standing still on four legs without its torso touching the ground, occurring mainly when the dog successfully finds the victim;
(b) walking—the dog moves at slow speed and its legs are moving one after another;
(c) trotting—the dog moves at a faster speed than walking and slower than running. This is the most frequent movement activity during the search and rescue operation; and
(d) running—the dog moves at a very fast speed, occurring mainly when the dog is released by its trainer at the beginning of the search and rescue operation.

In cases where it was not possible to identify the dog activity, either due to insufficient light during the night operation or when the dog was not clearly shown in camera, (e.g., it was behind an obstacle) a "missing" label was considered. These data were omitted for the Artificial Intelligence (AI) training procedure. Next, the audio recordings include only two classes, barking and nonbarking, as the barking is the required state that designates that the SaR dog spotted the "victim". Examples of the four dog activities are shown in Figure 6.

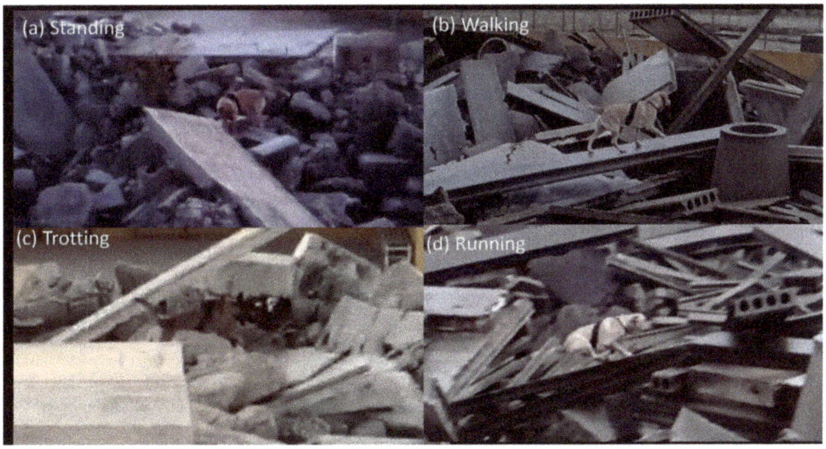

Figure 6. Instances of four activitie.

4.3. Details of the Created Dataset

The complete dataset comprises nine dog search and rescue sessions. After the labeling process, each session is segregated in various segments, where each segment comprises only one activity, considering a minimum segment duration of 2 s. Each second of raw data consists of 100 values for the two 3-axial sensors (3-axial accelerometer and 3-axial gyroscope) forming a total of 600 values. Next, each segment is segregated in samples with a 2 s length where a 50% overlap is considered. An example of samples for the four SaR dog activities from both the accelerometer and the gyroscope is illustrated in Figure 7. Evidently, the amplitude of the accelerometer and the gyroscope increase as the activity becomes more intense, which means that the lowest amplitude can be found in standing and the highest in running.

Further, the dataset details for all seven search and rescue testing sessions are tabulated in Table 4. Evidently, the most frequent activities are standing and trotting. This is expected, as during the search and rescue operation, on one hand the dog trots while searching for the "victim" between the ruins and on the other hand, when the "victim" is found, the dog remains in a standing position and barks. Moreover, only one of the K9s provided a sufficient amount of "running" examples (session 4), and only two canines sufficient amount of "standing" examples (session 4 and 6). Thus, by adopting a leave one subject out approach, it is impossible to check the model's generalizability on the classes "running" and "walking", and, as a result, we merged the motion activities "running", "walking" and "trotting" into one class, called "searching".

Turning our attention to the bark detection, similar to SaR dog activity detection, the labeling process was performed offline using the provided audio recordings and it was compared with the video recordings to verify the annotations. The annotated data were afterwards segmented into 2 s audio clips. This window size was selected to reduce the throughput to the developed model.

Another reason for selecting 2 s was to match the window size of the Inertial Measurement Unit (IMU) data and, also, to have a better understanding of the situation the SaR dog is into. For example, in the case of real-time inference and for e.g., a 4 s window, if the dog barks in the first second of the audio stream the model would still classify it as bark, despite the fact this occurred 3 s ago.

The dataset we built consists of 1761 examples (i.e., audio clips), where 258 are audio clips containing bark and 1503 do not, leading to an unbalanced dataset, which however reflects a real-world search and rescue operation. Before introducing the data in the Deep CNN, we split them into three subsets, namely training set, validation set, and test set, following the standard procedure of training an neural network. The train set contains around 74% of the data, the validation set around 10% of the data and the test set around 16% of the data. The split was performed based on the search and rescue sessions. i.e., audio signals recorded during a specific search and rescue session belong to the same dataset, avoiding in this way overlapping samples between the different sets or characteristic bark patterns.

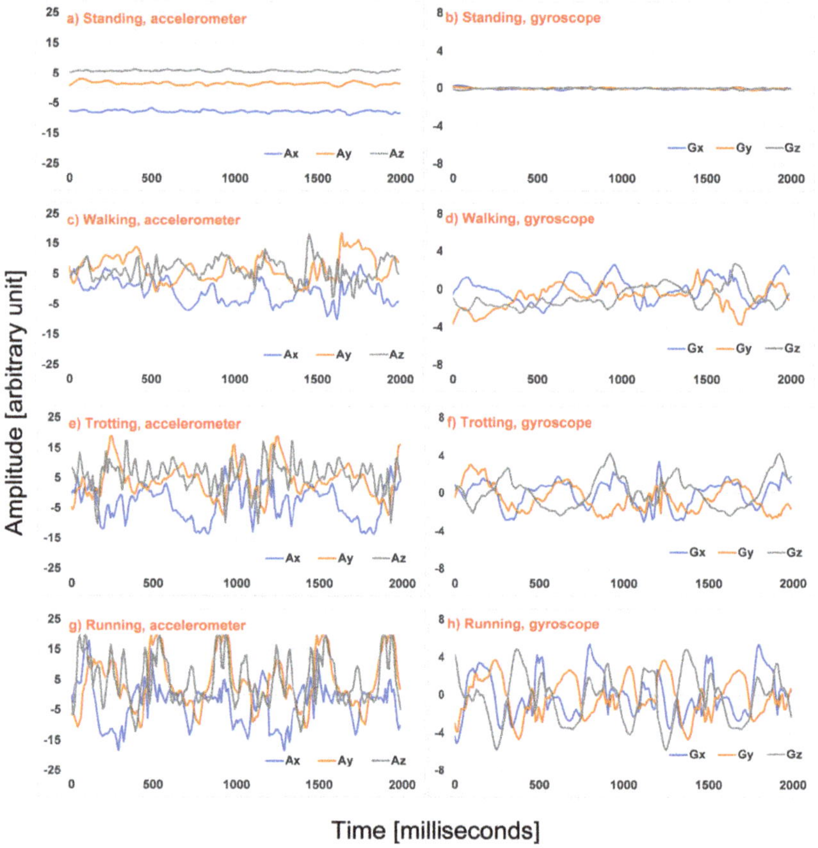

Figure 7. Sensor samples of 2 s duration for four activities.

Table 4. Number of samples for each search and rescue session for four monitored activities.

Session No.	Standing	Walking	Trotting	Running	Searching
1	32	0	38	0	38
2	44	0	28	0	28
3	37	4	20	0	24
4	22	23	80	23	126
5	18	0	10	0	10
6	47	38	27	4	69
7	34	0	13	0	13
Total (542)	234	65	216	27	308

4.4. Developed DL Algorithms

4.4.1. Activity Recognition

The employed Deep CNN for the dog activity recognition is a lightweight architecture to be deployed on the animal wearable (i.e., contains around 21,400 parameters), it is based on late sensor fusion [8] (i.e., the fist convolutional layers process the input signals individually) and consists of the following layers (Figure 8):

- layer 1: sixteen convolutional filters with a size of (1, 11), i.e., W_1 has shape (1, 11, 1, 16).
  This is followed by a ReLU activation function, a (1, 4) strided max-pooling operation and a dropout probability equal to 0.5.
- layer 2: twenty-four convolutional filters with a size of (1, 11), i.e., W_2 has shape (1, 11, 16, 24).
  Similar to the first layer, this is followed by a ReLU activation function, a (1,2) strided max-pooling operation and a dropout probability equal to 0.5.
- layer 3: thirty-two convolutional filters with a size of (2, 11), i.e., W_3 has shape (2, 11, 24, 32).

The 2D convolution operation is followed by a ReLU activation function, a 2D global max-pooling operation and a dropout probability equal to 0.5.

- layer 4: thirty-two hidden units, i.e., W_4 has shape (32, 1), followed by a sigmoid activation function.

Before feeding the algorithms with the collected data, we performed a preprocessing routine as follows. To acquire orientation independent features, we calculated a 3D vector (the l2-norm) from the sensors' individual axes [48]. The orientation-independent magnitude of the 3D-vector is defined as:

$$S(i) = \sqrt{s_x^2(i) + s_y^2(i) + s_z^2(i)} \tag{1}$$

where $s_x(i)$, $s_y(i)$, and $s_z(i)$ are the three respective axes of each sensor (accelerometer and gyroscope) for the ith sample. Then, the dataset is divided seven-fold (i.e., one per session). To obtain subject independent results and evaluate the generalization of the algorithms, we used five folds as a training set, one as a validation set, and one as a test set. Afterwards, a circular rotation between training, validation and test subsets was performed to ensure that the data from all sessions will be tested. Finally, each sensor's values (obtained by Equation (1)) were normalized by subtracting the mean value and dividing by the standard deviation (calculated by the examples included only in the training set), defined as:

$$Z(i) = \frac{S(i) - \mu}{\sigma} \tag{2}$$

where $S(i)$ denotes the ith sample of a particular sensor (e.g., accelerometer), $Z(i)$ its normalized representation and μ and σ denote their mean and standard deviation values, respectively.

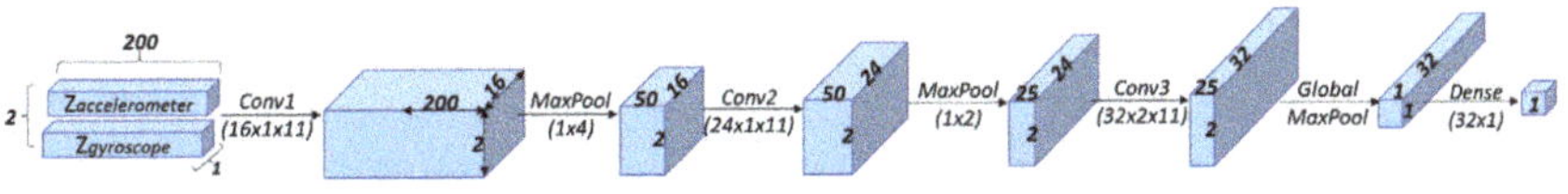

Figure 8. Overall architecture of developed Deep CNN for activity recognition task. Input tensor has two rows representing produced $Z(i)$ for accelerometer and gyroscope, each one of them containing 200 values and one channel. Every convolutional operation is followed by a ReLU activation function, and pooling layers are followed by a dropout equal to 0.5. Final dense layer outputs one value and is followed by a sigmoid operation that represents probability of SaR dog searching or standing.

4.4.2. Bark Detection

For the task of bark detection, we evaluated two different strategies. The first one is based on a large pretrained model where we applied transfer learning, i.e., we finetuned its weights using the dataset we collected. In particular, we selected the model introduced in [49] that achieved state-of-the-art results in the ESC dataset [41]. The code for reproducing the model is publicly available (https://github.com/anuragkr90/weak_feature_extractor, accessed on 12 September 2021). The latter was a custom lightweight (i.e., contains 10,617 parameters) Deep CNN architecture and consists of the following layers (Figure 9):

- layer 1: sixteen convolutional filters (i.e., kernels) with a size of (3, 3), i.e., W_1 has shape (3, 3, 1, 16)

This is followed by the ReLU activation function, a strided (2, 2) max-pooling operation and a dropout probability equal to 0.5.

- layer 2: twenty-four convolutional filters with a size of (3, 3), i.e., W_2 has shape (3, 3, 16, 24).

Similar to the first layer, this is followed by a ReLU activation function, a (2,2) strided max-pooling operation and a dropout probability equal to 0.5.

- layer 3: thirty-two convolutional filters with a size of (3, 3), i.e., W_3 has shape (3, 3, 24, 32).

The 2D convolution operation is followed by a ReLU activation function, a global max-pooling operation, and a dropout probability equal to 0.5.

- layer 4: thirty-two hidden units, i.e., W_4 has shape (32, 1), followed by a sigmoid activation function.

Before injecting the collected audio data in the CNN, we performed data normalization by dividing all the values with the max value included in the sample. Afterwards, the log-scaled mel-spectrograms were extracted from the audio clips having a window size of 1024, hop length of 512 and 128 mel-bands. Moreover, the segments of each clip overlapped 50% with the previous and the next one, and we discarded a lot of silent segments since they increased significantly the number of not-bark examples without, however, increasing the model's performance.

Figures 10 and 11 visualize the transformation of a clip containing bark and a clip including nonbarking activity, respectively. The comparative difference between the barking and the nonbarking state is obvious both in the raw data representation and in the mel-spectrogram.

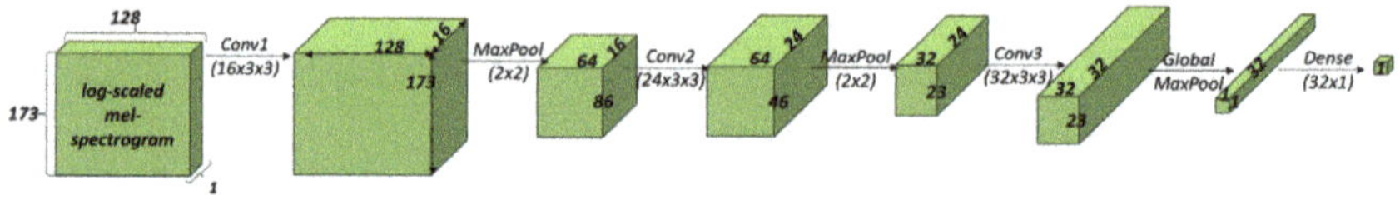

Figure 9. Overall architecture of developed Deep CNN for bark detection task. Input tensor is log-scaled mel-spectrogram, with 173 rows, each one of them containing 128 values (mels) and one channel. Every convolutional operation is followed by a ReLU activation function, and pooling layers are followed by a dropout equal to 0.5. Final dense layer outputs one value and is followed by a sigmoid operation that represents probability of SaR dog barking or not barking.

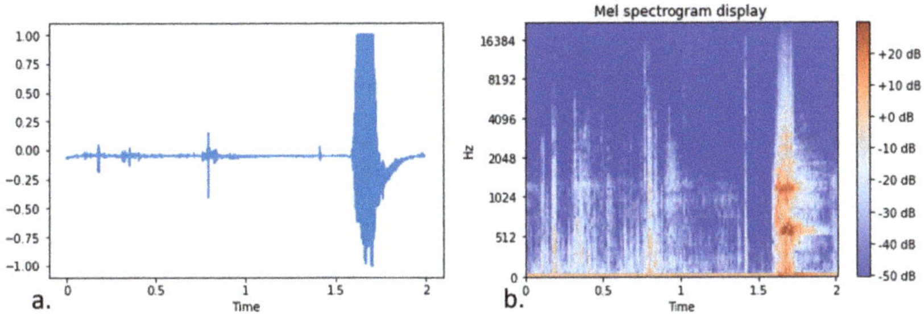

Figure 10. Raw representation (**a**) and log-scaled mel-spectrogram (**b**) of a dog barking audio signal.

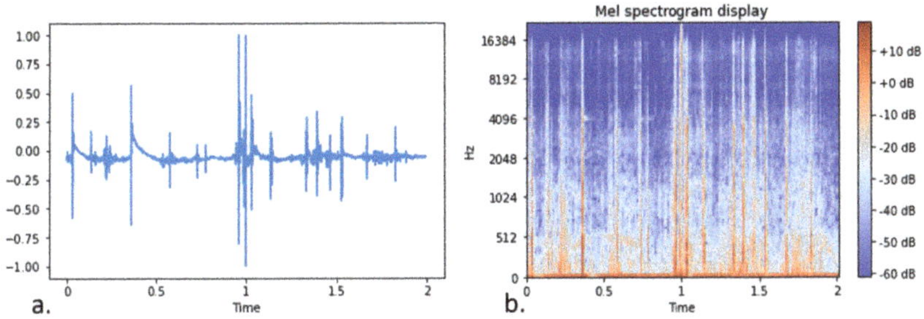

Figure 11. Raw representation (**a**) and log-scaled mel-spectrogram (**b**) of a dog not barking audio signal (dog running).

5. Results

5.1. Results on the Activity Recognition

In this section, we benchmark the proposed CNN against four other machine learning algorithms, namely Logistic Regression (LR), k-Nearest Neighbours (k-NN), Decision Tree (DT), and Random Forest (RF). For these algorithms we opted to extract the same seven time-dependent features for each sensor (accelerometer and gyroscope), resulting in 14 features in total (see Table 5). The ML experiments were executed on a computer workstation equipped with an NVIDIA GTX 1080Ti GPU, which has 11 gigabytes RAM, 3584 CUDA cores, and a bandwidth of 484 GB/s. Python was used as the programming language, and specifically the Numpy for matrix multiplications, data preprocessing, segmentation, and transformation and the Keras high-level neural networks library using as a backend the Tensorflow library. To accelerate the tensor multiplications, CUDA Toolkit in support with the cuDNN was used, which is the NVIDIA GPU-accelerated library for deep neural networks. The software is installed on a 16.04 Ubuntu Linux operating system.

The proposed CNN model was trained using the Adam optimizer [50] with the following hyper-parameters: learning rate = 0.001, $beta_1$ = 0.9, $beta_2$ = 0.999, epsilon = 10^{-8}, decay = 0.0. Moreover, we set the minimum number of epochs to 500; however, the training procedure terminated automatically whether the best training accuracy improved or not after a threshold of 100 epochs. The training epoch that achieved the lowest error rate on the validation set was saved, and its filters were used to obtain the accuracy of the model on the test set.

Table 6 presents the accuracy results that were obtained on applying the aforementioned algorithms and the developed Deep CNN architecture on the SaR dog activity recognition dataset. The presented results were obtained per dog having different folds in the test set (i.e., 5-fold cross-validation), while we made five runs for each to avoid reducing the dependency on different weights initializations and averaged them afterwards. The highest accuracy was achieved by the Deep CNN model (93.68%), which surpassed importantly the baseline algorithms, especially DT and k-NN. Moreover, having the algorithms achieved the best results (98.57% averaged accuracy) having dog five in the test set and the worst ones when they were evaluated on the dog seven examples (83.57% averaged accuracy). In addition to this, through the following table we can observe that k-NN had the biggest deviation in terms of accuracy among the seven subjects (i.e., dogs) ranging from 73.34% to 100%, while the RF was the smallest one, ranging from 84.34% to 100%.

Table 5. Description of selected features.

Feature	Description
Mean	Average value
Min	Minimum value
Max	Maximum value
Median	Median value
Standard deviation	Measure of dispersion
Skewness	The degree of asymmetry of the signal distribution
Kurtosis	The degree of peakedness of the signal distribution

Table 6. Per dog accuracy of each Machine Learning (ML) model on dog activity recognition dataset.

	Accuracy (%)							
Method	**Dog 1**	**Dog 2**	**Dog 3**	**Dog 4**	**Dog 5**	**Dog 6**	**Dog 7**	**Avg**
LR	91.43	90.28	96.72	95.27	100.0	87.93	87.23	92.69
k-NN	94.28	93.06	100.0	89.86	100.0	85.34	73.34	90.70
DT	90.57	86.11	90.49	89.32	92.85	82.24	79.14	87.25
RF	91.71	91.67	98.69	94.86	100.0	85.17	87.23	92.76
Deep CNN	91.14	93.06	100.0	95.00	100.0	84.66	91.91	93.68

Figure 12 displays the confusion matrix of the developed deep CNN averaged over the different test sets. The false positives (i.e., examples falsely predicted as "stand") are more than the false negatives (i.e., examples falsely predicted as "search"), which is somewhat unexpected since the "search" class contains more examples than the "stand" class. However, after performing error analysis on the obtained results we noticed that 11 out of the 65 walking activities, were falsely classified as "stand". This misclassification concerning the SaR dogs' low intense activities adds around 1.52 false positives, and without it, the portion of false-positive and negatives would be almost equal.

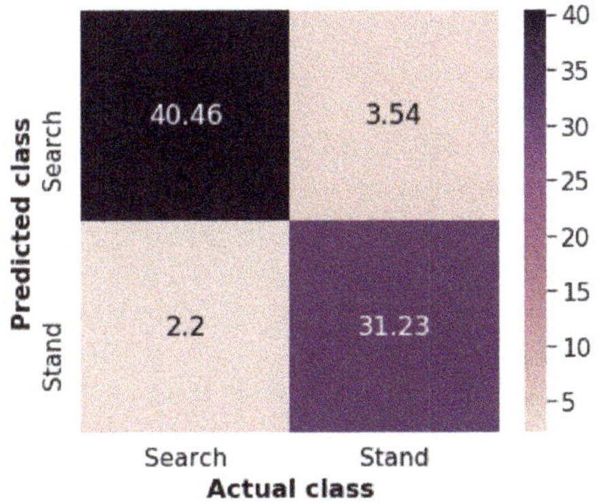

Figure 12. Confusion matrix (averaged over different test sets) of developed deep CNN.

5.2. Results on the Bark Detection

We followed the same experimental set-up that described in section for activity recognition regarding the workstation used, the libraries, and the optimizer. The hyperparameters of the Deep CNN were: learning rate = 0.001, $beta_1$ = 0.9, $beta_2$ = 0.999, epsilon = 10^{-8}, decay = 0.0, while Adam optimizer is also considered. Moreover, we set the minimum number of epochs to 1000; however, the training procedure terminated automatically whether the best training accuracy had improved or not, after a threshold of 100 epochs. Similar with the case of the CNN in the activity recognition, the training epoch that achieved the lowest error rate on the validation set was saved, and its filters were used to obtain the accuracy of the model on the test set.

The results on the test set of the developed search and rescue dataset are presented in Table 7 the best results were achieved exploiting the Deep CNN after applying transfer learning using the Deep CNN in [49] (named as Deep CNN TL). The attainable accuracy of our model is 99.13% and the F1-score is 98.41%, while the Deep CNN TL achieved 99.34% accuracy and 98.73% F1-score.

Furthermore, Figure 13 shows the confusion matrix for the bark and nonbark classes of the lightweight CNN model. Evidently, the model produced on average more false negatives (2.1 bark activity examples were classified and not bark) than false positives (0.4 not bark activity examples were classified and bark) probably due to the fact that the dataset is imbalanced, containing significantly more nonbarking examples (6/1 ratio).

Table 7. Performance of developed ML models on SaR dog bark detection dataset.

Method Name	Accuracy	F1-Score
Deep CNN TL [49]	99.34%	98.73%
Ours Deep CNN	99.13%	98.41%

Apart from the performance metrics, since we were interested in deploying the selected DL model on the wearable device, we measured the inference time of the models. Table 8 presents the response times for both DL models measured on (a) a workstation equipped with an Intel(R) Core(TM) i7-7700K CPU (4 cores) running on max turbo frequency equal to 4.20 GHz and (b) a Raspberry Pi 4 computing module (quad-core ARM Cortex-A72 processor). We converted the developed models to a TensorFlow Lite format. TensorFlow Lite is a set of tools that enables on-device machine learning such as mobile, embedded, and IoT devices. As a result, the TensorFlow models were converted in a special efficient portable format known as FlatBuffers (identified by the .tflite file extension), providing several advantages over TensorFlow's protocol buffer model format (identified by the .pb file extension) such as reduced size and faster inference time. The performance of the models was not decreased after the conversion to .tflite format.

For our measurement purposes, we ran the models 10,000 times and then computed the average inferencing time. The first inferencing run, which takes longer due to loading overheads, was discarded. As expected the inference time for the .tflite formats is significantly lower than those of the .pb formats. Moreover, since the objective was to deploy the model to a Raspberry Pi 4 we selected to use our Deep CNN. Even though it achieved a 0.32% lower F1-score, it is significantly faster (almost x7 times) than the Deep CNN TL model enabling real-time inference at the edge of the network.

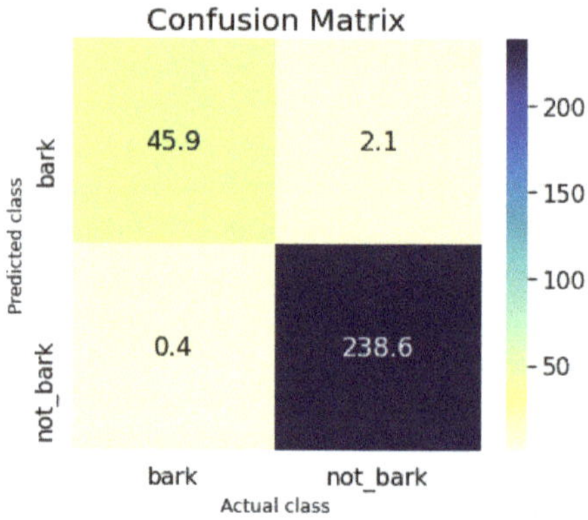

Figure 13. Confusion matrix of Deep CNN on test set of SaR dog search and rescue dataset.

Table 8. Mean inference time measure in milliseconds for each model.

Model	Intel I7-7700K CPU	Raspberry Pi 4
Deep CNN TL [49] .pb format	175.64 ms	839.59 ms
Ours Deep CNN .pb format	39.1 ms	116.88 ms
Deep CNN TL [49] .tflite format	25.59 ms	170.10 ms
Ours Deep CNN .tflite format	5.84 ms	25.53 ms

6. Validation of the Proposed Implementation

The proposed system was validated in an abandoned and demolished hospital southwest of Madrid, running two scenarios with the assistance of different SaR dogs. Similarly to the data collection process, a first responder had the role of the "victim", and was hidden somewhere in the arena among the ruins. Then, a SaR dog with the developed wearable mounted on its back started its SaR mission.

During this process we measured the accuracy and F1-scores of the developed bark detection and activity recognition models separately. Moreover, we estimated the overall F1-score for notifying the K9 handlers whether the victim was found or not. This is achieved by injecting an alert rule on the mobile that is triggered when the SaR dog is barking and standing simultaneously, which is what it is trained for denoting that it has found a missing person.

Table 9 presents the classes of the collected singals (IMU and audio). Not all of the motion signals were annotated. This is due to the fact that the SaR dog was missing (e.g., was behind the debris) or there was an overlap in the activities for a 2 s window (e.g., the SaR dog was searching for the first 800 ms and then stopped moving for the rest 1200 ms). Thus there are presented less examples than the total amount.

Table 9. Number of samples for two SaR evaluation scenarios.

Session No.	Standing	Searching	Barking	Not Barking	Duration (Sec)
1	57	98	17	258	275
2	167	170	40	555	595
Total	224	268	57	813	870

The obtained F1-scores and the corresponding accuracy results are presented in Table 10. The developed deep CNN activity recognition model achieved a F1-score equal to 91.21% and 91.26% accuracy, while the bark detection model acquired 99.08% F1-score and 99.77% accuracy. In particular, the latter provided only two false positives (i.e., the misclacified "not barking" as "barking"), and these, also, triggered the alert notification providing the same F1-score and accuracy metrics for the overall victim detection task.

Table 10. Obtained F1-score and accuracy results for tasks of activity recognition, bark detection, and victim found recognition regarding two evaluation SaR scenarios.

Task	Accuracy	F1-score
Activity recognition	91.26%	91.21%
Bark detection	99.77%	99.08%
Victim found recognition	99.77%	99.08%

Moreover, the developed solution was able to operate in real-time on the field, exploiting data processing at the edge, and it enabled the first responders to be aware of the K9 position and its behavior. Figures 14 and 15 display a summary plot of the outputs of the DL models and the received smartphone notifications with respect to the received KAFKA messages, respectively. A video displaying these results and the whole validation procedure can be found here (https://www.youtube.com/watch?v=704AV4mNfRA, accessed on 20 January 2022).

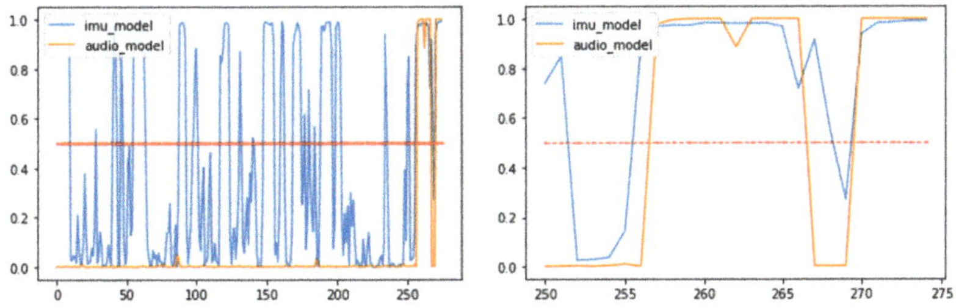

Figure 14. Plots displaying outputs of developed DL models during 275 s of 1st SaR scenario (**left**). Red line denotes threshold value (i.e., 0.5) for classifying an audio signal as "bark" and IMU signal as "stand". The final 25 s of this scenario are displayed on (**right**) plot.

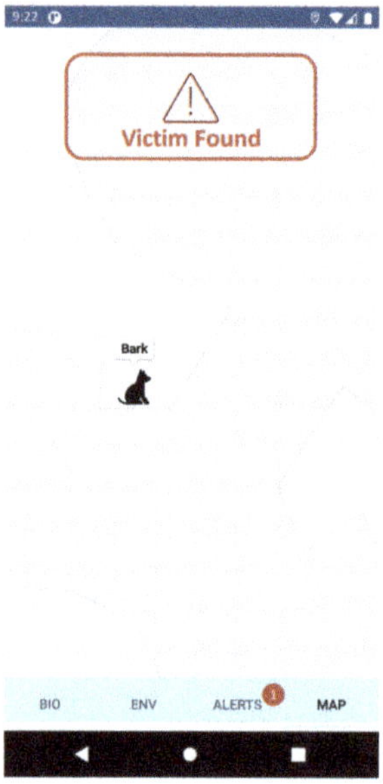


```
{
  "id": "K9A0103",
  "latitude": "40.35959868333333",
  "longitude": "-3.9208161833333333",
  "bark": false,
  "activity": "search",
  "time": 1634548969
}

{
  "id": "K9A0103",
  "latitude": "40.359579366666665",
  "longitude": "-3.9208374166666666",
  "bark": false,
  "activity": "stand",
  "time": 1634548970
}

{
  "id": "K9A0103",
  "latitude": "40.359579366666665",
  "longitude": "-3.9208374166666666",
  "bark": true,
  "activity": "stand",
  "time": 1634548971
}
```


Figure 15. Mobile screenshot displaying generated alert in 1st SaR scenario (**left**), and corresponding KAFKA messages, with last one triggering alert rule (**right**).

7. Discussion

One of the main advantages of the current work is that it exploits edge computing to process in real-time the generated data before transmitting them through the network. In particular, in the case where there is no Wi-Fi available and the RF module is not efficient to send streaming audio data since the maximum data rate is 250 kbits/s, and the necessary rate for a medium quality audio signal is equal to 192 kbit/s, let alone the need to transmit the IMU signal and the GPS coordinates. In addition to this, to expand the data transmission range we reduced the data rate to 10 kbit/s, making it impossible to transmit the produced raw signals.

Moreover, the inclusion of IMU sensors is significant since the included SaR dogs are trained to bark and stand still when identifying a missing/trapped person. Thus, it reduces the false positives (i.e., victim found recognition) in the case the algorithm outputs that the dog barks but it is not standing or the dog falsely produces a barking sound. Furthermore, micro movements where the dog is confused (e.g., makes small circles) or is sniffing are not noticeable (i.e., the displayed coordinates will indicate it as standing) though the GPS signal, due to its estimation error (could reach up to 5 m), but are classified as searching by our algorithm.

However, one limitation of the approach is the activity recognition algorithm's performance. Even though the overall accuracy is high, having an average of 7.32 misclafications in 100 s time span, for a critical mission application where even a second matters, this is not considered to be low, mainly due to the fact that the provided algorithm has not "seen" the examples of the dogs included in the test set. In other words, the behavioral patterns of some dogs are not close to the others and having more training data would be beneficial for the algorithm's performance [51], a case that will be explored in the future.

Another possible limitation is that of the activity recognition algorithm's generalizability in different dog breeds and environments. The SaR dogs included in training and evaluation were German Shepherds, American Labrador Retrievers, Golden Retrievers, Belgian Malinois, or mixed breeds (of the aforementioned) and ranged from 20 kg to 32 kg dogs. Moreover, the training and evaluation environments (arenas) were relative small areas with a lot of obstacles, such as debris. Thus, the algorithms performance on bigger

SaR dogs (e.g., Saint Bernard) and wide open areas was not tested (e.g., forest covered with snow).

Finally, the current work has followed the guidelines regarding the Ethics Code (https://escuelasalvamento.org/wp-content/uploads/2021/04/Codigo-Etico_vf.pdf, accessed on 5 August 2021) of K9 training and the participating SaR dogs did not undergo any extra training for the purposes of this paper.

8. Conclusions

In this paper, we proposed a novel implementation that performs dog activity recognition and bark detection in real-time to alert the dog handler (a) about the dog position and (b) whether it has found the victim during a search and rescue operation. The proposed solution can significantly aid the first aid responders in search and rescue missions, especially in places where the rescuers either are not possible to enter, e.g., below debris, or if they cannot have the rescue dog within their line of sight. To realize thins, the candidate implementation incorporates CNNs, which have the ability to extract features automatically, attaining the highest accuracy compared with other known ML algorithms. In particular, it attained an accuracy of more than 93% both in activity recognition and bark detection in the collected test datasets and managed in both discrete validation scenarios to classify and alert the rescuer at the time that the dog managed to find the victim.

Author Contributions: Conceptualization, P.K. and C.Z.P.; methodology, P.K. and D.U.; software, P.K., V.D. and C.G.; validation, P.K., V.D. and D.U.; formal analysis, P.K., V.D. and D.U.; investigation, P.K., S.I.F. and M.B.G.; data curation, P.K. and D.U.; resources, S.I.F. and M.B.G.; writing—original draft preparation, P.K., V.D. and D.U.; visualization, P.K. and D.U.; supervision, D.G.K. and C.Z.P.; project administration, D.G.K. and C.Z.P.; funding acquisition, C.Z.P. All authors have read and agreed to the published version of the manuscript.

Funding: This research was funded by the European Commission's H2020 program (under project FASTER) grant number 833507.

Institutional Review Board Statement: Not applicable.

Informed Consent Statement: Not applicable.

Acknowledgments: This research was funded by the European Commission's H2020 program (under project FASTER) grant number 833507.

Conflicts of Interest: The authors declare no conflict of interest.

Abbreviations

The following abbreviations are used in this manuscript:

DL	Deep Learning
CNN	Convolutional Neural Network
SaR	Search and Rescue
IMU	Inertial Measurement Unit
SIM	Secure IoT Middleware
PCOP	Portable Commmand Center
SVM	Support Vector Machines
LR	Logistic Regression
k-NN	k-Nearest Neighbours
DT	Decision Tree
RF	Random Forest
ANN	Artificial Neural Network
AAR	Animal Activity Recognition
DAR	Dog Activity Recognition

References

1. Doulgerakis, V.; Giannousis, C.; Kalyvas, D.; Feidakis, M.; Patrikakis, C.Z.; Bocaj, E.; Laliotis, G.P.; Bizelis, I. An Animal Welfare Platform for Extensive Livestock Production Systems. In Proceedings of the AmI, Rome, Italy, 13–15 November 2019.
2. Zeagler, C.; Byrne, C.; Valentin, G.; Freil, L.; Kidder, E.; Crouch, J.; Starner, T.; Jackson, M.M. Search and Rescue: Dog and Handler Collaboration through Wearable and Mobile Interfaces. In Proceedings of the Third International Conference on Animal-Computer Interaction (ACI '16), Milton Keynes, UK, 15–17 November 2016; Association for Computing Machinery: New York, NY, USA, 2016. [CrossRef]
3. Doull, K.E.; Chalmers, C.; Fergus, P.; Longmore, S.N.; Piel, A.K.; Wich, S.A. An Evaluation of the Factors Affecting 'Poacher' Detection with Drones and the Efficacy of Machine-Learning for Detection. *Sensors* **2021**, *21*, 4074. [CrossRef] [PubMed]
4. Valletta, J.J.; Torney, C.J.; Kings, M.; Thornton, A.; Madden, J.R. Applications of machine learning in animal behavior studies. *Anim. Behav.* **2017**, *124*, 203–220. [CrossRef]
5. Kamminga, J.W. Hiding in the Deep: Online Animal Activity Recognition Using Motion Sensors and Machine Learning. Ph.D. Thesis, University of Twente, NB Enschede, TheNetherlands, 2020.
6. Kumpulainen, P.; Cardó, A.V.; Somppi, S.; Törnqvist, H.; Väätäjä, H.; Majaranta, P.; Gizatdinova, Y.; Antink, C.H.; Surakka, V.; Kujala, M.V.; et al. Dog behavior classification with movement sensors placed on the harness and the collar. *Appl. Anim. Behav. Sci.* **2021**, *241*, 105393. [CrossRef]
7. Valentin, G.; Alcaidinho, J.; Howard, A.M.; Jackson, M.M.; Starner, T. Creating collar-sensed motion gestures for dog-human communication in service applications. In Proceedings of the 2016 ACM International Symposium on Wearable Computers, Heidelberg, Germany, 12–16 September 2016.
8. Kasnesis, P.; Patrikakis, C.Z.; Venieris, I.S. PerceptionNet: A deep convolutional neural network for late sensor fusion. In Proceedings of the SAI Intelligent Systems Conference, London, UK, 6–7 September 2018; Springer: Heidelberg, Germany, 2018; pp. 101–119.
9. Kasnesis, P.; Chatzigeorgiou, C.; Toumanidis, L.; Patrikakis, C.Z. Gesture-based incident reporting through smart watches. In Proceedings of the 2019 IEEE International Conference on Pervasive Computing and Communications Workshops (PerCom Workshops), Kyoto, Japan, 11–15 March 2019; pp. 249–254.
10. Bocaj, E.; Uzunidis, D.; Kasnesis, P.; Patrikakis, C.Z. On the Benefits of Deep Convolutional Neural Networks on Animal Activity Recognition. In Proceedings of the 2020 IEEE International Conference on Smart Systems and Technologies (SST), Osijek, Croatia, 4–16 October 2020; pp. 83–88.
11. Terrasson, G.; Llaria, A.; Marra, A.; Voaden, S. Accelerometer based solution for precision livestock farming: Geolocation enhancement and animal activity identification. In *IOP Conference Series: Materials Science and Engineering*; IOP Publishing: Bristol, UK, 2016; Volume 138, p. 012004.
12. Demir, G.; Erman, A.T. Activity recognition and tracking system for domestic animals. In Proceedings of the 2018 IEEE 26th Signal Processing and Communications Applications Conference (SIU), Izmir, Turkey, 2–5 May 2018; pp. 1–4.
13. Kleanthous, N.; Hussain, A.; Mason, A.; Sneddon, J.; Shaw, A.; Fergus, P.; Chalmers, C.; Al-Jumeily, D. Machine learning techniques for classification of livestock behavior. In Proceedings of the International Conference on Neural Information Processing, Siem Reap, Cambodia, 13–16 December 2018; Springer: Berlin/Heidelberg, Germany, 2018; pp. 304–315.
14. Kamminga, J.W.; Le, D.V.; Meijers, J.P.; Bisby, H.; Meratnia, N.; Havinga, P.J. Robust sensor-orientation-independent feature selection for animal activity recognition on collar tags. *Proc. ACM Interact. Mob. Wearable Ubiquitous Technol.* **2018**, *2*, 1–27. [CrossRef]
15. Debauche, O.; Elmoulat, M.; Mahmoudi, S.; Bindelle, J.; Lebeau, F. Farm animals' behaviors and welfare analysis with AI algorithms: A review. *Revue d'Intelligence Artificielle* **2021**, *35*, 243–253. [CrossRef]
16. Soltis, J.; Wilson, R.P.; Douglas-Hamilton, I.; Vollrath, F.; King, L.E.; Savage, A. Accelerometers in collars identify behavioral states in captive African elephants Loxodonta africana. *Endanger. Spec. Res.* **2012**, *18*, 255–263. [CrossRef]
17. Fehlmann, G.; O'Riain, M.J.; Hopkins, P.W.; O'Sullivan, J.; Holton, M.D.; Shepard, E.L.; King, A.J. Identification of behaviors from accelerometer data in a wild social primate. *Anim. Biotelem.* **2017**, *5*, 1–11. [CrossRef]
18. le Roux, S.; Wolhuter, R.; Niesler, T. An overview of automatic behavior classification for animal-borne sensor applications in South Africa. In Proceedings of the ACM Multimedia 2017 Workshop on South African Academic Participation, Mountain View, CA, USA, 23 October 2017; pp. 15–19.
19. Junior, R.L. IoT applications for monitoring companion animals: A systematic literature review. In Proceedings of the 2020 IEEE 14th International Conference on Innovations in Information Technology (IIT), Al Ain, United Arab Emirates, 17–18 November 2020; pp. 239–246.
20. De Seabra, J.; Rybarczyk, Y.; Batista, A.; Rybarczyk, P.; Lebret, M.; Vernay, D. Development of a Wearable Monitoring System for Service Dogs. 2014. Available online: https://docentes.fct.unl.pt/agb/files/service_dogs.pdf (accessed on 16 December 2021).
21. Ladha, C.; Hammerla, N.; Hughes, E.; Olivier, P.; Ploetz, T. Dog's life: Wearable activity recognition for dogs. In Proceedings of the 2013 ACM International Joint Conference on Pervasive and Ubiquitous Computing, Zurich, Switzerland, 8–12 September 2013; pp. 415–418.
22. den Uijl, I.; Álvarez, C.B.G.; Bartram, D.J.; Dror, Y.; Holland, R.; Cook, A.J.C. External validation of a collar-mounted triaxial accelerometer for second-by-second monitoring of eight behavioral states in dogs. *PLoS ONE* **2017**, *12*, e0188481. [CrossRef]

23. Massawe, E.A.; Michael, K.; Kaijage, S.; Seshaiyer, P. Design and Analysis of smart sensing system for animal emotions recognition. *ICAJ* 2017, 169, 46–50.
24. Wernimont, S.M.; Thompson, R.J.; Mickelsen, S.L.; Smith, S.C.; Alvarenga, I.C.; Gross, K.L. Use of accelerometer activity monitors to detect changes in pruritic behaviors: Interim clinical data on 6 dogs. *Sensors* **2018**, *18*, 249. [CrossRef]
25. Gerencsér, L.; Vásárhelyi, G.; Nagy, M.; Vicsek, T.; Miklósi, A. Identification of behavior in freely moving dogs (Canis familiaris) using inertial sensors. *PLoS ONE* **2013**, *8*, e77814. [CrossRef] [PubMed]
26. Brugarolas, R.; Latif, T.; Dieffenderfer, J.P.; Walker, K.; Yuschak, S.; Sherman, B.L.; Roberts, D.L.; Bozkurt, A. Wearable Heart Rate Sensor Systems for Wireless Canine Health Monitoring. *IEEE Sens. J.* **2016**, *16*, 3454–3464. [CrossRef]
27. Hansen, B.D.; Lascelles, B.D.X.; Keene, B.W.; Adams, A.K.; Thomson, A.E. Evaluation of an accelerometer for at-home monitoring of spontaneous activity in dogs. *Am. J. Vet. Res.* **2007**, *68*, 468–475. [CrossRef] [PubMed]
28. Aich, S.; Chakraborty, S.; Sim, J.S.; Jang, D.J.; Kim, H.C. The design of an automated system for the analysis of the activity and emotional patterns of dogs with wearable sensors using machine learning. *Appl. Sci.* **2019**, *9*, 4938. [CrossRef]
29. Chambers, R.D.; Yoder, N.C.; Carson, A.B.; Junge, C.; Allen, D.E.; Prescott, L.M.; Bradley, S.; Wymore, G.; Lloyd, K.; Lyle, S. Deep learning classification of canine behavior using a single collar-mounted accelerometer: Real-world validation. *Animals* **2021**, *11*, 1549. [CrossRef]
30. Piczak, K.J. Environmental sound classification with convolutional neural networks. In Proceedings of the 2015 IEEE 25th International Workshop on Machine Learning for Signal Processing (MLSP), Boston, MA, USA, 17–20 September 2015; pp. 1–6.
31. Hershey, S.; Chaudhuri, S.; Ellis, D.P.W.; Gemmeke, J.F.; Jansen, A.; Moore, R.C.; Plakal, M.; Platt, D.; Saurous, R.A.; Seybold, B.; et al. CNN architectures for large-scale audio classification. In Proceedings of the 2017 IEEE International Conference on Acoustics, Speech and Signal Processing (ICASSP), New Orleans, LA, USA, 5–9 March 2017; pp. 131–135.
32. Krizhevsky, A.; Sutskever, I.; Hinton, G.E. ImageNet classification with deep convolutional neural networks. *Commun. ACM* **2012**, *60*, 84–90. [CrossRef]
33. Simonyan, K.; Zisserman, A. Very Deep Convolutional Networks for Large-Scale Image Recognition. *arXiv* **2015**, *arXiv:1409.1556*.
34. Szegedy, C.; Vanhoucke, V.; Ioffe, S.; Shlens, J.; Wojna, Z. Rethinking the Inception Architecture for Computer Vision. In Proceedings of the 2016 IEEE Conference on Computer Vision and Pattern Recognition (CVPR), Las Vegas, NV, USA, 27–30 June 2016; pp. 2818–2826.
35. He, K.; Zhang, X.; Ren, S.; Sun, J. Delving Deep into Rectifiers: Surpassing Human-Level Performance on ImageNet Classification. In Proceedings of the 2015 IEEE International Conference on Computer Vision (ICCV), Santiago, Chile, 7–13 December 2015; pp. 1026–1034.
36. Gemmeke, J.F.; Ellis, D.P.W.; Freedman, D.; Jansen, A.; Lawrence, W.; Moore, R.C.; Plakal, M.; Ritter, M. Audio Set: An ontology and human-labeled dataset for audio events. In Proceedings of the 2017 IEEE International Conference on Acoustics, Speech and Signal Processing (ICASSP), New Orleans, LA, USA, 5–9 March 2017; pp. 776–780.
37. Salamon, J.; Bello, J.P. Unsupervised feature learning for urban sound classification. In Proceedings of the 2015 IEEE International Conference on Acoustics, Speech and Signal Processing (ICASSP), South Brisbane, Australia, 19–24 April 2015; pp. 171–175.
38. Coates, A.; Ng, A. Learning Feature Representations with K-Means. In *Neural Networks: Tricks of the Trade*; Springer: Berlin/Heidelberg, Germnay, 2012.
39. Kumar, A.; Raj, B. Deep CNN Framework for Audio Event Recognition using Weakly Labeled Web Data. *arXiv* **2017**, arXiv:1707.02530.
40. Salamon, J.; Bello, J.P. Deep Convolutional Neural Networks and Data Augmentation for Environmental Sound Classification. *IEEE Signal Process. Lett.* **2017**, *24*, 279–283. [CrossRef]
41. Piczak, K.J. ESC: Dataset for Environmental Sound Classification. In Proceedings of the 23rd ACM International Conference on Multimedia, Brisbane Australia, 26–30 October 2015.
42. Jackson, M.M.; Byrne, C.A.; Freil, L.; Valentin, G.; Zuerndorfer, J.; Zeagler, C.; Logas, J.; Gilliland, S.M.; Rapoport, A.; Sun, S.; et al. Technology for working dogs. In Proceedings of the Fifth International Conference on Animal-Computer Interaction, Atlanta, GA, USA, 4–6 December 2018.
43. Valentin, G.; Alcaidinho, J.; Howard, A.M.; Jackson, M.M.; Starner, T. Towards a canine-human communication system based on head gestures. In Proceedings of the 12th International Conference on Advances in Computer Entertainment Technology, Iskandar, Malaysia, 16–19 November 2015.
44. Pantazes, T. Wearable Canine and Feline Collar with Camera and Added Features. U.S. Patent 9,615,546, 30 March 2016.
45. David Lopez, B.V.C. Interactive Communication and Tracking Dog Collar. U.S. Patent 8,543,134 B2, April 2012.
46. Ferworn, A.; Wright, C.; Tran, J.; Li, C.; Choset, H. Dog and snake marsupial cooperation for urban search and rescue deployment. In Proceedings of the 2012 IEEE International Symposium on Safety, Security, and Rescue Robotics (SSRR), College Station, TX, USA, 5–8 November 2012; pp. 1–5.
47. Yu, Y.; Wu, Z.; Xu, K.; Gong, Y.; Zheng, N.; Zheng, X.; Pan, G. Automatic Training of Rat Cyborgs for Navigation. *Comput. Intell. Neurosci.* **2016**, *2016*, 6459251. [CrossRef]
48. Kamminga, J.W.; Bisby, H.C.; Le, D.V.; Meratnia, N.; Havinga, P.J. Generic online animal activity recognition on collar tags. In Proceedings of the 2017 ACM International Joint Conference on Pervasive and Ubiquitous Computing and Proceedings of the 2017 ACM International Symposium on Wearable Computers, Maui, HI, 11–15 September 2017; pp. 597–606.

49. Kumar, A.; Khadkevich, M.; Fügen, C. Knowledge Transfer from Weakly Labeled Audio Using Convolutional Neural Network for Sound Events and Scenes. In Proceedings of the 2018 IEEE International Conference on Acoustics, Speech and Signal Processing (ICASSP), Calgary, AB, Canada, 15–20 April 2018; pp. 326–330.
50. Kingma, D.P.; Ba, J. Adam: A method for stochastic optimization. *arXiv* **2014**, arXiv:1412.6980.
51. Hestness, J.; Narang, S.; Ardalani, N.; Diamos, G.F.; Jun, H.; Kianinejad, H.; Patwary, M.M.A.; Yang, Y.; Zhou, Y. Deep Learning Scaling is Predictable, Empirically. *arXiv* **2017**, arXiv:1712.00409.

sensors

MDPI

Article

E2DR: A Deep Learning Ensemble-Based Driver Distraction Detection with Recommendations Model

Mustafa Aljasim and Rasha Kashef *

Electrical, Computer, and Biomedical Engineering, Ryerson University, Toronto, ON M5B 2K3, Canada; mustafa.aljasim@ryerson.ca
* Correspondence: rkashef@ryerson.ca

Abstract: The increasing number of car accidents is a significant issue in current transportation systems. According to the World Health Organization (WHO), road accidents are the eighth highest top cause of death around the world. More than 80% of road accidents are caused by distracted driving, such as using a mobile phone, talking to passengers, and smoking. A lot of efforts have been made to tackle the problem of driver distraction; however, no optimal solution is provided. A practical approach to solving this problem is implementing quantitative measures for driver activities and designing a classification system that detects distracting actions. In this paper, we have implemented a portfolio of various ensemble deep learning models that have been proven to efficiently classify driver distracted actions and provide an in-car recommendation to minimize the level of distractions and increase in-car awareness for improved safety. This paper proposes E2DR, a new scalable model that uses stacking ensemble methods to combine two or more deep learning models to improve accuracy, enhance generalization, and reduce overfitting, with real-time recommendations. The highest performing E2DR variant, which included the ResNet50 and VGG16 models, achieved a test accuracy of 92% as applied to state-of-the-art datasets, including the State Farm Distracted Drivers dataset, using novel data splitting strategies.

Keywords: deep learning; stacking; ensemble learning; distracted driving

Citation: Aljasim, M.; Kashef, R. E2DR: A Deep Learning Ensemble-Based Driver Distraction Detection with Recommendations Model. *Sensors* **2022**, *22*, 1858. https://doi.org/10.3390/s22051858

Academic Editors: Andrei Velichko, Dmitry Korzun and Alexander Meigal

Received: 25 December 2021
Accepted: 23 February 2022
Published: 26 February 2022

1. Introduction

With the continuous growth of the population, new technologies and transportation methods need to emerge to serve people effectively and efficiently. Building an efficient and safe transportation system can positively affect economies, the environment, and human mental and physical health. The increasing number of accidents is a major issue in our current transportation system. According to the World Health Organization, road accidents are the eighth highest reason for death worldwide [1]. According to [2], 1.35 million people die every year in a car accident, and up to 50 million people are injured. This makes traffic safety a major concern worldwide. More than 80% of road accidents are caused by distracted driving, such as using a mobile phone, talking to passengers, and smoking [2]. Therefore, more attention has been directed to driver action analysis and monitoring. Many efforts have been made to tackle the problem of driver distraction with effective approaches using countermeasures for distracted driver actions [3]. The measures can be divided into three categories: (1) distraction prevention before distraction occurs, (2) distracting action detection (through alertness) after distraction occurs, and (3) collision avoidance when a potential collision is expected [3]. Imposing strict fines, government legislation, and raising public awareness are methods used to decrease the number of accidents caused by distracted driving through preventing distraction sources before it happens. When a potential collision is expected, collision avoidance systems are implemented in most newly manufactured cars through lane control, automatic emergency braking, and forward-collision warning. Distraction alertness is critical and can be more effective in preventing driver distraction; thus, accurate real-time driver action detection methods are essential for this driver distraction category. Distraction alertness can be approached with different modalities. A camera was used to detect distracted driving behavior while driving in many applications. A Controller Area Network Bus can assess the vehicle's performance, such as wheel angle and brake level. Moreover, the system can detect if the driver is distracted or focused on driving based on the in-car collected information. Finally, sensors, such as the electrocardiograph and the electroencephalograph, can be used to estimate the emotional and physiological states of a driver, which can be associated with the level of distraction and fatigue in drivers [4]; however, there is a lack of reflection on the fact that they are invasive sensors for a driver. The driver's action or behavior, such as gaze, head pose, and hand position, can be detected through deep learning models and the analysis of the car information [5]. Existing methods in detecting driver distraction fall short in providing accurate detection and recommendations in real-time. Ensemble learning has shown better classification performance compared to individual models, as it combines the benefits of multiple models while overcoming their drawbacks [6]. While authors in [6] used a fixed architecture of only three deep learning models including the residual network (ResNet), the hierarchical recurrent neural network (HRNN), and the Inception network, there is a research gap in the literature in using a scalable and incremental stacking-based ensemble learning with real-time recommendations to achieve high accuracy in detecting distracted driving activities with minimal computational overhead. Thus, in this paper, we have proposed a novel scalable model that uses ensemble learning, focusing on stacking that combines two or more baseline models and generates an ensemble with better performance than the adopted models. Our method aims to enhance generalization, reduce overfitting, increase performance, and provide real-time recommendations. This paper first examines the performance of several state-of-the-art image deep learning classification methods. An Ensemble-Based Distraction Detection with Recommendations model is designed, namely (E2DR), with the goal of improving the accuracy of distracted behavior detection. In the proposed E2DR model, two or more deep learning models are aggregated in a stacking ensemble. A recommendation layer is also provided for real-time recommendations to drivers in each case of the distracted behaviors to allow drivers or autonomous vehicles to take the best course of action when drivers are detected under distracted behaviors. Experimental results show that state-of-the-art image classification models achieve a test accuracy ranging between 82–88% in detecting driver distraction. Furthermore, results show an average improvement of 5–8% in detection accuracy when the proposed E2DR is used with a real-time data splitting based on the driver IDs. Similar results are obtained for other metrics such as Precision and F1 score. The rest of this paper is as follows: Section 2 discusses deep learning driver distraction detection systems and the related work. Sections 3 and 4 introduce the adopted and proposed models, respectively. Section 5 presents the experimental results and analysis. We conclude the paper with future directions in Section 6.

2. Related Work on Deep Learning Driver Distraction Detection

There are three main types of distracted driving: cognitive, visual, and manual distraction. Cognitive distraction occurs when the driver's mind is not entirely focused on driving. Driver gaze and talking to passengers are examples of cognitive distraction. Even drivers listening to music or the radio are at risk. The audio or music can shift the driver's attention from driving and overall surroundings. Visual distraction is when the driver is not looking at the road ahead. Drivers who observe shop signs and billboards on the side of the road are considered visually distracted. Looking at electronic devices such as GPS devices, smartphones, and digital entertainment devices while driving is under the category of visual distraction. Finally, manual distraction occurs when the driver, for any reason, takes their hands off the steering wheel. Drivers who smoke while driving, eat and drink in the car, or try to get something from anywhere in the vehicle are under the risk of manual distraction. Texting while driving is the most dangerous driver distraction as it combines all three types of distractions. When drivers take their eye off the road to send a message or check a notification, it is long enough to cover the length of a football field at 80 km/h [5]. Various research studies have been proposed to address the drivers' distraction detection problem. This section will survey the most recent state-of-the-art research work using Single-based vs. Hybrid-based deep learning to address this problem.

2.1. Single-Based Deep Learning Models

A gaze estimation model called X-Aware is introduced in [7] to analyze the driver's face along with contextual information. The model visually improves the fusion of the captured environment of the driver's face, where the contextual attention mechanism is directly attached to the output of convolutional layers of the InceptionResNetV2 networks. The accuracy of their best model outperformed the other baseline models in the literature. The dynamics of the driver's gaze and their use to understand other attentional mechanisms are addressed in [8]. The model is built based on two questions, where and what is the driver looking at. The model is trained through coarse-to-fine convolutional networks on short sequences from the DR(eye)VE dataset [8]. Their experiments showed that the driver's gaze could be learned to some extent, considering its highly subjective challenges and the scene's irreproducibility showing the driver's gaze for each sequence. The results showed that the model could achieve accurate results and could be integrated into practical applications. In [9], the authors proposed a deep learning model that detects drivers' behavior and actions during travel. The deep learning model classifies the driver actions into ten classes. The first class represents safe driving, and the other nine classes represent unsafe drivers' actions such as fixing makeup and texting. The driver receives an alert if an unsafe action is detected. They used Convolutional Neural Networks (CNNs) to perform training and detection. The core of the deep learning system is ResNet50. A dense net architecture followed the ResNet50 architecture to make classifications. The dataset used is the State Farm dataset and included images of different drivers' actions that cause distracted driving. The model achieved high accuracy in detecting the driver's actions. A facial expression recognition model in [10] monitors drivers' emotions and operates in low specification devices installed in cars. A Hierarchal Weighted Random Forest Classifier (HRFC) is used and trained on the similarity of sample data. Geometric features and facial landmarks are detected and extracted from input images. The features are vectorized and implemented in the Hierarchal Random-Forest Classifier to detect facial expressions. The method was evaluated on the MMI dataset, the Keimyung University Facial Expression of Drivers (KMU-FED) dataset and the Cohn-Kahnde dataset. The results showed that the proposed model had similar performance to other state-of-the-art methods. The study in [11] introduced a computationally efficient distracted driver detection system based on convolutional neural networks. The authors proposed a new architecture called mobileVGG. The architecture is based on depth-wise separable convolutions. The authors used a simplified version of the VGG16 model, allowing the proposed architecture to be suitable for real-time applications with decent classification accuracy. The datasets used are the State Farm dataset and the American University in Cairo Distracted Driver (AUCDD) detection dataset. The results showed that the proposed architecture outperformed other approaches while being computationally simple. The driver's face pose is detected by training CNNs [12]; the CNNs then identify if the driver's head position is considered under the category of distracted driving. The model consists of five CNNs followed by three fully connected layers. The results showed that the proposed model has better accuracy when compared to non-linear and linear embedding algorithms. In [13], the authors proposed a driver action recognition system called dilated and deformable Faster Region-Based Convolutional Neural Networks (R-CNN). It detects driver actions by detecting motion-specific objects exhibiting inter-class similarity and intra-class differences. The irregular and small features, such as cell phones and cigarettes, are extracted through the dilated and deformable residual block. Then, the region proposal optimization network algorithm decreases the number of features and improves the model's efficiency. Finally, the feature pooling module is replaced with a deformable one, and the R-CNN network is trained as the classifier of the network. The authors established the dataset and contained images of different driver actions. Results showed that the model demonstrates acceptable results. Authors in [14] implemented a driver distraction detection model that uses a light-weight octave-like convolutional neural network. The network consists of octave-like convolutional blocks called OLCMNet. The OCLM block splits the feature map into two branches through point-wise convolution. Average pooling and depth-wise convolution are performed on the feature map. A DC operator captures the fine details in the high-frequency branches. Lastly, the OCLMNet exchanges further information between layers. The model performed well on the Lilong Distracted Driving Behavior dataset while being implemented on a limited computation budget. A unique approach is proposed in [15] that uses both spatial and temporal information of electroencephalography (EEG) signals as an input to a deep learning model. The relationship between the driver distraction and the EEG signal in the time domain is mapped through gated recurrent units (GRUs) and CNNs. Twenty-four volunteers were tested while doing activities that cause a distraction while driving, and their EEG response was recorded. Then, the proposed deep learning network was trained based on the EEG information. The deep learning approach consisted of a temporal–spatial information network (TSIN), combining CNNs and GRUs to better detect spatial and temporal features from EEG signals. The authors of [16] proposed a modifier deep learning approach for distraction detection. They used the OpenPose library for a two-category problem of distraction detection. The library draws 43 points on the facial skeleton to detect the human face. The detection is sent to a deep neural network that uses the ResNet50 model. The results demonstrated good accuracy and outperformed other residual network architectures. The work in [17] introduced a new approach to distracted driver detection using wearable sensing and deep neural networks. The study included information from twenty participants through wearable motion sensors attached to their wrists. The participants performed five distraction activities under instructions in a driving simulator. The captured data were sent to a deep learning model that consisted of recurrent neural networks and long short-term memory (RNN-LSTM) which classified distraction tasks. The results showed a good potential for the wearable proposed sensing approach.

2.2. *Hybrid-Based Deep Learning Models*

A hybrid model is designed in [18] with an ensemble of weighted CNNs for driver posture classification. The authors proved that using a weighted ensemble classifier using the genetic algorithm resulted in a better confidence score for classification. Additionally, the effect of variable visual elements is analyzed, such as face and hands, in detecting distracted driver action through localization of face and hands. The dataset used is the Distracted Driver dataset, which contains ten classes of driver actions. The best model has an accuracy of 96%, and a smaller version of the ensemble model achieved an accuracy of 94.29%. In [19], a distracted driver detection technique using pose estimation is introduced. The model is an ensemble of ResNets and classifies drivers through pose estimation images. ResNet and HRnet are used to generate pose images. Then, ResNet50 and ResNet101 classify the original and pose estimation images. The grid search method identifies the optimum weight for predictions from both models. Classifying pose estimation images is useful when used with the original image classification model as it increases classification accuracy. The dataset used is the AUCDD dataset. The results showed that the introduced model achieved an accuracy of 94.28%. The study in [20] detected driver–vehicle volatilities using driving data to detect the occurrence of critical events and give appropriate feedback to drivers and surrounding vehicles through analyzing multiple real-time data streams such as vehicle movements, instability of driving, and driver distraction. The deep learning model consisted of a Convolutional Neural Network (CNN) model and a long short-term memory (LSTM) model. The data were collected from more than 3500 drivers and included 1315 severe and 7566 normal events. The model achieved high accuracy and was effective in detecting accidents. A CNNs-based model to identify driver's activities is introduced in [21]. The driving activities are divided into several classes, in which 4 are considered normal driving activities, and the other three are classified as distracted driving. The Gaussian mixture model detects the driver's body from the background before sending the image to the CNN model. The authors used transfer learning to fine-tune three pre-trained state-of-the-art CNN models: Restnet50, AlexNet, and GoogLeNet. The model was trained as a binary classifier to detect whether the driver was distracted or not. The authors collected the data from 10 drivers involved in the most common driving activities. The results showed that the model was effective as a binary classifier. In [22], a model for distracted driving action recognition is proposed using a hybrid of two convolutional neural network architectures, Xception and Inception V3, to detect 10 classes of driver actions. The authors used ImageNet weights for transfer learning. The performance of both models was analyzed under different weighting schemes. Using pre-trained weights helped the network learn basic shapes and edges without starting training from scratch, which allowed the model to achieve good results in under 10 epochs of training, applied to the State Farm Distracted Driver dataset. The results showed that the Inception model had a better performance compared to the Xception model. A distracted driver action recognition system is introduced in [23] based on the Discriminative Scale Space Tracking (DSST) and Deep Predictive Coding Network (PCN) algorithms, dynamic face tracking, location, and face detection. Then, the YOLOv3 object detection model detects distracting behavior around the driver's face, such as phone calls and smoking. The dataset used is a self-built dataset of people making phone calls and smoking. The results demonstrated that the model could detect a driver's behavior with high accuracy. A hybrid driver distraction detection model is presented in [24]. The model uses CNNs and Bidirectional Long Short-Term Memory (BiLSTM). The proposed model captures the spatio-spectral features of the images and consists of two steps: (1) detect the spatial features of different postures using CNNs automatically, and (2) the spectral components from the stacked feature map are extracted through the BiLSTMs. They used the AUCDD dataset. Results showed that their model performed better than most state-of-the-art models. The work in [25] used deep learning to detect driver inattentive and aggressive behavior. They classified inattentive driver behavior into driver fatigue, downiness, driver distraction, and other risky driver behavior such as driving aggressiveness. All these risky driving behaviors are associated with various factors that include driving age, experience, illness, and gender. The authors used CNNs, RNNs and LSTMs. They showed that the CNNs achieved the best performance. The algorithm in [26] detects driver manual distraction using two modules; in the first module, the bounding boxes of the driver's right ear and right hand are detected from RGB images through YOLO, a deep learning object detection model. Then, the bounding boxes are taken as an input by the second module, a multi-layer perceptron, to predict the distraction type. The dataset consisted of 106,677 frames extracted from a video obtained from 20 participants in a driving simulator. The proposed algorithm achieved comparable results with other models in the same field. Table 1 provides a comparative study of the recent work in driver distraction detection systems. There is a research gap in the literature in using stacking-based ensemble learning to achieve high accuracy in detecting distracted driving activities with minimal computational overhead. Thus, in this paper, we have proposed a framework that uses ensemble learning, focusing on stacking that combines two baseline models and generates an ensemble with better performance than the adopted models.

Table 1. Comparative Analysis of Driver Distraction detection systems.

Paper	Model (Type)	Dataset	Validation	Pros	Cons
[7]	Deep learning Gaze estimation system	Driver Gaze in the Wild dataset	Accuracy	High performance	It can be only accurate to an extent
[8]	Deep learning Gaze estimation driver-assistant system	DR(eye)VE dataset	Ground truth	Provide suggestion	Driver gaze is subjective
[9]	Deep learning distracted driver detection	Distracted driver dataset	Accuracy, Recall, Precision, F1 score	Computationally efficient	Few epochs for training
[10]	Hierarchical, weighted random forest (WRF) model	The Keimyung University Facial Expression of Drivers (KMU-FED) and the Cohn-Kahnde datasets	Accuracy	Requires low amount of memory and computing operations	Not accurate when the face is rotated
[11]	Driver distraction detection using CNNs	State farm dataset and the AUC distracted driver dataset	Accuracy, sensitivity	Computationally efficient	Not enough validation metrics
[12]	Deep learning distracted driver detection using pose estimation	AUC Distracted Driver Dataset	Accuracy, F1 score	Pose estimation improves accuracy	Low-resolution images affected training
[13]	Driver action recognition using R-CNN	images of different driver actions	Accuracy and log loss	Effective feature representation	Small dataset
[14]	Driver Distraction recognition Using Octave-Like CNN	Lilong Distracted Driving Behavior data	Accuracy, training duration	Lightweight network	Not enough validation metrics
[15]	Temporal–Spatial Deep Learning driver distraction detection	EEG signals from 24 participants	Precision, Recall, F1 score	Unique approach	Drivers' individual differences need to be considered
[16]	Optimized Residual Neural Network Architecture	The State Farm Distracted Driver dataset	Accuracy, training time	Enhanced model	Only detects head movement
[17]	Wearable sensing and deep learning driver distraction detection	Wearable sensing information from 20 participants	Recall, Precision, F1 score	Good potential	Small dataset
[18]	Hybrid Distraction detection model using deep learning	State farm dataset	Accuracy	Computationally expensive	Not enough validation
[19]	Triple-Wise Multi-Task Learning	AUC Distracted Driver Dataset	Accuracy, sensitivity	High detection accuracy	High computational cost
[20]	Safety-critical events prediction	Driving events from 3500 drivers	Accuracy, Recall, Precision, F1 score	Can detect potential car accidents	Hard to get enough data
[21]	CNN driver action detection system	10 drivers' data with driving activities	Accuracy	Accurate	It does not detect the driver action
[22]	CNN driver action detection system	Distracted driver dataset	Accuracy and loss	Computationally simple	Not enough training
[23]	Distracted driver behavior detection using deep learning	Self-built dataset of drivers making phone calls and smoking	Recall, Precision, Speed	Real-time	Only trained to detect 2 driver actions
[24]	hybrid driver distraction detection model	(AUC) Distracted Driver Dataset	Accuracy and loss	High Performance	Complex
[25]	Driver Inattentiveness detection	NA	Accuracy	Comprehensive analysis of deep learning models	Not effective in detecting aggressive behavior
[26]	Deep learning manual distraction detection model	106,677 frames extracted from a video that was taken from 20 participants in a driving simulator	Accuracy, Recall, Precision, F1 score	Novel approach	Only detects manual distraction

3. Adopted Deep Learning Models

3.1. ResNet50 Model

ResNet50 is a 50-layer deep convolutional neural network (Figure 1) [27]. The pre-trained version of the network can be imported from the ImageNet database [28], trained on over a million photos. The network is trained to classify images into 1,000 different object categories, including pencils, tables, mice, and various animals and objects. As a result, the network has learned a variety of rich feature representations for a large variety of images [29]. In the final classification model, ResNet50 is used as the convolutional base, and the pre-trained model is used to learn the patterns in the data. ResNet50 requires the size of the input images to be 224 × 224 (width, height) [29]. All the experiments were conducted with color images. The dimensions of each image sent to the classification model were (224, 224, 3), where 3 indicates the number of channels in the images. The three channels indicated are color channels composed of Green, blue, and red.

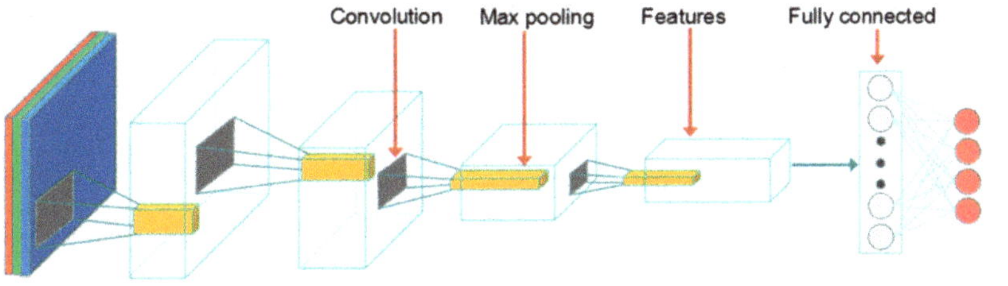

Figure 1. The ResNet50 blocks [27].

3.2. VGG16 Model

Oxford's VGG16 architecture from the Visual Geometry Group (VGG) (Figure 2) has an advantage over AlexNet by replacing large kernel-sized filter 5 and 100 in the second and first convolutional layers, respectively, with several kernel-sized filters of size 3 × 3 one after another [30]. Similar to the ResNet50 model, the input to the network is a 224 × 224 × 3 image, where 3 indicates the RGB channels. The image is passed through a series of convolutional layers with small receptive field filters with a size of 3 × 3 [31]. This filter size is the smallest to capture center, up/down and left/right notions. Additionally, the configuration utilizes 1 × 1 convolutional filters that can be considered a linear transformation of the input channel [32].

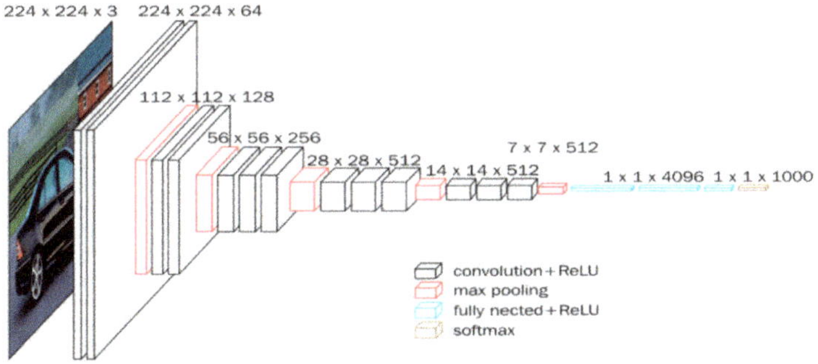

Figure 2. The VGG16 blocks [33].

3.3. Inception Model

The Inception model (Figure 3) is a significant milestone in the evolution of CNN classifiers. Inception changed the traditional approach of adding more and deeper convolutional layers to improve performance [34]. Inception went through several versions and developed with time. Inception V1 [35] uses multiple filters that operate simultaneously, making the network wider rather than deeper. Then, the authors introduced Inception V2 and V3 [36]. Inception V2 significantly improved performance and computational speed by using two 3 × 3 convolutional operations instead of a single 5 × 5 convolution which is 2.78 times more computationally expensive [37]. Inception V3, the model used in the experiment, includes all upgrades in Inception V2 and factorized 7 × 7 convolutions, which improved performance even more, and added Label Smoothing to decrease the chances of overfitting [38]. The main contribution of Inception V4 is adding reduction blocks to change the width and height of the grid [39].

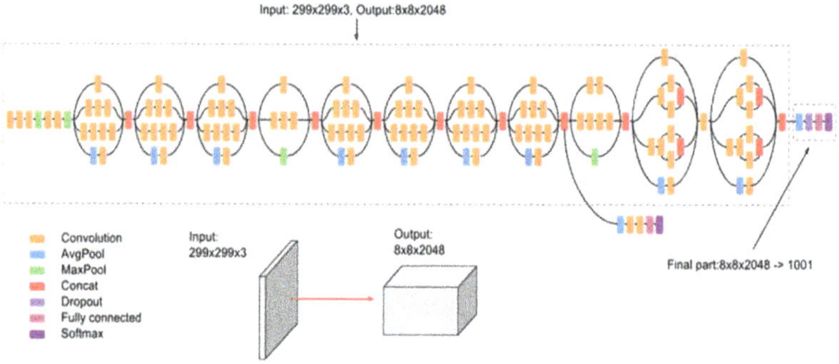

Figure 3. The Inception v3 architecture [39].

3.4. *MobileNet Model*

MobileNet (Figure 4) is the first mobile computer vision model based on TensorFlow [40]. The name Mobile implies the ability of the model to function in mobile applications [41]. MobileNet is based on separable depth-wise convolutions, which significantly reduces the number of parameters, especially when compared to networks with regular convolutions that have the same depth of the nets. This makes MobileNet a lightweight deep neural network suitable for mobile applications [42]. The depth-wise separable convolution is made from two primary operations: depth-wise convolution and point-wise convolution. The depth-wise convolution came from the idea that the filter's spatial and depth dimensions can be separated. The filter is separated by its height and width dimensions, and then the depth dimension is separated from the horizontal (width×height) dimension. The point-wise convolution is a 1 × 1 convolution that changes the dimension of the previous layer.

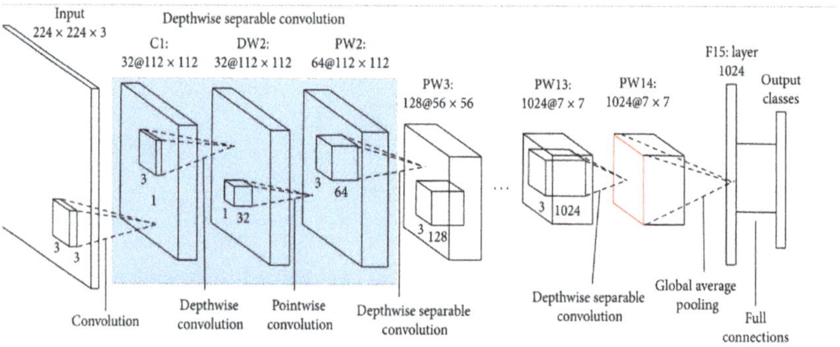

Figure 4. The MobileNet Architecture [43].

4. The Proposed E2DR Model

Existing driver distraction detection systems in the literature only use a single model trained for classification. Moreover, most recent work uses a single state-of-the-art classifier or a network of convolutional neural layers to get the best performance. In this paper, an Ensemble-Based Distraction Detection with Recommendations system is designed, namely

E2DR, to improve the accuracy of driver distraction detection and provide recommendations. In the proposed E2DR model, two deep learning models are aggregated in a stacking ensemble. A recommendation layer is also provided for real-time recommendations in each case of distracted behaviors. The E2DR model enhances the generalization of the detection process and reduces overfitting. The E2DR model allows drivers or autonomous vehicles, depending on the technology in the vehicle, to take the best action when drivers are detected under distracted behaviors.

4.1. The Ensemble-Based Distraction Detection with Recommendations Model (E2DR)

Stacked generalization (SG) was first introduced in [44]; it was shown that stacking reduces the bias of the single model concerning the training set, where bias is the average difference between actual and predicted results [44]. The deduction results from the stacking model's ability to harness the capabilities of more than one well-performing model on a regression or classification task to generate better performance and predictions than base classifiers in the ensemble, which reduces the error and bias. Inspired by the theory of stacking generalization, the E2DR model combines two or more detection models to provide better and more accurate predictions than individual models. The stacking algorithm takes the output of the base model as an input to another model, sometimes called a meta-learner, which learns how to combine the predictions of base models to generate better predictions. In more detail, the stacking architecture has two levels. The first level contains the base models, and the second level includes a meta-learner that concatenates the outcomes of base models to provide final predictions. Figure 5 shows the pair-wise stacking in the E2DR architecture (i.e., only two base models are combined).

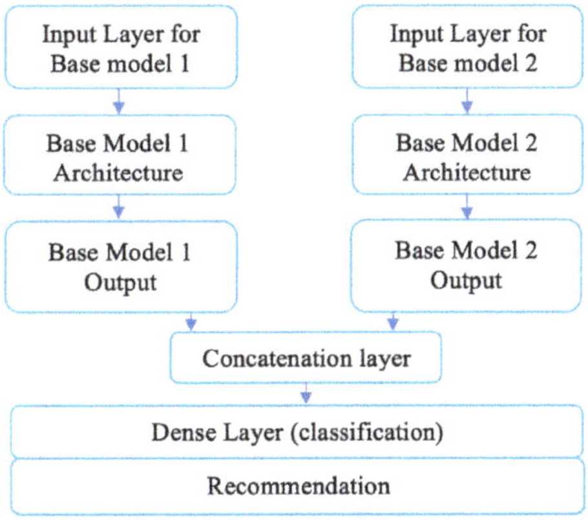

Figure 5. The E2DR (Pair-wise stacking) Architecture.

4.2. E2DR Variants

In this paper, six models are developed using variants of base model 1 and base model 2, such as E2DR (A1, A2) where A1 and A2 $\in$ {ResNet, VGG16, MobileNet, Inception}. The E2DR model combines 2 of the mentioned models using the Stacked Generalization (SG) ensemble method. The SG ensemble method uses the outputs from the pre-trained base models, concatenates them, and sends them to a meta-learner model at level 2 consisting of a dense layer for classification. Once the distracted behavior is classified, a set of recommended actions are provided to ensure safety. We calculate an assessment measure for each E2DR (A1, A2) using Accuracy, Loss, F-measure, Precision, and Recall.

4.3. Computational Complexity

Assume T_{A1} and T_{A2} are the computational time taken by both base models A1 and A2, respectively. Assume the meta learner needs overhead of T_M and the recommendation layer needs O(k) to retrieve recommendations based on the output classification, where k is the number of recommendations. We assume a linear search algorithm for recommendations extraction. The overall computational complexity of the E2DR model is computed as the maximum of T_{A1} and T_{A2} in addition to the overhead of concatenation and recommendation retrieval, as shown in Equation (1).

$$T_{E2DR} = O(Max(T_{A1}, \text{and } T_{A2}) + T_M + O(k) \quad (1)$$

4.4. Adopted Base Model Architectures

All adopted architectures use CNNs, a deep learning model that learns from spatial features of images by creating feature maps using filters and kernels (sliding windows). Many variations of CNNs have been studied recently to detect driving postures and actions. The models adopted in this paper are among the highest-performing CNN models. For all models, we used a learning rate of 0.001 and Categorical Cross Entropy as the loss function. The models are explained in detail in Section 3.

ResNet50 Model: When building the CNN model, the classification top of the ResNet50 Model (Figure 6), which was originally designed to classify 1000 classes [45], was dropped from the network to adapt the new CNN architecture to the dataset used that included only 10 classes. To avoid the problem of overfitting, a drop-out layer was added, and performance on the validation set was observed after every epoch. The hyperparameters, such as batch size, learning rate, and the number of neurons, were adjusted to optimize the model's performance and enhance the model's generalizability. We used different batch sizes: 128, 64, 32, and 16 to understand the significance of selecting the batch size as well as its effect on the network, with 32 as the best performing batch size.

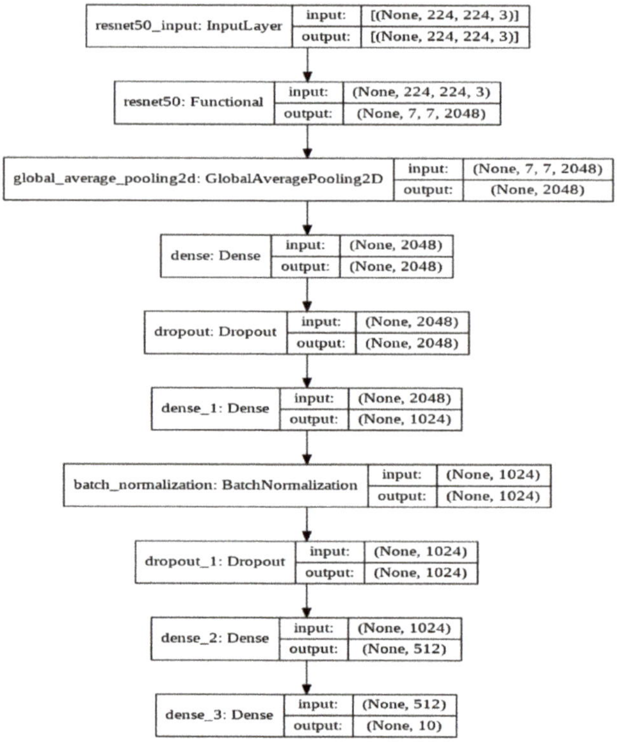

Figure 6. ResNet50 Architecture.

VGG16 Model: The VGG16 model (Figure 7) is among the largest models with many parameters. The padding is 1 pixel for 3×3 convolutional layers to preserve the spatial padding after undergoing convolution. The five-max pooling layers carry out the spatial pooling that follows some convolutional layers [46]. The max pooling is applied through a 2 × 2 pixel widow that has a stride value of 2. The same filter size is applied several times, allowing the network to represent complex features [47]. This "blocks" concept became more common after VGG was introduced [46]. As with the ResNet50, the classification layer (top layer) is adapted to the used dataset with 10 classes. The hyperparameter was chosen to optimize performance and training time with a batch size equals to 32.

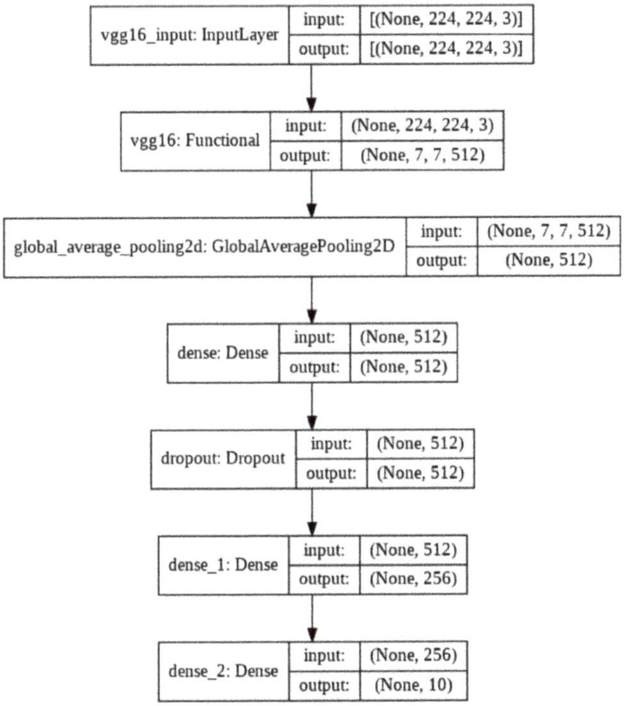

Figure 7. Dense net architecture (VGG16).

Inception model: The Inception model (Figure 8) is a widely-used image classification model with medium complexity. Its continual evolution resulted in the creation of multiple versions of the model. The one used in the experiments is the third version of the network, which has similar parameters to the ResNet50 model discussed earlier. The batch size equals 32, and the model is trained for 5 epochs. The model uses smaller convolutions which can be significant in decreasing computational time. In addition, factorizing convolutions reduces the number of parameters. Therefore, the Inception model has a lower training time compared to the ResNet50 and VGG16 models.

MobileNet model: we used the MobileNet architecture (Figure 9) to classify drivers' actions to examine its performance, considering it is the smallest state-of-the-art image classification network in terms of size and number of parameters. The main difference compared to other models is that MobileNet uses a 3 × 3 depth-wise convolution and 1 × 1 point-wise convolution instead of the traditional 3 × 3 convolution layer in most CNN models. The dense network is similar to the ResNet and Inception model networks discussed earlier. The batch size is 32, and the model was trained for 5 epochs. The top layer was removed from the network as with other models to modify the classifications according to the dataset used.

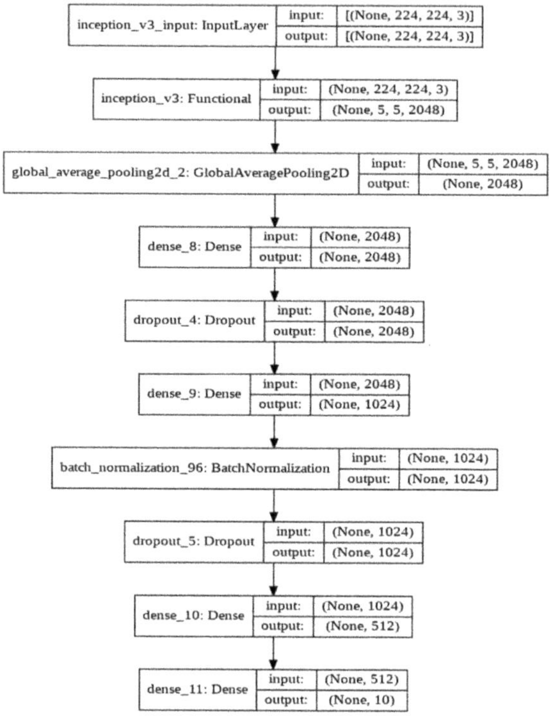

Figure 8. The Inception Model Architecture.

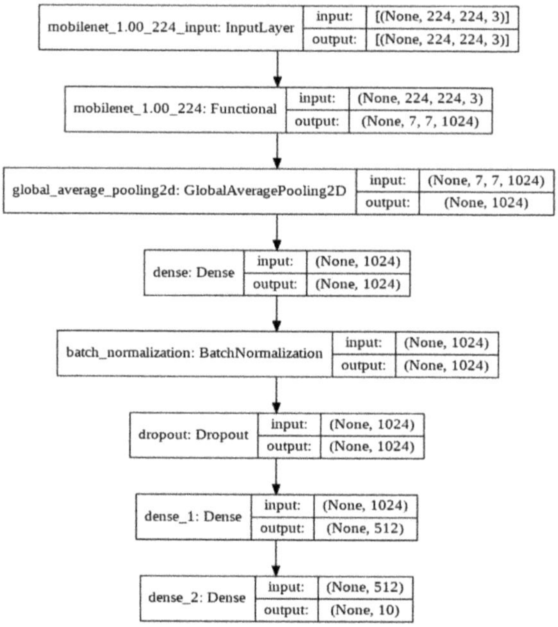

Figure 9. Model Architecture (MobileNet).

4.5. Recommendations

Adding a recommendation after the classification of each class can be a great improvement to the distracted driver detection implementations. In most cases, the best action to consider, especially in driving, is as easy as keeping the driver's focus on the road with no distraction. Reminding drivers is the best action to consider avoiding losing their attention during driving. An alert system can be effective with alternatives and actions to remind drivers of options to ensure their safety, especially drivers that need to take an important phone call or send an urgent text. In the case of autonomous vehicles, the recommendations can be sent to the vehicle to perform the best course of action. However, this is limited by the technology available in the vehicle. Table 2 provides the list of recommended actions as alertness signals to the driver based on the class of distracting activities while driving. The category of the distracting activities is retrieved from the ensemble classification layer in the E2DR model.

Table 2. Recommendations for distracted drivers.

Class Number	Class	Recommendation
C0	Safe driving	-
C1	Texting—Right	"Please avoid texting in all cases or make a stop"
C2	Talking on the phone—Right	"Please use a hands-free device"
C3	Texting—Left	"Please avoid texting in all cases or make a stop"
C4	Talking on the phone—Left	"Please use a hands-free device"
C5	Adjusting Radio	"Please use steering control"
C6	Drinking	"Please keep your hands at the steering wheel or make a stop"
C7	Reaching Behind	"Please keep your eyes on the road make a stop"
C8	Hair and Makeup	"Please make a stop"
C9	Talking to passenger	"Please keep your eyes on the road while talking"

5. Experimental Analysis and Results

5.1. Dataset

The dataset used in the experiment is the State Farm Distracted Drivers dataset [48]. There are 22,424 images of drivers in distracted positions that can be used for training and testing. The images in the dataset were taken with the contribution of 26 unique subjects in different cars (random numbering (i.e., not in consecutive order)). The dataset has 10 classes: safe driving, texting—right, talking on the phone—right, texting—left, talking on the phone—left, operating the radio, drinking, reaching behind, hair and makeup, and talking to a passenger. A representation of each class in the dataset is shown in Figure 10.

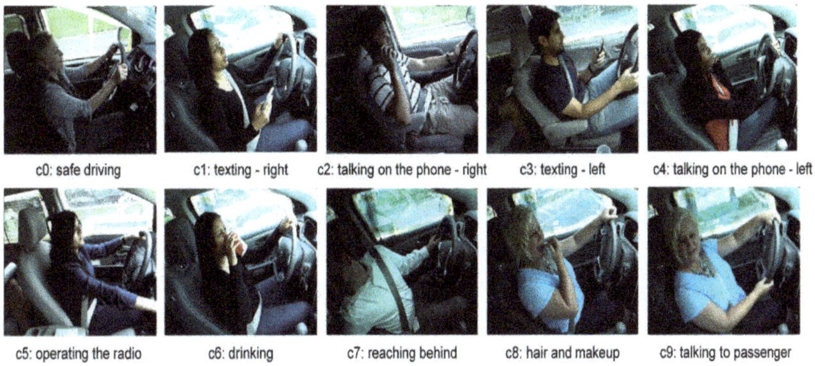

Figure 10. State Farm Distracted Driver dataset class representation [47].

5.2. Experimental Setup

A MacBook Pro and Google collab (Pro) are used to train and test the models.

5.3. Preprocessing and Splitting Strategy

The Distracted Driver dataset is ingested, then preprocessed as follows: (1) the images and the driver_imgs_list.csv file are stored, (2) the images are loaded, converted from BGR to RGB, and resized to 244 × 244 × 3 as this is the size used by most models and architectures for transfer learning, (3) the data are split into training, validation, and test sets; the validation and test set was created based on the subject (Driver ID); the subjects chosen for validation were: p18, p27, and p39, and the subjects chosen for testing were: p015, p022, p050, and p056. Finally, the labels were converted into categorical values. As a result, the training set had 15,963 images, the validation set had 2769 images and the test set had 3692 images.

5.4. Evaluation Metrics

Precision, Recall, F1 score, and Accuracy [49–54] are the most well-known evaluation metrics to assess the performance of a classifier. Precision finds pertinent instances among the gathered instances. It can be defined as the ratio between the True Positives (TP) and the sum of True Positives and False Positives (FP) as shown in Equation (2).

$$\text{Precision} = (\text{TP})/(\text{TP} + \text{FP}) \tag{2}$$

Recall, also known as Sensitivity, is defined as the ratio of True Positives and the sum of True Positives and False Negatives (FN).

$$\text{Recall} = (\text{TP})/(\text{TP} + \text{FN}) \tag{3}$$

F1 score: It is defined as the harmonic mean of Precision and Recall as shown in Equation (4).

$$\text{F1} - \text{Score} = (2 * \text{Precision} \times \text{Recall})/(\text{Precision} + \text{Recall}) \tag{4}$$

Accuracy finds the correct predictions among the total predictions. It is defined as the ratio between the sum of True Positives and True Negatives and the sum of True Positives, False Negatives, True Negatives, and False Negatives.

$$\text{Accuracy} = (\text{TP} + \text{TN})/(\text{TP} + \text{FP} + \text{TN} + \text{FN}) \tag{5}$$

5.5. Performance Evaluation: Base Models

The performance of all base models is shown in Table 3. ResNet50 performs best with the highest accuracy and recall on the test set. The VGG16 performs just as well as the ResNet50 model, but the training time was significantly longer than ResNet50 and all other tested models since it has many variables. The Inception model had a test accuracy of 0.83, lower than ResNet50 and VGG16. The Inception model had the highest loss, and the training time was close to the ResNet50 model. Finally, the MobileNet had a similar performance to the Inception model with a lower loss and significantly faster training time. This is because MobileNet is a low-power, low-latency, light model parameterized to meet the constraints of computational and time resources of various applications. Choosing which optimum model to use depends on the trade-off between performance and computational complexity. ResNet50 and VGG16 can be used when powerful and robust computational resources and flexible time constraints are available. The MobileNet can be used for faster training and decent accuracy, which is not as good as VGG16 and ResNet50 but is still a good choice for limited computational resources. The Inception model did not perform well and lagged other models in most aspects, making it not favorable compared to the other tested models. Figure 11 shows how each model performed on the training, validation, and test sets. As shown in Figure 11, all models have a gradual increase in validation accuracy with the increasing number of epochs except for the MobileNet model, which has the highest validation accuracy at the third epoch and decreases afterwards. Similarly, the loss of all models decreases as epochs increase except for the MobileNet, which had the lowest loss value at epoch number three, which shows that the model was overfitting after epoch three. We even increased the number of epochs up to one, and we observed that the individual baseline models suffered from overfitting and could not show an increase in performance even when training was continued for a larger number of epochs. The performance report (Figure 12) shows how each model performs for each class. All models perform well for classes 1–5 and perform poorly for class 8, which is "hair and makeup", because it is a challenging class to be detected and usually confused with class 7, as shown in the confusion matrices in Figure 13. Moreover, the data quality for this class might not be on the same level as other classes.

Table 3. Deep learning image classification models performance.

Model	Training Accuracy	Validation Accuracy	Test Accuracy
ResNet	0.89	0.88	0.88
VGG16	0.94	0.86	0.87
Mobile Net	0.88	0.84	0.82
Inception	0.83	0.84	0.83

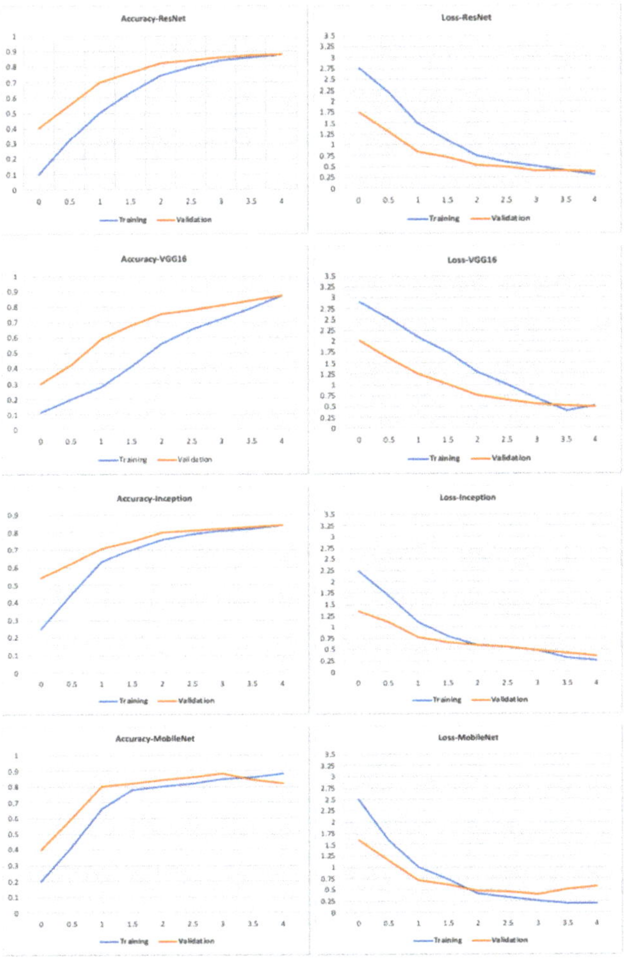

Figure 11. Accuracy and loss graphs for the models on the training and validation sets.

	precision	recall	f1-score	support
0	0.86	0.80	0.83	412
1	0.84	0.97	0.90	339
2	0.95	0.96	0.96	348
3	0.95	0.99	0.97	399
4	0.97	0.92	0.94	396
5	0.91	0.97	0.94	403
6	0.82	0.97	0.89	392
7	0.87	0.96	0.91	334
8	0.74	0.57	0.64	332
9	0.84	0.66	0.74	337
accuracy			0.88	3692
macro avg	0.88	0.88	0.87	3692
weighted avg	0.88	0.88	0.88	3692

(a) Resnet50

	precision	recall	f1-score	support
0	0.82	0.84	0.83	412
1	0.93	0.87	0.90	339
2	0.96	0.79	0.87	348
3	0.98	0.98	0.98	399
4	0.99	0.83	0.91	396
5	0.92	0.95	0.94	403
6	0.79	0.94	0.86	392
7	0.90	0.99	0.94	334
8	0.63	0.73	0.68	332
9	0.83	0.75	0.79	337
accuracy			0.87	3692
macro avg	0.88	0.87	0.87	3692
weighted avg	0.88	0.87	0.87	3692

(b) VGG16

	precision	recall	f1-score	support
0	0.66	0.79	0.72	412
1	0.98	0.94	0.96	339
2	0.88	0.97	0.92	348
3	0.89	0.98	0.93	399
4	0.98	0.73	0.84	396
5	0.85	0.96	0.90	403
6	0.89	0.78	0.83	392
7	0.69	0.98	0.81	334
8	0.69	0.43	0.53	332
9	0.84	0.68	0.75	337
accuracy			0.83	3692
macro avg	0.83	0.82	0.82	3692
weighted avg	0.84	0.83	0.82	3692

(c) Inception

	precision	recall	f1-score	support
0	0.87	0.78	0.82	412
1	0.94	0.86	0.90	339
2	0.83	0.85	0.84	348
3	0.86	0.97	0.91	399
4	0.98	0.70	0.82	396
5	0.99	0.95	0.97	403
6	0.83	0.85	0.84	392
7	0.72	0.93	0.81	334
8	0.48	0.57	0.52	332
9	0.79	0.72	0.75	337
accuracy			0.82	3692
macro avg	0.83	0.82	0.82	3692
weighted avg	0.84	0.82	0.82	3692

(d) MobileNet

Figure 12. Performance reports for deep learning models on the test set.

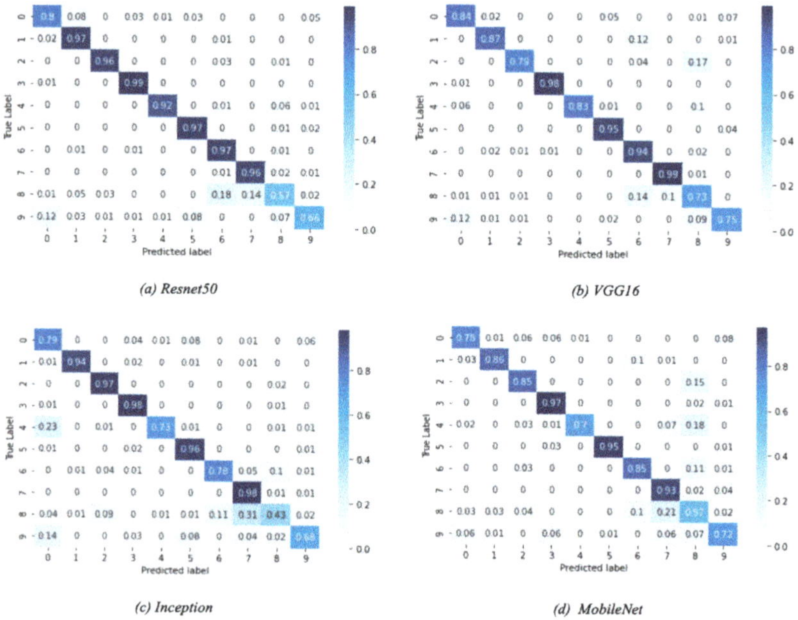

Figure 13. Confusion matrices for the deep learning models.

5.6. The E2DR Performance Evaluation

5.6.1. Settings

In the first layer of the E2DR model, the individual models were trained. Their layers are executed in parallel (after optimizations) when loaded in the ensemble, so their weights are not altered during training. Each of the two base models has 10 outputs representing each class in the dataset. The output of the base models is sent to a concatenation layer, which is then sent to a dense layer with 10 neurons (equal to the number of classes).

A SoftMax activation function is used to perform classification. A learning rate of 0.001 and Adam optimizer are used to compile the model with a batch size equal to 32. The loss function used is the Categorical Cross Entropy loss function. The E2DR was trained for five epochs similar to base models.

5.6.2. Results and Discussion

The results of the E2DR models showed a remarkable improvement in performance compared to the individual models. The best performing E2DR model was the stacked ensemble combination of ResNet and VGG16 with a test accuracy of 92%. The lowest-performing E2DR model with a test accuracy of 88% was the MobileNet–Inception E2DR variant, which was also expected, as the base models did not perform very well individually. The performance of each variant of the E2DR model is shown in Table 4. The improvement in accuracy was around 5–8%, which is a significant improvement considering that the base models could not exceed the late 80% in their accuracy. The fact that E2DR models reached accuracies exceeding 90% proves that the E2DR models effectively improved generalization compared to the individual base models. Other metrics, such as Precision, Recall, and F1 scores, showed similar results and improvements to accuracy, which further validates the model's performance. The loss function used in all experiments is the Categorical Cross Entropy function, representing the confidence of predictions made by the model. The loss of the base models and the E2DR variants were in the same range with a small improvement in the E2DR models. This is because the classification confidence did not significantly improve, which means that despite making more correct classifications, which led to an increase in accuracy, the model did not have high certainty in making those predictions. Although the ensemble model in [6] achieved a higher performance with the traditional percentage-based data split, our method provides further credibility as it was tested on completely new data, which simulates real-world scenarios. This was performed by choosing subjects (Driver IDs) that are not included in the training set when constructing the validation and test sets, allowing the model to be tested on data it had not seen before. This approach is not followed in other implementations. The batch size used when recording the training duration is 32. The performance and confusion matrix of the highest performing E2DR model, which includes ResNet50 and VGG16, is presented in Figure 14. When looking at the performance report of this E2DR variant, the strongest classes from the ResNet50 model were 0 and 6, while the VGG16 performed best for classes 3 and 4. However, after analyzing the performance report of the E2DR model, our method combined the strong classes from each model in a single robust model. This is one of the most useful advantages of the E2DR model, where the model combines the skills and strong points of different models into one model, allowing the base models to complement each other in terms of performance. Similarly, Figure 15 shows the performance report and the confusion matrix of the lowest-performing E2DR variant that uses MobileNet and Inception as base models. Although it is the lowest-performing variant, it still showed a huge performance boost compared to the base models' performance. The E2DR model effectively addressed the weak points of the Inception model (classes 0 and 7) and MobileNet model (classes 2 and 9) by boosting the classification performance for those classes in the E2DR model. Comparing the confusion matrices of the base models and the E2DR variants also improves classification performance, especially for class 8, where the confusion rate with class 7 has decreased compared to the base models. Figures 16–18 visualize the performance evaluation across different metrics for the base models and the E2DR variants. The E2DR variants outperform the baseline models measured by the test Accuracy, Precision, Recall, F1 score, and Loss value, as shown in Figures 16–18. As recorded in Equation (1), the computational time to fully develop the E2DR models would be the maximum training duration of the combined base models in addition to the overhead of concatenation and recommendation retrieval. The execution of the E2DR models after training can be applied in real time. The additional overhead in training the E2DR models is shown in Figure 19. It can be observed that there is an average overhead of 7% in using the E2DR models, as illustrated in Figure 19. However, due to the limited GPU computational power in the experimental hardware used as discussed in Section 5.2., we anticipate that this overhead will be significantly reduced if additional GPUs are used in the training phase. Using the baseline models, the recognition time of one image is 14.45 ms on average with 15.21 ms (on average) when using the ensemble E2DR models.

Table 4. E2DR models performance on the test set.

E2DR Model	Accuracy	Precision	Recall	F1 score	Loss
MobileNet–Inception	0.88	0.89	0.88	0.88	0.55
ResNet50–Inception	0.88	0.89	0.88	0.88	0.47
ResNet50–MobileNet	0.90	0.91	0.9	0.9	0.43
VGG16–Inception	0.90	0.91	0.9	0.9	0.39
VGG16–MobileNet	0.91	0.92	0.91	0.91	0.42
ResNet50–VGG16	0.92	0.92	0.92	0.92	0.37

	precision	recall	f1-score	support
0	0.87	0.96	0.91	412
1	1.00	0.98	0.99	339
2	0.98	0.97	0.98	348
3	1.00	0.99	0.99	399
4	0.99	0.86	0.92	396
5	0.96	0.99	0.98	403
6	0.93	0.89	0.91	392
7	0.90	0.99	0.94	334
8	0.65	0.80	0.72	332
9	0.93	0.72	0.81	337
accuracy			0.92	3692
macro avg	0.92	0.91	0.91	3692
weighted avg	0.92	0.92	0.92	3692

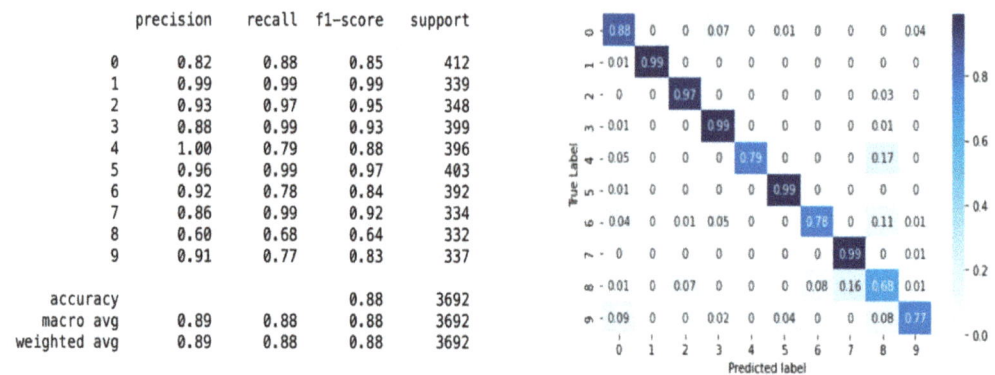

a) Best performing E2DR model classification report

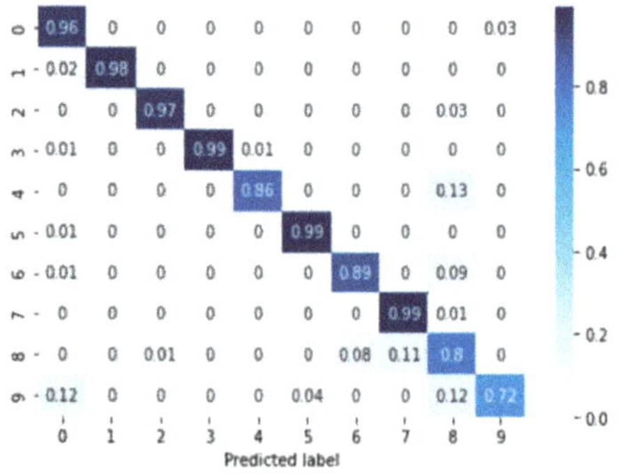

(b) Best performing E2DR model Confusion matrix

Figure 14. Best performing E2DR model classification report and confusion matrix.

	precision	recall	f1-score	support
0	0.82	0.88	0.85	412
1	0.99	0.99	0.99	339
2	0.93	0.97	0.95	348
3	0.88	0.99	0.93	399
4	1.00	0.79	0.88	396
5	0.96	0.99	0.97	403
6	0.92	0.78	0.84	392
7	0.86	0.99	0.92	334
8	0.60	0.68	0.64	332
9	0.91	0.77	0.83	337
accuracy			0.88	3692
macro avg	0.89	0.88	0.88	3692
weighted avg	0.89	0.88	0.88	3692

a) Lowest performing E2DR model classification report

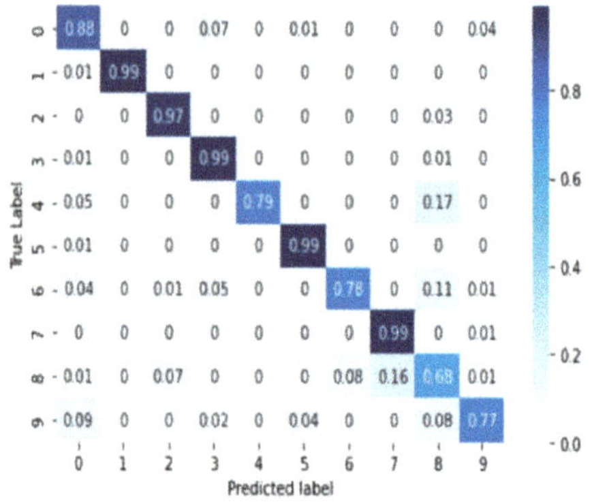

(b) Lowest performing E2DR model Confusion matrix

Figure 15. Lowest performing E2DR model classification report and confusion matrix.

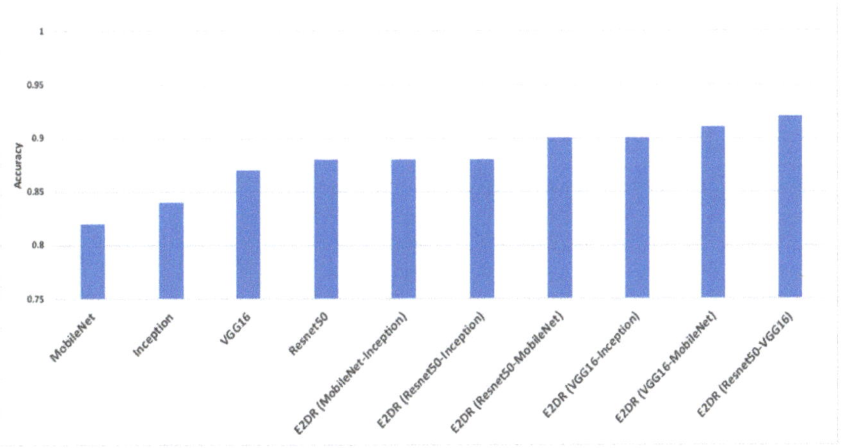

Figure 16. Accuracy of base models and E2DR models.

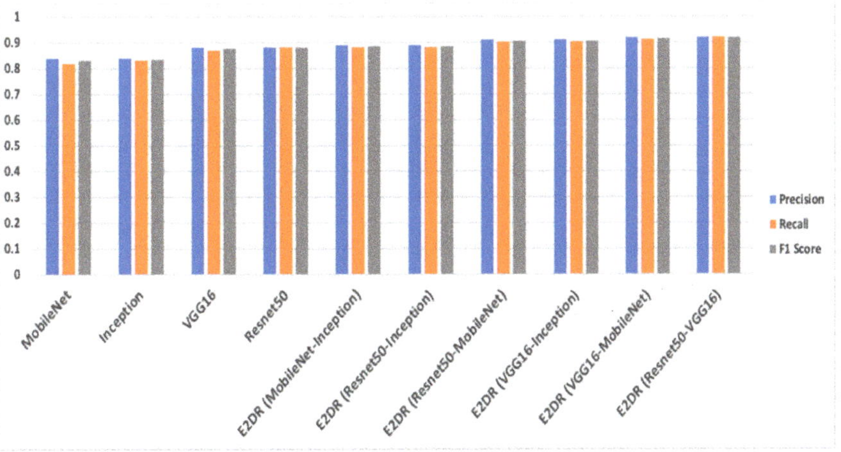

Figure 17. The Precision, Recall, and F1 score of base models and E2DR models.

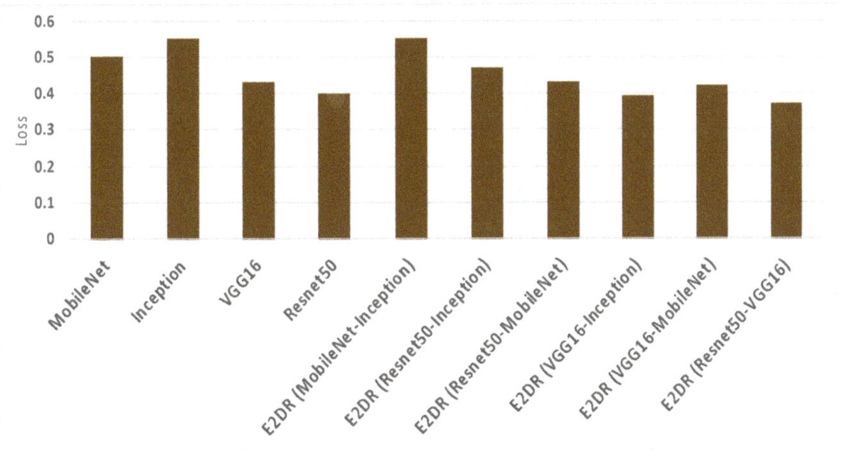

Figure 18. The Loss of base models and E2DR models.

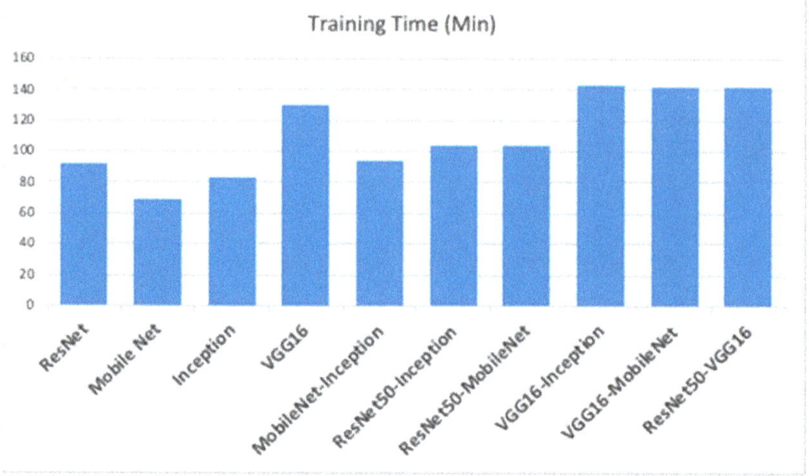

Figure 19. Training Time (Proposed E2DR vs. baseline deep learning models).

6. Conclusions and Future Directions

This paper examines different deep learning classification models for distracted driver classification [55–59] and proposes a model that improves performance and provides recommendations. We explored the performance of different models: ResNet50, VGG16, MobileNet, and Inception. All models provided viable means in detecting distracted driver actions. This paper proposes E2DR, a new model that uses stacking ensemble methods to improve accuracy, enhance generalization and reduce overfitting. Additionally, a set of recommendations are added by the model. The highest performing E2DR variant, which included the ResNet50 and VGG16 models, achieved an accuracy of 92%, while the highest performing single model was the ResNet50 with 88% accuracy. The lowest-performing E2DR model was the MobileNet–Inception variant, which achieved an accuracy of 88%, and the lowest-performing individual model was the MobileNet, with an accuracy of 82%. The accuracy difference between the highest and lowest performing models for the E2DR models and the individual models shows a significant increase in performance when using our proposed E2DR model. Other metrics were recorded and presented to evaluate the classification performance of the tested base models and E2DR variants such as Recall, Precision, and F1 score, which showed a similar increase in performance. Furthermore, the performance reports and confusion matrices showed that the E2DR models effectively addressed the weak points of the base models and boosted their classification performance. The computational complexity when developing the E2DR models from scratch is considered a limitation. Since computational speed is important in real-time applications, a light model such as MobileNet can be integrated with ResNet50 or VGG16, which in our experiment showed a significant boost in performance without adding much computational complexity.

For future work, the performance of more than two models combined in the stacking ensemble method can be examined; it was infeasible to test multiple combinations with the limited computational resources used to conduct the experiments. Furthermore, the model can be associated with the police departments to fine violators and identify drivers' actions in case of accidents. The model can also be integrated with face recognition and alarm systems [60,61] capabilities that can allow the model to be used in a wide range of applications, such as driver authentication and theft prevention. Finally, the model can be developed and used in autonomous vehicles to detect critical conditions or situations that might endanger the driver's health and safety, such as strokes, heart attacks, and other sicknesses. The model can recommend the vehicle to ensure the safety and health of the driver and others.

Author Contributions: Conceptualization, M.A. and R.K.; methodology, M.A. and R.K.; software, M.A.; validation, M.A. and R.K.; formal analysis, M.A. and R.K.; investigation, M.A. and R.K.; resources, M.A.; data curation, M.A.; writing—original draft preparation, M.A. and R.K.; writing—review and editing, M.A. and R.K.; visualization, M.A. and R.K.; supervision, R.K.; project administration, R.K.; funding acquisition, R.K. All authors have read and agreed to the published version of the manuscript.

Funding: This paper was funded by Ryerson University.

Institutional Review Board Statement: Not applicable.

Informed Consent Statement: Not applicable.

Data Availability Statement: The State Farm Distracted Drivers dataset can be accessed in [47].

Conflicts of Interest: The authors declare no conflict of interest.

References

1. The World Health Organization. Global Status Report on Road Safety. 2018. Available online: https://www.who.int/publications/i/item/9789241565684 (accessed on 15 January 2020).
2. Yanbin, Y.; Lijuan, Z.; Mengjun, L.; Ling, S. Early warning of traffic accident in Shanghai based on large data set mining. In Proceedings of the 2016 International Conference on Intelligent Transportation, Big Data & Smart City (ICITBS), Changsha, China, 17–18 December 2016; pp. 18–21.
3. Engstörm, J.; Victor, T.W. Real-Time Distraction Countermeasures. In *Driver Distraction: Theory, Effects, and Mitigation*; CRC Press: Boca Raton, FL, USA, 2008; pp. 465–483.
4. Kang, H.B. Various approaches for driver and driving behavior monitoring: A review. In Proceedings of the IEEE International Conference on Computer Vision Workshops, Washington, DC, USA, 2–8 December 2013; pp. 616–623.
5. Krajewski, J.; Trutschel, U.; Golz, M.; Sommer, D.; Edwards, D. Estimating fatigue from predetermined speech samples transmitted by operator communication systems. In Proceedings of the Fifth International Driving Symposium on Human Factors in Driver Assessment, Training and Vehicle Design, Big Sky, MT, USA, 24 June 2009; pp. 468–473.
6. Alotaibi, M.; Alotaibi, B. Distracted driver classification using deep learning. *Signal. Image Video Process.* **2019**, *14*, 617–624. [CrossRef]
7. Stappen, L.; Rizos, G.; Schuller, B. X-aware: Context-aware human-environment attention fusion for driver gaze prediction in the wild. In Proceedings of the 2020 International Conference on Multimodal Interaction, Virtual, 25–29 October 2020; pp. 858–867.
8. Palazzi, A.; Solera, F.; Calderara, S.; Alletto, S.; Cucchiara, R. Learning where to attend like a human driver. *IEEE Int. Veh. Symp.* **2017**, 920–925. [CrossRef]
9. Methuku, J. In-Car driver response classification using Deep Learning (CNN) based Computer Vision. *IEEE Trans. Intell. Veh.* **2020**.
10. Jeong, M.; Ko, B.C. Driver's Facial Expression Recognition in Real-Time for Safe Driving. *Sensors* **2018**, *18*, 4270. [CrossRef] [PubMed]
11. Baheti, B.; Talbar, S.; Gajre, S. Towards Computationally Efficient and Realtime Distracted Driver Detection with Mobile VGG Network. *IEEE Transact. Intell. Veh.* **2020**, *5*, 565–574. [CrossRef]
12. Kumari, M.; Hari, C.; Sankaran, P. Driver Distraction Analysis Using Convolutional Neural Networks. In Proceedings of the 2018 International Conference on Data Science and Engineering (ICDSE), Kochi, India, 7–9 August 2018; pp. 1–5. [CrossRef]
13. Lu, M.; Hu, Y.; Lu, X. Driver action recognition using deformable and dilated faster R-CNN with optimized region proposals. *Appl. Intell.* **2019**, *50*, 1100–1111. [CrossRef]
14. Li, P.; Yang, Y.; Grosu, R.; Wang, G.; Li, R.; Wu, Y.; Huang, Z. Driver Distraction Detection Using Octave-Like Convolutional Neural Network. *IEEE Trans. Intell. Transp. Syst.* **2021**, 1–11. [CrossRef]
15. Li, G.; Yan, W.; Li, S.; Qu, X.; Chu, W.; Cao, D. A Temporal-Spatial Deep Learning Approach for Driver Distraction Detection Based on EEG Signals. *IEEE Trans. Autom. Sci. Eng.* **2021**, 1–13. [CrossRef]
16. Abbas, T.; Ali, S.F.; Khan, A.Z.; Kareem, I. optNet-50: An Optimized Residual Neural Network Architecture of Deep Learning for Driver's Distraction. In Proceedings of the 2020 IEEE 23rd International Multitopic Conference (INMIC), Bahawalpur, Pakistan, 5–7 November 2020. [CrossRef]
17. Xie, Z.; Li, L.; Xu, X. Recognition of driving distraction using driver's motion and deep learning. *IIE Ann. Conf. Proc.* **2020**, 949–954.
18. Abouelnaga, Y.; Eraqi, H.M.; Moustafa, M.N. Real-time distracted driver posture classification. *arXiv* **2017**, arXiv:1706.09498.
19. Koay, H.; Chuah, J.; Chow, C.-O.; Chang, Y.-L.; Rudrusamy, B. Optimally-Weighted Image-Pose Approach (OWIPA) for Distracted Driver Detection and Classification. *Sensors* **2021**, *21*, 4837. [CrossRef]
20. Arvin, R.; Khattak, A.J.; Qi, H. Safety critical event prediction through unified analysis of driver and vehicle volatilities: Application of deep learning methods. *Accid. Anal. Prev.* **2020**, *151*, 105949. [CrossRef] [PubMed]
21. Xing, Y.; Lv, C.; Wang, H.; Cao, D.; Velenis, E.; Wang, F.-Y. Driver Activity Recognition for Intelligent Vehicles: A Deep Learning Approach. *IEEE Trans. Veh. Technol.* **2019**, *68*, 5379–5390. [CrossRef]

22. Varaich, Z.A.; Khalid, S. Recognizing actions of distracted drivers using inception v3 and xception convolutional neural networks. In Proceedings of the 2019 2nd International Conference on Advancements in Computational Sciences (ICACS), Lahore, Pakistan, 18–20 February 2019; pp. 1–8.
23. Mao, P.; Zhang, K.; Liang, D. Driver Distraction Behavior Detection Method Based on Deep Learning. *IOP Conf. Series. Mater. Sci. Eng.* **2020**, *782*, 22012. [CrossRef]
24. Mase, J.M.; Chapman, P.; Figueredo, G.P.; Torres, M.T. A Hybrid Deep Learning Approach for Driver Distraction Detection. In Proceedings of the International Conference on Information and Communication Technology Convergence (ICTC), Jeju, Korea, 21–23 October 2020. [CrossRef]
25. Alkinani, M.H.; Khan, W.Z.; Arshad, Q. Detecting Human Driver Inattentive and Aggressive Driving Behavior Using Deep Learning: Recent Advances, Requirements and Open Challenges. *IEEE Access* **2020**, *8*, 105008–105030. [CrossRef]
26. Li, L.; Zhong, B.; Hutmacher, C., Jr.; Liang, Y.; Horrey, W.J.; Xu, X. Detection of driver manual distraction via image-based hand and ear recognition. *Accid. Anal. Prevent.* **2020**, *137*, 105432. [CrossRef] [PubMed]
27. Springer Link. Available online: https://link.springer.com/article/10.1007/s00330-019-06318-1/figures/1 (accessed on 19 March 2021).
28. ImageNet. Available online: http://www.image-net.org/ (accessed on 17 March 2021).
29. He, K.; Zhang, X.; Ren, S.; Sun, J. Deep residual learning for image recognition. In Proceedings of the IEEE Conference on Computer Vision and Pattern Recognition, Las Vegas, NV, USA, 27–30 June 2016; pp. 770–778.
30. Simonyan, K.; Zisserman, A. Very Deep Convolutional Networks for Large-Scale Image Recognition. *arXiv* **2014**, arXiv:1409.1556.
31. Alex, K.; Sutskever, I.; Hinton, G.E. ImageNet classification with deep convolutional neural networks. *Commun. ACM* **2017**, *60*, 84–90. [CrossRef]
32. LeCun, Y.; Bengio, Y.; Hinton, G. Deep learning. *Nature* **2015**, *521*, 436. [CrossRef]
33. VGG16—Convolutional Network for Classification and Detection. Available online: https://neurohive.io/en/popular-networks/vgg16/ (accessed on 19 March 2021).
34. A Simple Guide to the Versions of the Inception Network. Available online: https://towardsdatascience.com/a-simple-guide-to-the-versions-of-the-inception-network-7fc52b863202 (accessed on 19 March 2021).
35. Szegedy, C.; Liu, W.; Jia, Y.; Sermanet, P.; Reed, S.; Anguelov, D.; Erhan, D.; Vanhoucke, V.; Rabinovich, A. Going deeper with con-volutions. In Proceedings of the IEEE Conference on Computer Vision and Pattern Recognition, Boston, MA, USA, 7–12 June 2015; pp. 1–9.
36. Bose, S.R.; Kumar, V.S. Efficient inception V2 based deep convolutional neural network for real-time hand action recognition. *IET Image Process.* **2020**, *14*, 688–696. [CrossRef]
37. Szegedy, C.; Vincent, V.; Sergey, I.; Jon, S.; Wojna, Z. Rethinking the inception architecture for computer vision. In Proceedings of the IEEE Conference on Computer Vision and Pattern Recognition, Las Vegas, NV, USA, 27–30 June 2016; pp. 2818–2826.
38. Szegedy, C.; Ioffe, S.; Vanhoucke, V.; Alemi, A.A. Inception-v4, inception-resnet and the impact of residual connections on learning. In Proceedings of the Thirty-First AAAI Conference on Artificial Intelligence, San Francisco, CA, USA, 12 February 2017.
39. Inception-v3. Available online: https://paperswithcode.com/method/inception-v3 (accessed on 20 March 2021).
40. Howard, A.G.; Zhu, M.; Chen, B.; Kalenichenko, D.; Wang, W.; Weyand, T.; Adam, H. Mobilenets: Efficient convolutional neural networks for mobile vision applications. *arXiv* **2017**, arXiv:1704.04861.
41. Image Classification With MobileNet. Available online: https://medium.com/analytics-vidhya/image-classification-with-mobilenet-cc6fbb2cd470 (accessed on 26 March 2021).
42. Kim, W.; Jung, W.-S.; Choi, H.K. Lightweight Driver Monitoring System Based on Multi-Task Mobilenets. *Sensors* **2019**, *19*, 3200. [CrossRef] [PubMed]
43. An Overview on MobileNet: An Efficient Mobile Vision CNN. Available online: https://medium.com/@godeep48/an-overview-on-mobilenet-an-efficient-mobile-vision-cnn-f301141db94d (accessed on 15 July 2021).
44. Wolpert, D.H. Stacked generalization. *Neural Networks* **1992**, *5*, 241–259. [CrossRef]
45. ResNet and ResNetV2. Available online: https://keras.io/api/applications/resnet/#resnet50-function (accessed on 17 July 2021).
46. Ciresan, D.C.; Meier, U.; Masci, J.; Gambardella, L.M.; Schmidhuber, J. Flexible, high performance convolutional neural networks for image classification. In Proceedings of the Twenty-Second international joint conference on Artificial Intelligence, Barcelona, Spain, 16–22 July 2011.
47. He, K.; Sun, J. Convolutional neural networks at constrained time cost. In Proceedings of the IEEE Conference on Computer Vision and Pattern Recognition, Boston, MA, USA, 7–12 June 2015; pp. 5353–5360.
48. State Farm Distracted Driver Detection. Available online: https://www.kaggle.com/c/state-farm-distracted-driver-detection (accessed on 25 July 2021).
49. Close, L.; Kashef, R. Combining Artificial Immune System and Clustering Analysis: A Stock Market Anomaly Detection Model. *J. Intell. Learn. Syst. Appl.* **2020**, *12*, 83–108. [CrossRef]
50. Kashef, R. Enhancing the Role of Large-Scale Recommendation Systems in the IoT Context. *IEEE Access* **2020**, *8*, 178248–178257. [CrossRef]
51. Yeh, T.-Y.; Kashef, R. Trust-Based Collaborative Filtering Recommendation Systems on the Blockchain. *Adv. Int. Things* **2020**, *10*, 37–56. [CrossRef]
52. Ebrahimian, M.; Kashef, R. Detecting Shilling Attacks Using Hybrid Deep Learning Models. *Symmetry* **2020**, *12*, 1805. [CrossRef]

53. Li, M.; Kashef, R.; Ibrahim, A. Multi-Level Clustering-Based Outlier's Detection (MCOD) Using Self-Organizing Maps. *Big Data Cogn. Comput.* **2020**, *4*, 24. [CrossRef]
54. Tobin, T.; Kashef, R. Efficient Prediction of Gold Prices Using Hybrid Deep Learning. In *International Conference on Image Analysis and Recognition*; Springer: Cham, The Netherlands, 2020; pp. 118–129.
55. Ledezma, A.; Zamora, V.; Sipele, O.; Sesmero, M.; Sanchis, A. Implementing a Gaze Tracking Algorithm for Improving Advanced Driver Assistance Systems. *Electronics* **2021**, *10*, 1480. [CrossRef]
56. Liu, D.; Yamasaki, T.; Wang, Y.; Mase, K.; Kato, J. TML: A Triple-Wise Multi-Task Learning Framework for Distracted Driver Recognition. *IEEE Access* **2021**, *9*, 125955–125969. [CrossRef]
57. Kumar, A.; Sangwan, K.S. A Computer Vision Based Approach forDriver Distraction Recognition Using Deep Learning and Genetic Algorithm Based Ensemble. *arXiv* **2021**, arXiv:2107.13355.
58. Eraqi, H.M.; Abouelnaga, Y.; Saad, M.H.; Moustafa, M.N. Driver Distraction Identification with an Ensemble of Convolutional Neural Networks. *J. Adv. Transp.* **2019**, *2019*, 1–12. [CrossRef]
59. Gite, S.; Agrawal, H.; Kotecha, K. Early anticipation of driver's maneuver in semiautonomous vehicles using deep learning. *Prog. Artif. Intell.* **2019**, *8*, 293–305. [CrossRef]
60. Magán, E.; Ledezma, A.; Sesmero, P.; Sanchis, A. Fuzzy Alarm System based on Human-centered Approach. *VEHITS* **2020**, 448–455. [CrossRef]
61. Sipele, O.; Zamora, V.; Ledezma, A.; Sanchis, A. Advanced Driver's Alarms System through Multi-agent Paradigm. In Proceedings of the 2018 3rd IEEE International Conference on Intelligent Transportation Engineering(ICITE), Singapore, 3–5 September 2018; pp. 269–275.

sensors

MDPI

Article

CNN Architectures and Feature Extraction Methods for EEG Imaginary Speech Recognition

Ana-Luiza Rusnac * and Ovidiu Grigore *

Department of Applied Electronics and Information Engineering, Faculty of Electronics, Telecommunications and Information Technology, Polytechnic University of Bucharest, 060042 Bucharest, Romania
* Correspondence: ana_luiza.dumitrescu@upb.ro (A.-L.R.); ovidiu.grigore@upb.ro (O.G.)

Abstract: Speech is a complex mechanism allowing us to communicate our needs, desires and thoughts. In some cases of neural dysfunctions, this ability is highly affected, which makes everyday life activities that require communication a challenge. This paper studies different parameters of an intelligent imaginary speech recognition system to obtain the best performance according to the developed method that can be applied to a low-cost system with limited resources. In developing the system, we used signals from the Kara One database containing recordings acquired for seven phonemes and four words. We used in the feature extraction stage a method based on covariance in the frequency domain that performed better compared to the other time-domain methods. Further, we observed the system performance when using different window lengths for the input signal (0.25 s, 0.5 s and 1 s) to highlight the importance of the short-term analysis of the signals for imaginary speech. The final goal being the development of a low-cost system, we studied several architectures of convolutional neural networks (CNN) and showed that a more complex architecture does not necessarily lead to better results. Our study was conducted on eight different subjects, and it is meant to be a subject's shared system. The best performance reported in this paper is up to 37% accuracy for all 11 different phonemes and words when using cross-covariance computed over the signal spectrum of a 0.25 s window and a CNN containing two convolutional layers with 64 and 128 filters connected to a dense layer with 64 neurons. The final system qualifies as a low-cost system using limited resources for decision-making and having a running time of 1.8 ms tested on an AMD Ryzen 7 4800HS CPU.

Keywords: imaginary speech; convolutional neural network; electroencephalography; signal processing; Kara One database

Citation: Rusnac, A.-L.; Grigore, O. CNN Architectures and Feature Extraction Methods for EEG Imaginary Speech Recognition. *Sensors* **2022**, *22*, 4679. https://doi.org/10.3390/s22134679

Academic Editors: Andrei Velichko, Dmitry Korzun, Alexander Meigal and Raffaele Bruno

Received: 4 April 2022
Accepted: 17 June 2022
Published: 21 June 2022

1. Introduction

Communication is the basis of interpersonal relationships and is one of the most important ways to connect with other people and to express your needs and feelings. The most common forms of communication are writing or speaking, but the latter is the most natural mechanism involved in the transmission of thoughts. This relatively easy to gain ability is often taken for granted; however, it hides a complex mechanism. Speaking involves translating thoughts into the desired words and transmitting them with the help of motor neurons to a large number of muscles and joint components of the vocal tract that must be positioned differently for each spoken sound. This is why speech takes a large part of cortical motor homunculus [1].

Unfortunately, there are cases when this ability is lost, or the speech cannot be articulated due to some affections such as cerebral stroke, lock-down syndrome, amyotrophic lateral sclerosis, cerebral palsy, etc. In order to overcome this dysfunction, a series of alternative methods were proposed. The purpose of the research in this field was to find an easy and natural way of communication.

The activity of the brain can be measured using different methods such as electroencephalography (EEG), magnetoencephalography (MEG), electrocorticography (ECoG), functional magnetic resonance imaging (fMRI) and stereoelectroencephalography (sEEG). However, when it comes to developing brain computer interface systems (BCI), the most common methods for brain activity recording are EEG and MEG due to their considerable advantages of being non-invasive techniques and more accessible for signal acquisition. The ECoG signals are also widely used in BCI systems, even though they are invasive. The major advantage of the ECoG signals is the quality of the brain activity measurements by recording the signals directly from the cortex, eliminating in this way the attenuation given by the tissues between the cortex and the electrodes in comparison to EEG. fMRI signals are harder to acquire and more expensive than EEG and MEG, even though it is also a non-invasive method. Nevertheless, the best quality of brain activity measurements is collected using the sEEG technique because the electrodes are implanted deep into the brain. This method is the least used method for BCI due to the invasive approach.

In our study, we chose to focus on the EEG signals for their advantages in developing a low-cost, non-invasive portable device.

2. State of the Art

One of the first studies that tried to reconstruct the speech from EEG signals dates back to 1967 when the scientist Edmond M. Dewan [2] discovered that we can voluntarily control the alpha wave of the EEG signal. Starting from this point, the scientist used morse code in his developed system in order to obtain letters and, finally, conduct words.

Later studies also focused on creating words from letters for subjects to silently communicate with the computer. For example, in 2000, P. R. Kennedy et al. [3] used implanted neurotrophic electrodes on patients with amyotrophic lateral sclerosis (ALS) or brain stroke and obtained a functional system that uses the movement of a cursor as a form of communication. One of the system paradigms was to form words from letters by moving a cursor on the monitor and choosing the desired letter. Another similar approach was presented in [4] that concentrated on finding the trigger of P300 event-related potential (ERT) when the desired line and column of a matrix with letters and numbers were highlighted. Both methods work properly; however, these approaches represent an inconvenient way to communicate since it takes a long time to form a word.

Recent studies focused on finding patterns in EEG signals acquired during imaginary speaking of words or phonemes rather than finding a trigger, trying to obtain a more cursive way of communicating the thoughts. One attempt at unspoken speech recognition was made by Marek Wester in 2006 [5] for his PhD thesis, with results that reached 50% accuracy in multiple class classification. However, the group later revealed in [6] that the experiment process favored the results because the signal acquisition protocol assumed to speak or think the exact stimulus multiple consecutive times, and this accidentally creates temporal correlation in EEG signals. This was an important discovery in data acquisition protocol for further created databases.

In 2015, an open-source database acquired by Schunan Zhao and Frank Rudzicz at the Toronto Rehabilitation Institute was released [7]. The database contains signals collected from 14 healthy subjects during thinking and speaking of seven phonemes: /iy/, /uw/, /piy/, /diy/, /tiy/, /m/, /n/ and four words: "pat", "pot", "knew", "gnaw". This stimulus was chosen to have a relatively even number of vowels, plosives, and nasals as well as voiced and unvoiced phonemes. The researchers further created five binary classification tasks: consonant versus vocals (C/V), presence or absence of nasal (±Nasal), presence or absence of bilabial (±Bilabial), presence or absence of /iy/ phoneme (±/iy/) and presence or absence of /uw/ phoneme (±/uw/). In the conducted study, the researchers computed various statistical features over 10% of the segment windows with 50% overlap, including mean, median, standard deviation, variance, etc. (the details are specified in Table 1). They used the SVM-quad classifier and obtained maximum accuracy over the /uw/ phoneme: 79.16% and the minimum accuracy when classifying consonants versus vocals: 18.08%.

Later, in 2017, using the same database, the researchers Pengfei Sun and Jun Qin [8] conducted an experimental evaluation of three neural networks based on EEG-speech (NES) with the purpose of recognizing all the eleven phonemes. The three neural network models were: imagined EEG-speech (NES-I), biased imagined-spoken EEG-speech (NES-B) and gated imagined-speech (NES-G), with the last two introducing the EEG signals acquired during actual speech. The best results in this multi-classification problem were obtained using the NES-G network with an overall accuracy of 41.5%.

Another approach for the Kara One database binary task classification was proposed by Pramit Saha and Sidney Fels at the University of British Columbia [9]. In the developed study, the researchers used a mixed deep neural network strategy composed of a convolutional neural network (CNN), a long-short term network (LSTM) and a deep autoencoder. The hierarchical deep neural network used the cross-covariance matrix as the input feature matrix, with this method of feature extraction aiming to encode the connectivity of the electrodes. The obtained results increased the overall accuracy of the above binary tasks by 22.5%, achieving an average accuracy of 77.9% across the five known tasks [7].

However, when it comes to multi-classification of the phonemes and words, the results decrease significantly. In 2018 [10], a group of researchers introduced methods of speech recognition in their imaginary speech recognition from EEG signals using mel-cepstral coefficients (MFCC) as feature extraction and SVM classifier for recognition and broke the ice with an average accuracy of 20.80%—this value rising by 9% over the chance level. The results slightly improved when using MFCC for feature extraction and CNN as a classifier in the study [11]. The CNN neural network improved the overall accuracy, obtaining 24.19%.

Nevertheless, the highest accuracy over the multi-class classification of the Kara One phonemes and words was also obtained by the researchers from the University of British Columbia [12]. In their study, the researchers used the cross-covariance matrix (CCV) as feature extraction and a hierarchical combination of deep neural networks. In the first level of the final architecture of the classifier, a CNN was used to extract the spatial features from the covariance matrix. In parallel with CNN, they applied a temporal CNN (TCNN) to explore the hidden temporal features of the electrodes. Further, the latest fully connected layers from the CNN and TCNN were concatenated to compose a single feature vector, which was introduced to the second level of hierarchy consisting of a deep autoencoder (DAE). In the third level of hierarchy, they introduced the latent vector of DAE into an extreme gradient boost classification layer. The final neural network was first used to train the network for all six phonological tasks of Kara One and then to combine the gained information to further predict individual phonemes from all eleven categories.

Recent studies reported more encouraging results on the multi-class classification system of imaginary speech recognition. Developing an impressive database of eight different Russian words acquired from 270 subjects, the researchers [13] obtained a maximum accuracy of 85% when classifying the nine collected words and 88% for binary classification. The results were obtained using the frequency-domain of the signals and were classified with ResNet18 + 2GRU (gated recurrent unit).

Significant results for the imaginary speech recognition community were also obtained by using MEG signals. In 2020, Debadatta Dash, Paul Ferrari and Jun Wang [14] conducted a study based on MEG signals in order to recognize imagined and articulated speech of three different phrases of the English language. To achieve the final goal, the researchers used the discrete wavelet transform (DWT) in the feature extraction stage using a Daubechies (db)-4 wavelet with a seven-level decomposition. Further, they compared artificial neural networks (ANNs) and different configurations of CNNs. The best results were recorded using Spatial Spectral Temporal CNN, reaching an accuracy for the specific three classes of imaginary speech of 93.24%.

ECoG signals were also used for speech recognition and synthesis by Christian Herff et al. in [15]. The researchers managed to synthesize the vocal signals after analyzing motor, premotor and inferior frontal cortices and obtained an accuracy of 66.1% ± 6% in the correct identification of the word of 55 volunteered subjects. This approach offered very encouraging results for a real-time system; however, the brain signals were acquired in articulated speech (not imaginary speech), and the signals were collected using an invasive method.

Another recent study published in 2022 on ECoG signals for imaginary speech recognition was conducted by Thimotheé Proix et al. [16]. For binary classification using an SVM classifier, they managed to obtain an accuracy of over 60% for a patient-specific system. In the feature extraction stage, they used the analytic Morlet wavelet transform. The bands of interest were theta (4–8 Hz), low-beta (12–18 Hz), low-gamma (25–35 Hz) and broadband high-frequency activity (80–150 Hz).

An important role in the research community for EEG signal classification was also taken by the long-short term memory (LSTM) neural networks. LSTM neural networks are considered an improvement of the recurrent neural networks (RNN) due to the inclusion of the "gates" in the algorithm. These "gates" have the purpose of resolving the gradient problem, and they allow more precise control over the information that is kept in its memory [17]. Considering the highly dynamic behavior of the EEG signals, often the LSTM networks offered significantly better performance over different applications of EEG signals, such as emotion recognition, confusion detection and decision-making predictions [18–20]. A great success of LSTM neural networks for articulated speech recognition from EEG signals was presented in [21] for an automatic speech recognition (ASR) system. The researchers used MFCC as features and predicted the coefficients using different types of recognition systems: generative adversarial neural networks (GAN), Wasserstein generative adversarial neural network (WGAN) and LSTM Regression. The results showed an average of the root mean square (RMS) of 0.126 for the LSTM regression compared with 0.193 and 0.188 registered for the GAN and WGAN networks, respectively.

The most significant results from the state-of-the-art, regarding the imaginary speech recognition systems using surface EEG of the Kara One Database are presented in Table 1, along with the most relevant characteristics of the systems: pre-processing method, feature extractions and the classifier used.

This paper contains a study of EEG signals with the main purpose of recognizing seven phonemes and four words acquired during the development of the Kara One database. Our study was conducted on eight different subjects and is meant to be a subject's shared system. By a subject's shared system, we mean a system that can only be used by subjects in the database. However, it is not a subject-specific device that would require different training for each new subject but assumes that only a fine-tuning will be performed when adding a new subject.

This paper also aims to develop a study of two different features computed over different windows of a signal. We used as feature extraction the cross-covariance over the channels in time and frequency domains for data reduction and to encode the variability of the electrodes during the imaginary speech. This hypothesis is based on the fact that speaking is a complex mechanism, implying the connectivity of different areas of the brain during the entire process. We also studied the results obtained after applying a mean filter over the spectrum band with different window dimensions (3 and 5 samples).

Another study conducted in this paper was based on analyzing three different time-frames: 0.25, 0.5 and 1 s. Regarding this study, we aimed to determine the best analysis window dimension for EEG imaginary speech phoneme and word recognition. In a time series, the statistics of the entire signal is different from the statistics of smaller windows—a fact that can lead to a significant impact on the final results of the system.

In the second part of the study, we focused on different CNN architectures for feature classification in order to determine which one fits our data best.

Table 1. State-of-the-art EEG speech recognition of Kara One database phonemes and words.

Source	Task	Pre-Processing Method	Feature Extraction	Classification Method	Accuracy
[7]	Imagined speech: Vocal vs. Consonant (C/V) Presence of nasal (±Nazal) Presence of bilabial (±bilabial) Presence of /iy/ (±/iy/) Presence of /uw/ (±/uw/)	Eliminating ocular artifacts using Blind Source Separation (BSS) Band-pass filter 1–50 Hz	Features of window 10%/50% overlap: mean, median, standard deviation, variance, maximum, minimum, maximum ± minimum, sum, spectral entropy, energy, skewness and kurtosis	SVM-quad; Leave-one-out	C/V: 18.08% ±Nazal: 63.50% ±Bilabial: 56.64% ±/iy/: 59.60% ±/uw/: 79.16%
[9]	Imagined speech; Vocal vs. Consonant (C/V) Presence of nasal (±Nazal) Presence of bilabial ±bilabial) Presence of /iy/ (±/iy/) Presence of /uw/ (±/uw/)	Eliminating ocular artifacts using Blind Source Separation (BSS) Band-pass filter 1–50 Hz Subtraction of mean value from each channel	Cross-Covariance Matrix (CCV)	CNN + LTSM + Deep Autoencoder; Random shuffled data in train-validation-testing: 80-10-10; Cross-validation method	C/V: 85.23% ±Nazal: 73.45% ±Bilabial: 75.55% ±/iy/: 73.30% ±/uw/: 81.99%
[10]	Multi-class classification: /iy/, /uw/, /piy/, /tiy/, /diy/, /m/, /n/ + "gnaw", "knew", "pat", "pot"	Band-pass filter 1–50 Hz Laplacian filter over each channel Window 500 ms + 250 overlap ICA for noise removal	Linear features: mean, absolute mean, standard deviation, sum, median, variance, max, absolute max, min, absolute min, max + min, max − min Non-linear features: Hurst exponent, Higuchi's algorithm of fractal dimension, spectral power, spectral entropy, magnitude and phase MFCC coefficients	Decision tree; SVM; 5-fold Cross-validation; Patient specific	Multi-class: MFCC + decision tree: 19.69% Linear features + decision tree: 15.91% Non-linear features + decision tree: 14.67% MFCC + SVM: 20.80%
[11]	Multi-class classification: /iy/, /uw/, /piy/, /tiy/, /diy/, /m/, /n/ + "gnaw", "knew", "pat", "pot"	Notch filter 60 Hz Band-pass filter 0.5–100 Hz Visual analysis of signals and eliminating noisy ones	MFCC coefficients	CNN Random shuffled data in train-validation-testing: 80-10-10;	Multi-class accuracy: 24.19%
[8]	Imagined speech and spoken EEG signals; Multi-class classification: /iy/, /uw/, /piy/, /tiy/, /diy/, /m/, /n/ + "gnaw", "knew", "pat", "pot"	Band-pass filter 1–200 Hz, Subtraction of mean value from each channel	Imagined-EEG signals and phonemes and spoken EEG signals	NES-G model; Leave-One-Out	Multi-class accuracy: 41.5%
[12]	Imagined speech: Vocal vs. Consonant (C/V) Presence of nasal (±Nazal) Presence of bilabial (±bilabial) Presence of /iy/ (±/iy/) Presence of /uw/ (±/uw/) Multi-class classification: /iy/, /uw/, /piy/, /tiy/, /diy/, /m/, /n/ + "gnaw", "knew", "pat", "pot"	Eliminating ocular artifacts using blind source separation (BSS) Band-pass filter 1–50 Hz Subtraction of mean value from each channel	Cross-covariance matrix (CCV)	Three hierarchical levels: 1. CNN + TCNN 2. DAE 3. Extreme gradient boost leave-one-out	C/V: 89.16% ±Nazal: 78.33% ±Bilabial: 81.67% ±/iy/: 87.20% ±/uw/: 85.00% Multi-class accuracy (without phonological features): 28.08% Multi-class accuracy (with phonological features): 53.34%
[This study]	Multi-class classification: /iy/, /uw/, /piy/, /tiy/, /diy/, /m/, /n/ + "gnaw", "knew", "pat", "pot"	Notch filter 60 Hz Visual analysis of signals	Cross-covariance matrix in time-domain Cross-covariance matrix in frequency-domain Windows length: 0.25 s, 0.5 s and 1 s	CNN with different architectures 50%/50% of windows for training/testing	Best multi-class accuracy: 37.06%

3. Materials and Methods

3.1. Preparing Database

In this paper, we used the Kara One database described in [7]. The database contains signals acquired from 12 healthy subjects in 14 sessions during rest, speaking and thinking eleven different stimuli from which seven are phonemes (/iy/, /uw/, /piy/, /tiy/, /diy/, /m/, /n/) and four are words ("gnaw", "knew", "pat", "pot"). Each prompt was presented 12 times, meaning a total of 132 recorded signals for each subject, except for the subjects MM05 and P02, with a total of 165 trials.

The signals were acquired following a given protocol in order to obtain repeatability in the database signals. The protocol started with a 5 s state of rest in which the subject needed to relax for the next stage. Afterward, the stimulus appeared on the prompt for 2 s, and the utterance of the prompt was heard by the subject. This was followed by a 5 s stage in which the subject was instructed to imagine speaking the prompt. Finally, the subject was also asked to speak the prompt aloud.

Our goal was to identify the imagined speech, so in this paper, we only used the signals corresponding to the 5 s state of imaginary speaking of the prompt. Next, we eliminated the first and last 0.5 s of the signal, considering that these intervals correspond to a transition state, obtaining a 4 s signal in the end.

The signals resulting from the database were visually analyzed by an expert. In the first step of visual data analysis, it was discovered that six of the fourteen sessions presented signals with high noises or unattached ground wires. This situation was also discussed by the developers of the database, Shunan Zhao and Frank Rudzicz, in their paper [7]. Considering that discovery, we discarded all signals from the six contaminated sessions. Afterward, the expert visually analyzed all signals corresponding to thinking indexes and eliminated from the study the ones with high noise contamination. After this process of data analysis, we finally obtained a database with 624 signals to work with during the study. All signals from the database were collected using the 10-20 system for electrode positioning. In this paper, we used 62 electrodes. The electrodes and their position in the 10-20 system used are detailed in [7]. Finally, the signals were filtered using a notch filter in order to remove the 60 Hz power line artifact and all multiples of 60 Hz smaller than the Nyquist frequency.

3.2. Feature Extraction

In the feature extraction stage, we aimed to analyze the performance of the system when using the time- versus frequency-domain feature extraction methods for silent speech recognition. Another comparison study conducted in this stage was based on computing the features using different timeframes: 0.25, 0.5 and 1 s without overlapping. During this study, we aimed to find the time window in which the signal is quasi-stationary, but also contains all the needed information regarding the utterance.

All signals were segmented using these timeframes, and 50% of the timeframes from each recording were randomly distributed in the training set and 50% in the testing set.

EEG data usually produce a high-dimension time series due to the multiple electrodes. To decrease the dimension of EEG data, usually a data compression stage is conducted based on feature selection in order to extract the essential information from the signals [10] or to reduce the number of channels based on their informational relevance in relation to the system goal [22]. A new approach to reducing the data dimension of the EEG signals was presented by Pramit Saha and Sidney Fels in their study [9], where they computed the cross-covariance between the channels in the time domain in order to encapsulate the variability of the electrodes. In this study, we also used this technique of feature extraction and expanded it in the frequency domain.

The cross-covariance between two channels (c1 and c2) was defined in this study as:

$$\mathrm{Cov}\left(X^{c1}(t), X^{c2}(t)\right) = \mathrm{E}\Big[\big[X^{c1}(t) - \mathrm{E}(X^{c1}(t)\big]\big[X^{c2}(t) - \mathrm{E}(X^{c2}(t)\big]\Big], \quad (1)$$

where $X^{c1}(t)$ represents the EEG signal acquired for channel c1, $X^{c2}(t)$ is the EEG signal acquired for channel c2, and $E[X^{ch}(t)]$ represents the expected value (where ch corresponds to the specific channel c1 or c2) and is computed as:

$$E(X^{ch}(t)) = \frac{1}{W} \sum_{i=0}^{W-1} x_i^{ch} \tag{2}$$

The W value of Equation (2) corresponds to the window dimension for which the features are computed.

The second method of feature extraction analyzed in this paper assumes the transformation of the time domain series of EEG signals into the frequency domain using the Fast Fourier Transform (FFT). The Fourier transform is a method used to decompose the signal into sinus and cosine waves.

The FFT of a channel was computed using the following:

$$FX^{ch}(f) = \sum_{t=0}^{n-1} X_t^{ch} e^{-\frac{j2\pi ft}{n}} \tag{3}$$

where X_t^{ch} represents the EEG signal acquired for channel ch.

After computing the signals corresponding to the frequency-domain of desired channels using Equation (3), we computed the cross-covariance between the Fourier transform of the channels.

Figures 1 and 2 present examples of a 2D feature matrix with a 62 × 62 dimension, corresponding to the time and frequency domain, respectively, for a 0.25 s window timeframe.

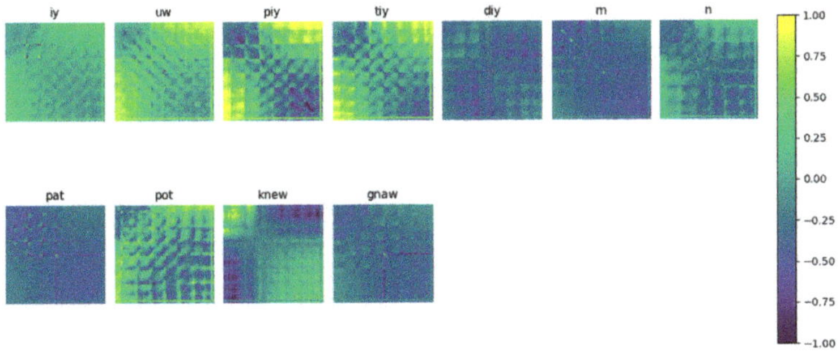

Figure 1. Example of a 2D feature matrix computed in the time domain for 0.25 s time window.

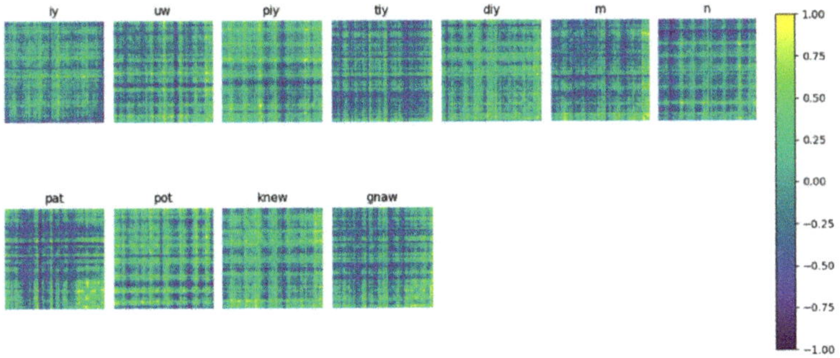

Figure 2. Example of a 2D feature matrix computed in the frequency domain for a 0.25 s time window.

3.3. Classification

Convolutional neural networks (CNN) are powerful networks when applied to images. They have the power to understand the image content and to extract the deep information encoded in the input data. Nowadays, many systems are based on this type of neural network. CNN showed a great success in understanding biomedical images for classification, segmentation, detection and localization [23] for different types of input images, offered a great false prediction rate in seizure prediction systems based on EEG signals [24], and is widely used in BCI systems for imaginary motion recognition [25–27] and assisting in the diagnosis of Parkinson's disease [28]. In the imaginary speech recognition domain, the CNN was a great resource for EEG signal classification [9,27].

The great success of CNN is due to the design of the hidden convolutional layers working as a decoder for the disguised essential information of the two-dimension matrix offered as input. It has the power to extract features and feed them to the dense layers designed to classify these computed features. The component of a CNN starts with an input layer that receives the given data. Then, it continues with the hidden layers corresponding to the convolutional layers in the first phase, which interprets the data received from the input. The output of the last convolutional layer is flattened and introduced into one or multiple dense layers having the purpose of learning the extracted features. Finally, the neural network contains an output layer, which usually has the role of classifying the data into the desired classes [29–31]. A general CNN block diagram is presented in Figure 3.

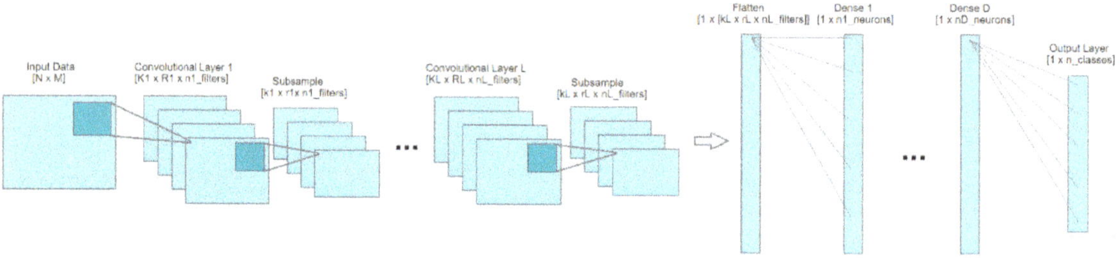

Figure 3. Block diagram of general convolutional neural networks.

In our research, we tested different architectures of the CNN neural network with the purpose of finding the one offering the best performance with respect to the complexity, memory, and the running time. We started with a low complexity architecture with one convolutional layer and one dense layer, and we increased the complexity up to three convolutional layers and one dense layer, having a larger number of filters and neurons.

In the training phase, we used a learning rate of 0.0001, categorical cross-entropy as loss and Adam as optimizer. We divided the training set into 75% training and 25% validation and used k-fold cross-validation in order to obtain a more accurate performance result. Figure 4 presents an example of the architecture used in the classification stage, with two convolutional layers of 64 and 128 filters, respectively, and one dense layer with 64 neurons.

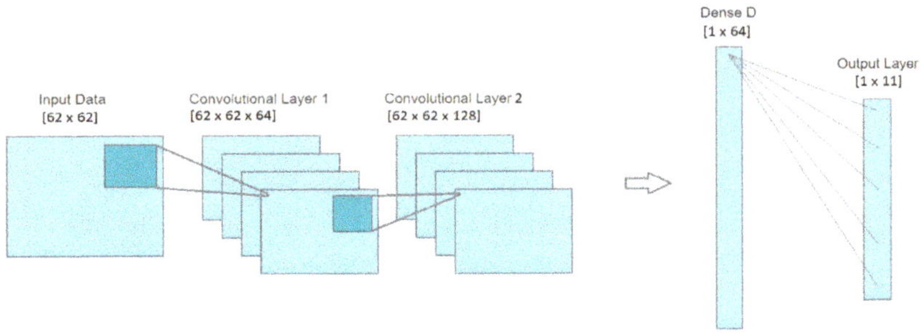

Figure 4. Block diagram of the CNN architecture used in the classification stage.

4. Results

During the development of the system, we aimed to study five different variables capable of influencing the performance of the imaginary speech recognition. Our study of system performance analysis included: (a) the influence of CNN hyperparameters; (b) modification of the network architecture; (c) the impact of the different activation functions that can be used in the CNN; (d) different features capable of encoding the speech hidden information by computing the covariance of the signals over the channels in time and frequency (B0) domain; (e) different window dimensions for the feature extraction method; (f) average filter of three (B3) and five (B5) dimension kernels over the computed spectrum of the data.

For further simplification of displaying the results of different architecture models, we used the abbreviation explained in Table 2. As an example, the architecture Conv2D (64, 128, 64)-Dense (64) corresponds to a CNN network with three convolutional layers, with 64, 128, and 64 filters, respectively, and one dense layer with the number of neurons in the layer equivalent to 64. For all architectures, after the dense layer was introduced, the output layer with 11 neurons corresponded to the 11 different classes.

Table 2. Convolutional Neural Network architecture abbreviations.

Architecture	Abbreviation
Conv2D (64)-Dense (64)	C64/D64
Conv2D (64, 64)-Dense (64)	C64-64/D64
Conv2D (128)-Dense (128)	C128/D128
Conv2D (64, 128)-Dense (64)	C64-128/D64
Conv2D (128, 64)-Dense (64)	C28-64/D64
Conv2D (64, 128, 64)-Dense (64)	C64-128-64/D64
Conv2D (64, 128, 64)-Dense (128)	C64-128-64/D128
Conv2D (128, 256, 128)-Dense (128)	C128-256-128/D128
Conv2D (512, 256, 128)-Dense (128)	C512-256-128/D128

The Kara One database does not show a significant class imbalance. The number of the samples from each class starts from a minimum of 83 (phoneme \m\) and reaches a maximum of 95 (word "pot") out of a total of 993. The a priori probability rises from 0.083 for \m\ phoneme to 0.095 for the word "pot".

4.1. Comparison of Activation Function: Tanh vs. Relu

The results obtained over the test set using different architectures of the CNN and different activation functions for the convolutional layers (hyperbolic tangent vs. rectified linear unit) using the covariance of the spectrum without an average filter (B0) computed over 0.5 s windows are detailed in Table 3.

Table 3. Results obtained using different CNN architectures for the covariance of spectrum features computed over a 0.5 s window comparing the hyperbolic tangent activation function of convolutional layers with the rectified linear unit.

Data characteristics: Features: Covariance of Spectrum Window: 0.5 s Bands: B0	Convolution Layer—Tanh Dense Layer—Tanh Output Layer—Softmax		Convolution Layer—Relu Dense Layer—Tanh Output Layer—Softmax	
	Loss	**Accuracy**	**Loss**	**Accuracy**
C64/D64	1.9344 ± 0.022	0.2974 ± 0.003	1.7929 ± 0.015	0.3465 ± 0.006
C64-64/D64	1.9549 ± 0.020	0.2939 ± 0.007	1.9581 ± 0.135	0.3698 ± 0.008
C128/D128	1.9146 ± 0.059	**0.3169 ± 0.004**	1.7818 ± 0.028	0.3471 ± 0.008
C64-128/D64	1.9459 ± 0.020	0.2932 ± 0.004	1.9514 ± 0.078	**0.3758 ± 0.004**
C128-64/D64	1.9374 ± 0.033	0.2954 ± 0.003	2.0107 ± 0.063	0.3697 ± 0.002
C64-128-64/D64	1.9634 ± 0.052	0.2901 ± 0.008	2.1169 ± 0.034	0.3747 ± 0.001
C64-128-64/D128	1.9882 ± 0.105	0.3035 ± 0.006	2.3308 ± 0.042	0.3693 ± 0.001
C128-256-128/D128	2.0120 ± 0.105	0.2989 ± 0.011	2.4393 ± 0.107	0.3705 ± 0.003

4.2. *Comparison of Features: Time vs. Frequency*

Further in our study, we also compared the differences between the features computed over the signal in the time and frequency domains. The results obtained using different tested architectures are presented in Table 4. It is easy to observe a significant accuracy decrease when using time-domain cross-covariance versus frequency-domain features. The difference between the accuracy of the two feature extraction methods increases to approximately 16%, with the accuracy of frequency features reaching a maximum of 37% and the maximum accuracy of the time-domain features decreasing to 21%. These differences imply that information of speech is more easily decoded by the neural network in the frequency domain rather than in the time domain. The main advantage of the covariance in the frequency domain is given by the elimination of the possible delays of the stimulus propagation over the channels, starting from the source activation of the specific imaginary articulation of the phoneme.

A study of different architectures of the neural network shows (Figure 5) that a CNN with three convolutional layers with 64 and 128 filters and connected with a dense layer with 64 neurons works best for the frequency-domain features (the features that provided the best accuracy rate), obtaining a performance of 37% accuracy. When it comes to the time domain, the best results were obtained using less complex architectures, and the best performance of the system was recorded using only one convolutional layer with 64 filters and one dense layer with 64 neurons.

Table 4. The results obtained after computing the different feature extractions: in the time domain and frequency domain over windows of 0.25 s.

Data Characteristics: Activation Functions: Relu-Tanh-Softmax Window: 0.25 s	**Time**		**Frequency**	
	Loss	**Accuracy**	**Loss**	**Accuracy**
C64/D64	2.3402 ± 0.027	**0.2140 ± 0.001**	1.7929 ± 0.015	0.3465 ± 0.006
C64-64/D64	2.4682 ± 0.075	0.2128 ± 0.003	1.9581 ± 0.135	0.3698 ± 0.008
C128/D128	2.5216 ± 0.155	0.2115 ± 0.002	1.7818 ± 0.028	0.3471 ± 0.008
C64-128/D64	2.3019 ± 0.031	0.2051 ± 0.001	1.9514 ± 0.078	**0.3758 ± 0.004**
C128-64/D64	2.5804 ± 0.324	0.2071 ± 0.010	2.0107 ± 0.063	0.3697 ± 0.002
C64-128-64/D64	2.5197 ± 0.184	0.2038 ± 0.004	2.1169 ± 0.034	0.3747 ± 0.001
C64-128-64/D128	3.2871 ± 0.402	0.2039 ± 0.002	2.3308 ± 0.042	0.3693 ± 0.001
C128-256-128/D128	3.0037 ± 0.571	0.1981 ± 0.001	2.4393 ± 0.107	0.3705 ± 0.003

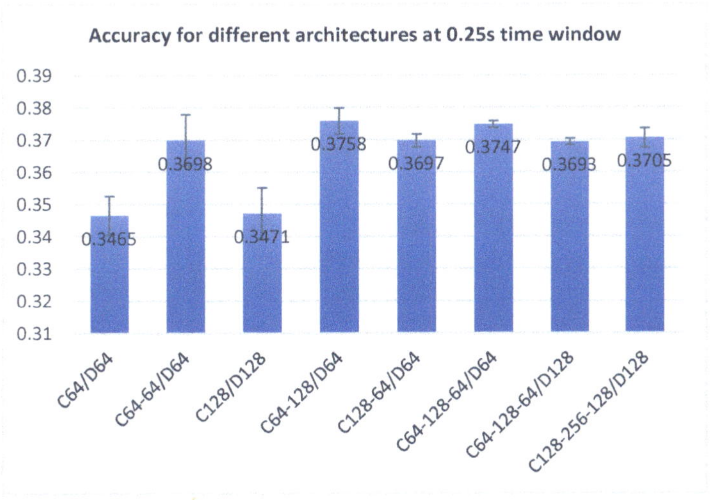

Figure 5. Accuracy for different architectures with a 0.25 s time window.

The mean confusion matrices for all k-folds for the time and frequency features are presented in Figure 6. In both images, we can see a distinction between phonemes and words. The system has a difficult time recognizing one phoneme against the other but makes a clearer distinction between them and the words. We can also observe that phoneme \diy\ is often confused with similar phonemes such as \iy\ and \piy\. It can also be seen that there is no significant imbalance in the recognition of any of the phonemes and words; however, the words have a higher accuracy rate of recognition.

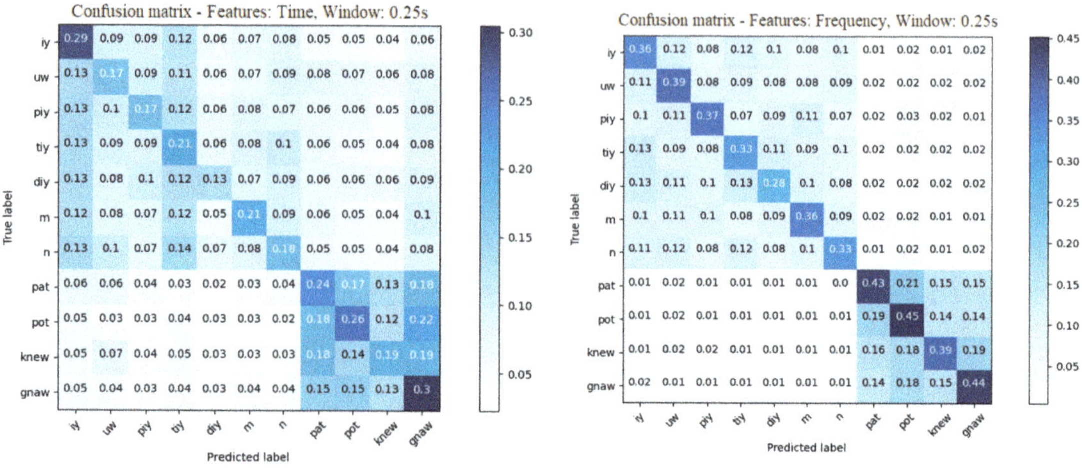

Figure 6. Mean of k-fold confusion matrix in the time and frequency domains.

4.3. Comparison of Time Window Length: 0.25, 0.5 and 1 s

After we concluded that the system works better with a rectified linear unit as an activation function for the convolutional layers in the frequency domain, we tested the network with different window lengths for the input data. The results are presented in Table 5.

Table 5. Comparison of different window length (0.25, 0.5, 1 s) results for the covariance of spectrum features without an average filter (B0).

Data Characteristics: Features: Covariance of Spectrum Activation Functions: Relu-Tanh-Softmax Bands: B0	0.25 s		0.5		1 s	
	Loss	Accuracy	Loss	Accuracy	Loss	Accuracy
C64/D64	1.7929 ± 0.015	0.3465 ± 0.006	1.9221 ± 0.023	0.3243 ± 0.005	2.0960 ± 0.033	0.2808 ± 0.011
C64-64/D64	1.9581 ± 0.135	0.3698 ± 0.008	1.9642 ± 0.019	0.3514 ± 0.004	2.2721 ± 0.087	0.2939 ± 0.007
C128/D128	1.7818 ± 0.028	0.3471 ± 0.008	1.8257 ± 0.017	0.3400 ± 0.004	2.0517 ± 0.025	0.2857 ± 0.004
C64-128/D64	1.9514 ± 0.078	**0.3758 ± 0.004**	1.9957 ± 0.065	0.3588 ± 0.003	2.1825 ± 0.087	**0.2980 ± 0.002**
C128-64/D64	2.0107 ± 0.063	0.3697 ± 0.002	1.9903 ± 0.053	**0.3620 ± 0.003**	2.3020 ± 0.126	0.2964 ± 0.006
C64-128-64/D64	2.1169 ± 0.034	0.3747 ± 0.001	2.1737 ± 0.080	0.3566 ± 0.002	2.3971 ± 0.091	0.2922 ± 0.003
C64-128-64/D128	2.3308 ± 0.042	0.3693 ± 0.001	2.2874 ± 0.212	0.3457 ± 0.007	2.6291 ± 0.135	0.2938 ± 0.013
C128-256-128/D128	2.4393 ± 0.107	0.3705 ± 0.003	2.4186 ± 0.142	0.3504 ± 0.005	2.6111 ± 0.325	0.2925 ± 0.006
C512-256-128/D128	2.5051 ± 0.086	0.3680 ± 0.005	2.1755 ± 0.101	0.3136 ± 0.007	2.6600 ± 0.2066	0.2871 ± 0.008

The 4 s EEG signal containing imaginary speech includes multiple imaginations of the specific stimulus. It is hard to precisely determine the moment containing the desired signal in the whole four seconds of recording, which is why we chose to segment the signal over different window lengths and observe the system behavior. Table 5, as well as Figure 7, shows that the best analysis window is 0.25 s, reaching an accuracy of 37%. Looking at the 0.5 and 1 s window lengths, we can observe that the 0.5 s offered an accuracy close to the 0.25 s window, meaning that the signals are still easier to decode compared to the 1 s window in which the accuracy significantly dropped to 29%. The mean confusion matrices for the 0.5 s window and 1 s window are presented in Figure 8.

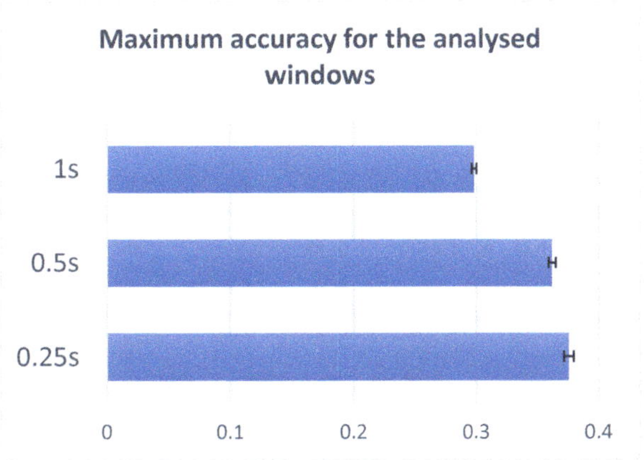

Figure 7. Maximum accuracy for the analyzed windows.

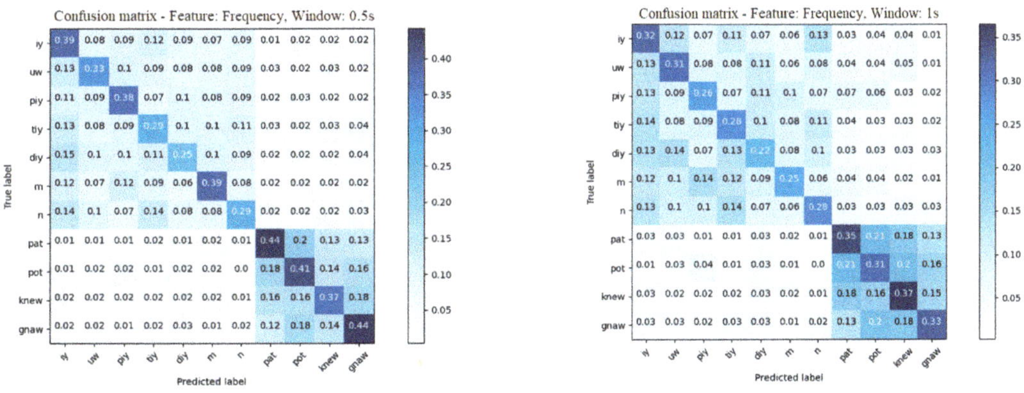

Figure 8. Mean of k-fold confusion matrix in the frequency domain for 0.5 s and 1 s windows.

4.4. Comparison of Mean Filter Kernel: B0, B3 and B5

Another study conducted in this paper focused on applying different average filter lengths over the spectrum before computing the covariance matrix. We tested two different filter lengths: three samples and five samples. We will further refer to the spectrum without a mean filter as B0, the spectrum with an applied mean filter length of three samples as B3, and the spectrum with an applied mean filter length of five samples as B5. The obtained results can be seen in Table 6. The main motivation for this approach was developed on the assumption that the analysis of multiple values of the spectrum, as opposed to analyzing only the local values, can offer a better perspective of the frequency distribution regarding different classes. This assumption did not stand up because, as can be seen in Table 6 and in Figure 9, the better accuracy results were obtained using the unmodified spectrum. These results imply that every frequency is important for the phoneme and word recognition problem.

Table 6. Comparison between the results obtained after applying different kernels for the average filter of the spectrum. The analysis window is 0.5 s.

Data Characteristics: Features: Covariance of Spectrum Activation Functions: Relu-Tanh-Softmax Window: 0.25 s	**B0**		**B3**		**B5**	
	Loss	**Accuracy**	**Loss**	**Accuracy**	**Loss**	**Accuracy**
C64/D64	1.7929 ± 0.015	0.3465 ± 0.006	2.0423 ± 0.011	0.2864 ± 0.003	2.0479 ± 0.023	0.2809 ± 0.003
C64-64/D64	1.9581 ± 0.135	0.3698 ± 0.008	2.4141 ± 0.185	0.2837 ± 0.007	2.3275 ± 0.023	0.2841 ± 0.003
C128/D128	1.7818 ± 0.028	0.3471 ± 0.008	2.0203 ± 0.041	**0.2886 ± 0.004**	1.9876 ± 0.025	0.2825 ± 0.003
C64-128/D64	1.9514 ± 0.078	**0.3758 ± 0.004**	2.2003 ± 0.121	0.2838 ± 0.003	2.3150 ± 0.119	**0.2863 ± 0.002**
C128-64/D64	2.0107 ± 0.063	0.3697 ± 0.002	2.2907 ± 0.150	0.2771 ± 0.005	2.3421 ± 0.215	0.2804 ± 0.005
C64-128-64/D64	2.1169 ± 0.034	0.3747 ± 0.001	2.5577 ± 0.244	0.2755 ± 0.003	2.5767 ± 0.171	0.2786 ± 0.007
C64-128-64/D128	2.3308 ± 0.042	0.3693 ± 0.001	2.4874 ± 0.226	0.2753 ± 0.001	2.5579 ± 0.3141	0.2707 ± 0.007
C128-256-128/D128	2.4393 ± 0.107	0.3705 ± 0.003	2.9467 ± 0.197	0.2758 ± 0.006	2.8533 ± 0.259	0.2707 ± 0.006

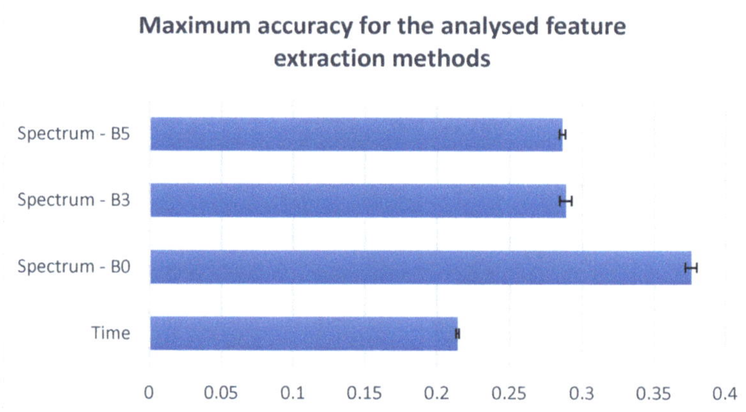

Figure 9. Maximum accuracy for the feature extraction methods analyzed.

4.5. Performance Evaluation Metrics

For a better understanding of the recorded results and the system performance, we introduced the computed values for all extracted features: the balanced accuracy, kappa and recall [32]. The obtained values are presented in Table 7.

Table 7. The obtained result for all features of balanced accuracy, kappa and recall.

	Time—Window Length 0.25 s	**Frequency—Window Length 0.25 s**	**Frequency—Window Length 0.5 s**	**Frequency—Window Length 1 s**
Balanced accuracy	0.2131 ± 0.001	0.3749 ± 0.004	0.3615 ± 0.003	0.2980 ± 0.001
Kappa	0.1349 ± 0.001	0.3132 ± 0.004	0.2980 ± 0.004	0.2278 ± 0.002
Recall	0.2140 ± 0.001	0.3750 ± 0.004	0.3620 ± 0.003	0.2980 ± 0.002

According to Table 7, the balanced accuracy and recall are not significantly different from the computed accuracies for the features, and only the kappa score dropped to a value of approximately 0.7 for all features.

4.6. Complexity and Memory Measurements

This paper aimed to develop a low-cost system working with limited resources. To achieve this goal, we tested different architectures of CNN networks for different types of features and windows. This research helped us to determine the best CNN architecture, features and window frame that can be implemented on a device with limited resources.

Given the application, the most significant resource consumer is the neural network. For the CNN neural network architecture, the complexity of the algorithm can be estimated as $O(k \times N \times M \times nF^{L-1} \times nF^{L})$, where k is the kernel matrix, N is the number of lines of the input matrix, M is the number of columns of the input matrix, nF^{L-1} is the number of filters from the anterior CNN layers and nF^{L} is the number of filters from the current layer. In our case, the input matrix has the same number of lines and columns (M = N = 62), and we can write the complexity as $O(k \times N^2 \times nF^{L-1} \times nF^{L})$. The details of the complexity, memory and time for the feature extraction stage and the best performance CNN architecture are presented in Table 8.

Table 8. Detailed complexity, memory and time computation for the system with the best results.

System Stages		Complexity	Memory	Time (s)
Feature Extraction	FFT	O(NxMlogM)	968 KB	3.12×10^{-4}
	COV	$O(N^2)$	88 KB	4.84×10^{-4}
CNN	Conv2D-64	$O(k \times N^2 \times 64)$	976 KB	1.7×10^{-3}
	Conv2D-128	$O(k \times N^2 \times 64 \times 128)$	2.81 MB	
	Dense-64	$O(k \times N^2 \times 128 \times 64)$	7.8 MB	
	Dense-11	$O(64 \times 11)$	748 B	

Using an AMD Ryzen 7 4800HS CPU with 16 GB memory RAM and 2.9 GHz clock frequency, we managed to obtain an average time per recognized input vector of 1.8×10^{-3} s starting from the feature extraction stage up to the decision making. The time was estimated (Table 8) using the characteristics of the best system in terms of performance, meaning computing the output for the 0.25 s window vector with the C64-128/D64 neural network architecture (Table 5).

A comparison of the methods in terms of execution time, as can be observed in Table 9, show that there are no significant differences between the execution of the different features; however, there is approximately an order of magnitude between the best performance architectures and the most complex one tested.

Table 9. Execution time for all tested architectures and features.

Architecture	Features			
	Time—Window Length 0.25 s	Frequency—Window Length 0.25 s	Frequency—Window Length 0.5 s	Frequency—Window Length 1 s
C64/D64	5.4×10^{-4}	6.4×10^{-4}	6.3×10^{-4}	7.3×10^{-4}
C64-64/D64	1.1×10^{-3}	1.2×10^{-3}	1.2×10^{-3}	1.3×10^{-3}
C128/D128	1.5×10^{-3}	1.8×10^{-3}	1.6×10^{-3}	1.7×10^{-3}
C64-128/D64	1.7×10^{-3}	1.8×10^{-3}	1.9×10^{-3}	1.9×10^{-3}
C128-64/D64	2×10^{-3}	2.1×10^{-3}	2.2×10^{-3}	2.3×10^{-3}
C64-128-64/D64	2.7×10^{-3}	2.8×10^{-3}	2.9×10^{-3}	2.9×10^{-3}
C64-128-64/D128	2.8×10^{-3}	2.9×10^{-3}	3×10^{-3}	3.1×10^{-3}
C128-256-128/D128	9.2×10^{-3}	10^{-2}	10^{-2}	8.9×10^{-3}

5. Discussion

This paper aims to compare different parameters of an intelligent imaginary speech recognition subject's shared system to observe the performance variation when using different mechanisms of feature extraction and different architectures of CNN in the classification stage.

We used the Kara One database in our study, designed and conducted at the Toronto Rehabilitation Institute by Shunan Zhao and Frank Rudzicz [7], which contains signals acquired during speech and imaginary speech of seven phonemes and four words.

During the recognition process, we pre-processed the signals, and after the visual inspection, eliminated all data from subjects containing electrodes with bad connectivity and the signals with high noise. Furthermore, in the pre-processing stage, we applied a notch filter to remove the 60Hz power line artifact and all multiples of 60Hz smaller than the Nyquist frequency. It is worth mentioning that, in our study, we kept all high-frequency information.

5.1. Time vs. Frequency Features

After the pre-processing stage, we went through a feature extraction stage where we focused on comparing the feature extraction based on cross-covariance over the channels in the time and frequency domains. The cross-covariance method is based on the fact that speech is a complex mechanism, requiring thinking of the speech stimulus, preparing the vocal tract for the actual vocalization and giving the signal to all components of the vocal tract involved in the actual speaking of the stimulus. For different stimuli, there are different positions and components involved in the process. This mechanism demands the activation of multiple areas of the brain that communicates in a very short time. The connections of different areas are best highlighted by the cross-covariance between the channels. The results presented in Table 4 show that there is a considerable difference between the results obtained using time-domain feature extractions versus frequency-domain feature extractions. When using frequency-domain features, the accuracy increases by approximately 16% to a value of 0.37 compared to 0.21 obtained when using features in the time-domain. This difference is given by the fact that the signal spectrum eliminates the delays of the stimulus propagation over the channels, starting from the activation focus of the specific imaginary articulation of the phoneme.

5.2. Time-Window Analysis

Another study conducted in this paper aims to compare different sizes of the analysis window in order to observe the signal statistics of different time gaps. During this study, we aimed to find the time window in which the signal is quasi-stationary but also contains all the needed information regarding the utterance. We compared three analysis window sizes: 0.25, 0.5 and 1 s. The obtained results can be seen in Table 5. Comparing the window dimensions, we observed that the best time window length was 0.25 s. The accuracy of the results is significantly higher when using 0.25 s, increasing to a value of 0.37, compared to 0.29 when using a 1 s window. The difference between the accuracy of the 0.25 s window and the 0.5 s window is 1%, which is not very significant. This means that for a 0.5 s window, the utterance of the phonemes and words are still captured by the frame.

Analyzing the results in Table 5 also shows that the maximum accuracy for all time-frame windows was obtained using a low-complex architecture for the CNN.

5.3. Mean Filter over the Spectrum Analysis

During our research for improvement, we also tried to average the spectrum of the signals with a filter of three and five samples. The main motivation for this approach was developed on the assumption that the analysis of multiple values of the spectrum, compared to analyzing only the local values, can offer a better perspective of the frequency distribution regarding different classes. The details of this research are presented in Table 6. As can be seen, applying an average filter over the spectrum did not increase the accuracy;

on the contrary, the accuracy dropped by approximately 9% when using filters with three and five samples.

5.4. CNN Architectures Analysis

In our final study, we tested different architectures for the CNN network to observe the system performance and shape the way for the future development of similar systems. We concluded that when it comes to the frequency-domain features (the features that provided the best accuracy rate), the best architecture is two convolutional layers with 64 and 128 filters connected to a dense layer with 64 neurons. More complex architectures do not improve the performance of the system, and on the contrary, the performance decreases.

6. Conclusions

This paper analyses the EEG signals for imaginary speech recognition of seven phonemes and four words. To accomplish our purpose, we developed an intelligent subject's shared system using a processing chain applied to the Kara One database [7]. The first stage in the analysis chain started with pre-processing the input signals in order to obtain better quality data. Further in the feature extraction stage, we compared the results obtained after computing the cross-covariance over the channels in the time and frequency domains. During our research, we also studied different time window lengths: 0.25, 0.5 and 1 s to find the time window in which the signal is quasi-stationary but also contains all the information needed regarding the utterance. We also studied the system behavior when applying a mean filter with kernel sizes of three and five samples assuming that the analysis of multiple values of the spectrum, compared to analyzing only the local values, can offer a better perspective of the frequency distribution regarding different classes. Finally, in the classification stage, we tested multiple architectures of the CNN neural network to determine the best performance of the system.

The best results were obtained using the cross-covariance over channels in the frequency domain using a 0.25 s window length. The best performance of the system was recorded when using a CNN with two convolutional layers and 64 and 128 filters, connected to a dense layer with 64 neurons. With these system characteristics, we achieved an accuracy of 37%, a significant improvement compared to using the Mel-Cepstral Coefficients for feature extraction, where the best accuracy recorded was 20.80% when using an SVM as the classifier [10] and 24.19% when using a CNN as the classifier [11]. During our study, we also showed that cross-covariance in the frequency domain offers a better understanding of the imaginary speech, reporting a better accuracy in comparison to the study made by Pramit Saha, Muhammad Abdul-Mageed and Sidney Fels in [12] where, using the cross-covariance in time and hierarchical deep learning (without phonological features), the best reported accuracy was 28%. However, when using phonological features, the accuracy increased to 54%, but this compromised the complexity and the memory of the system and is more difficult to implement in a low-complexity portable device.

The main limitation of our proposed system includes the acquisition of new data for each new subject before being able to wear the system. The collected data must be included in the database for which a fine-tuning of the network training must be applied. However, this limitation can be overcome in time by enriching the database with new examples.

In this study, we proposed a feature extraction method based on cross-covariance in the frequency domain that offered a significant improvement for the system performance compared to features computed in the time domain. We are confident that these features can be further exploited to obtain even more precise systems for imaginary speech recognition.

In this paper, we achieved our goal of highlighting the importance of using frequency in the feature extraction stage in contrast to the time domain. The advantage of using the frequency domain is given by the elimination of the delays caused by the propagation of the stimulus from one channel to another during the imaginary articulation of the speech. We also showed that a quicker analysis of the signal offers a better understanding of the thinking speech.

Finally, we can say that the proposed system qualifies as a portable, low-cost system using limited resources for decision making. The running time for the best performance CNN architecture was 1.8 ms tested on an AMD Ryzen 7 4800HS CPU.

Author Contributions: Conceptualization, O.G.; Data curation, A.-L.R.; Methodology, A.-L.R. and O.G.; Software, A.-L.R.; Supervision, O.G.; Writing – original draft, A.-L.R.; Writing – review & editing, O.G. All authors have read and agreed to the published version of the manuscript.

Funding: This research received no external funding.

Institutional Review Board Statement: Ethical approval was obtained from both the University of Toronto and the University Health Network, of which Toronto Rehab is a member.

Informed Consent Statement: Informed consent was obtained from all subjects involved in the study.

Data Availability Statement: http://www.cs.toronto.edu/~complingweb/data/karaOne/karaOne.html. (accessed on 16 June 2022).

Conflicts of Interest: The authors declare no conflict of interest.

References

1. Dronkers, N.; Ogar, J. Brain areas involved in speech production. *Brain* **2004**, *127*, 7. [CrossRef]
2. Dewan, E.M. Occipital Alpha Rhythm Eye Position and Lens Accommodation. *Nat. Publ. Group* **1967**, *214*, 975–977. [CrossRef]
3. Kennedy, P.R.; Bakay, R.A.E.; Moore, M.M.; Adams, K.; Goldwaithe, J. Direct control of a computer from the human central nervous system. *IEEE Trans. Rehab. Eng.* **2000**, *8*, 2. [CrossRef]
4. Jayabhavani, G.N.; Rajaan, N.R. Brain enabled mechanized speech synthesizer using Brain Mobile Interface. *Int. J. Eng. Technol.* **2013**, *5*, 1.
5. Wester, M.; Schultz, T. *Unspoken Speech—Speech Recognition Based on Elecroencephalography*; Universitat Karlsruhe: Karlsruhe, Germany, 2006.
6. Porbadnigk, A.; Wester, M.; Calliess, T.S.J.P. EEG-Based Speech Recognition—Impact of Temporal Effects. In Proceedings of the International Conference on Bio-inspired Systems and Signal Processing, Porto, Portugal, 13 February 2009; pp. 376–381. [CrossRef]
7. Zhao, S.; Rudzicz, F. Classifying phonological categories in imagined and articulated speech. In Proceedings of the 2015 IEEE International Conference on Acoustics, Speech and Signal Processing (ICASSP), South Brisbane, QL, Australia, 19–24 April 2015; pp. 992–996. [CrossRef]
8. Sun, P.; Qin, J. Neural Networks based EEG-Speech Models. *arXiv* **2017**, arXiv:1612.05369.
9. Saha, P.; Fels, S.; Abdul-Mageed, M. Deep Learning the EEG Manifold for Phonological Categorization from Active Thoughts. In Proceedings of the ICASSP 2019—2019 IEEE International Conference on Acoustics, Speech and Signal Processing (ICASSP), Brighton, UK, 12–17 May 2019; pp. 2762–2766. [CrossRef]
10. Cooney, C.; Folli, R.; Coyle, D. Mel Frequency Cepstral Coefficients Enhance Imagined Speech Decoding Accuracy from EEG. In Proceedings of the 2018 29th Irish Signals and Systems Conference (ISSC), Belfast, UK, 21 June 2018; pp. 1–7. [CrossRef]
11. Rusnac, A.-L.; Grigore, O. Generalized Brain Computer Interface System for EEG Imaginary Speech Recognition. In Proceedings of the 2020 24th International Conference on Circuits, Systems, Communications and Computers (CSCC), Chania, Greece, 19–22 July 2020; pp. 184–188. [CrossRef]
12. Saha, P.; Abdul-Mageed, M.; Fels, S. SPEAK YOUR MIND! Towards Imagined Speech Recognition with Hierarchical Deep Learning. In Proceedings of the INTERSPEECH 2019, Graz, Austria, 15–19 September 2019.
13. Vorontsova, D.; Menshikov, I.; Zubov, A.; Orlov, K.; Rikunov, P.; Zvereva, E.; Flitman, L.; Lanikin, A.; Sokolova, A.; Markov, S.; et al. Silent EEG-Speech Recognition Using Convolutional and Recurrent Neural Network with 85% Accuracy of 9 Words Classification. *Sensors* **2021**, *21*, 6744. [CrossRef]
14. Dash, D.; Ferrari, P.; Wang, J. Decoding Imagined and Spoken Phrases from Non-invasive Neural (MEG) Signals. *Front. Neurosci.* **2020**, *14*, 290. [CrossRef] [PubMed]
15. Herff, C.; Diener, L.; Angrick, M.; Mugler, E.; Tate, M.C.; Goldrick, M.A.; Krusienski, D.J.; Slutzky, M.W.; Schultz, T. Generating Natural, Intelligible Speech From Brain Activity in Motor, Premotor, and Inferior Frontal Cortices. *Front. Neurosci.* **2019**, *13*, 1267. [CrossRef] [PubMed]
16. Proix, T.; Delgado Saa, J.; Christen, A.; Martin, S.; Pasley, B.N.; Knight, R.T.; Tian, X.; Poeppel, D.; Doyle, W.K.; Giraud, A.L.; et al. Imagined speech can be decoded from low- and cross-frequency intracranial EEG features. *Nat. Commun.* **2022**, *13*, 48. [CrossRef]
17. Tsiouris, K.M.; Pezoulas, V.C.; Zervakis, M.; Konitsiotis, S.; Koutsouris, D.D.; Fotiadis, D.I. A Long Short-Term Memory deep learning network for the prediction of epileptic seizures using EEG signals. *Comput. Biol. Med.* **2018**, *99*, 24–37. [CrossRef] [PubMed]
18. Xing, X.; Li, Z.; Xu, T.; Shu, L.; Hu, B.; Xu, X. SAE + LSTM: A New Framework for Emotion Recognition From Multi-Channel EEG. *Front. Neurorobot.* **2019**, *13*, 37. [CrossRef] [PubMed]

19. Ni, Z.; Yuksel, A.C.; Ni, X.; Mandel, M.I.; Xie, L. Confused or not Confused? Disentangling Brain Activity from EEG Data Using Bidirectional LSTM Recurrent Neural Networks. In Proceedings of the 8th ACM International Conference on Bioinformatics, Computational Biology, and Health Informatics, Boston, MA, USA, 20–23 August 2017; pp. 241–246. [CrossRef]
20. Xu, G.; Ren, T.; Chen, Y.; Che, W. A One-Dimensional CNN-LSTM Model for Epileptic Seizure Recognition Using EEG Signal Analysis. *Front. Neurosci.* **2020**, *14*, 578126. [CrossRef]
21. Krishna, G.; Han, Y.; Tran, C.; Carnahan, M.; Tewfik, A.H. State-of-the-art Speech Recognition using EEG and Towards Decoding of Speech Spectrum from EEG. *arXiv* **2019**, arXiv:1908.05743.
22. Sharon, R.A.; Narayanan, S.; Sur, M.; Murthy, H.A. An Empirical Study of Speech Processing in the Brain by Analyzing the Temporal Syllable Structure in Speech-input Induced EEG. In Proceedings of the ICASSP 2019—2019 IEEE International Conference on Acoustics, Speech and Signal Processing (ICASSP), Brighton, UK, 12–17 May 2019; pp. 4090–4094. [CrossRef]
23. Sarvamangala, D.R.; Kulkarni, R.V. Convolutional neural networks in medical image understanding: A survey. *Evol. Intel.* **2021**, *15*, 1–22. [CrossRef]
24. Chen, R.; Parhi, K.K. Seizure Prediction using Convolutional Neural Networks and Sequence Transformer Networks. In Proceedings of the 2021 43rd Annual International Conference of the IEEE Engineering in Medicine & Biology Society (EMBC), Jalisco, Mexico, 19 November 2021; pp. 6483–6486. [CrossRef]
25. Huang, J.-S.; Liu, W.-S.; Yao, B.; Wang, Z.-X.; Chen, S.-F.; Sun, W.-F. Electroencephalogram-Based Motor Imagery Classification Using Deep Residual Convolutional Networks. *Front. Neurosci.* **2021**, *15*, 774857. [CrossRef]
26. Milanes, D.; Codorniu, R.T.; Baracaldo, R.L.; Zamora, R.S.; Rodriguez, D.D.; Albuerne, Y.L.; Alvarez, J.R.N. Shallow Convolutional Network Excel for Classifying Motor Imagery EEG in BCI Applications. *IEEE Access* **2021**, *9*, 98275–98286. [CrossRef]
27. Zhang, J.; Yan, C.; Gong, X. Deep convolutional neural network for decoding motor imagery based brain computer interface. In Proceedings of the 2017 IEEE International Conference on Signal Processing, Communications and Computing (ICSPCC), Xiamen, China, 22–25 October 2017; pp. 1–5. [CrossRef]
28. Lee, S.; Hussein, R.; Ward, R.; Jane Wang, Z.; McKeown, M.J. A convolutional-recurrent neural network approach to resting-state EEG classification in Parkinson's disease. *J. Neurosci. Methods* **2021**, *361*, 109282. [CrossRef] [PubMed]
29. Lin, J.; Yao, Y. A Fast Algorithm for Convolutional Neural Networks Using Tile-based Fast Fourier Transforms. *Neural Process Lett.* **2019**, *50*, 1951–1967. [CrossRef]
30. Scott Gray, A.L. Fast Algorithms for Convolutional Neural Networks. *arXiv* **2015**, arXiv:1509.09308v2.
31. Jun Zhang, T.L.; Shuangsang Fang, Y.Z.; Wang, P. Implementation of Training Convolutional Neural Networks. *arXiv* **2015**, arXiv:1506.01195v2.
32. Grandini, M.; Bagli, E.; Visani, G. Metrics for Multi-Class Classification: An Overview. *arXiv* **2020**, arXiv:2008.05756.

sensors

MDPI

Article

Diagnosis and Prognosis of COVID-19 Disease Using Routine Blood Values and LogNNet Neural Network

Mehmet Tahir Huyut [1,*] and Andrei Velichko [2,*]

[1] Department of Biostatistics and Medical Informatics, Faculty of Medicine, Erzincan Binali Yıldırım University, 24000 Erzincan, Turkey
[2] Institute of Physics and Technology, Petrozavodsk State University, 33 Lenin Str., 185910 Petrozavodsk, Russia
* Correspondence: tahir.huyut@erzincan.edu.tr (M.T.H.); velichko@petrsu.ru (A.V.)

Abstract: Since February 2020, the world has been engaged in an intense struggle with the COVID-19 disease, and health systems have come under tragic pressure as the disease turned into a pandemic. The aim of this study is to obtain the most effective routine blood values (RBV) in the diagnosis and prognosis of COVID-19 using a backward feature elimination algorithm for the LogNNet reservoir neural network. The first dataset in the study consists of a total of 5296 patients with the same number of negative and positive COVID-19 tests. The LogNNet-model achieved the accuracy rate of 99.5% in the diagnosis of the disease with 46 features and the accuracy of 99.17% with only mean corpuscular hemoglobin concentration, mean corpuscular hemoglobin, and activated partial prothrombin time. The second dataset consists of a total of 3899 patients with a diagnosis of COVID-19 who were treated in hospital, of which 203 were severe patients and 3696 were mild patients. The model reached the accuracy rate of 94.4% in determining the prognosis of the disease with 48 features and the accuracy of 82.7% with only erythrocyte sedimentation rate, neutrophil count, and C reactive protein features. Our method will reduce the negative pressures on the health sector and help doctors to understand the pathogenesis of COVID-19 using the key features. The method is promising to create mobile health monitoring systems in the Internet of Things.

Keywords: COVID-19; biochemical and hematological biomarkers; routine blood values; feature selection method; LogNNet neural network; Internet of Medical Things; IoT

Citation: Huyut, M.T.; Velichko, A. Diagnosis and Prognosis of COVID-19 Disease Using Routine Blood Values and LogNNet Neural Network. *Sensors* **2022**, *22*, 4820. https://doi.org/10.3390/s22134820

Received: 24 May 2022
Accepted: 23 June 2022
Published: 25 June 2022

1. Introduction

The new severe acute respiratory syndrome coronavirus (SARS-CoV-2), first identified in 2019, has rapidly affected the world and caused a pandemic [1,2]. The disease, identified as coronavirus 2019 (COVID-19), can cause severe pneumonia and fatal acute respiratory distress syndrome (ARDS) [3–6]. While the disease may be asymptomatic, severe ARDS is thought to be caused by an inflammatory cytokine storm that may be encountered during the disease period [6,7]. The pathogen can cause a serious respiratory disorder that requires special intervention in intensive care units (ICUs) and, in some cases, may cause death [6,7]. Moreover, the symptoms of COVID-19 induced by the new SARS-CoV-2 are difficult to distinguish from known infections in the majority of patients [6,8,9].

Previous studies have demonstrated the clinical importance of changes in routine blood parameters (RBV) in the diagnosis and prediction of prognosis of infectious diseases [1–4,10–12]. Similarly, many abnormalities have been reported in the peripheral blood of patients infected with COVID-19 [6,7,11]. However, Jiang et al. [13] and Zheng et al. [14] emphasized that information on early predictive factors for particularly severe and fatal COVID-19 cases is relatively limited and further research is needed. Huyut et al. [6] and Lippi et al. [15] described that the rapid spread of disease in pandemics overwhelms health systems and raises concerns about the need for intensive care treatment [6,15]. In addition, the detection of severe and mild patients in COVID-19 is an important and clinically difficult process in terms of morbidity and mortality [6]. Despite these clinical features of COVID-19, studies with large samples representing laboratory abnormalities of patients are needed [3,16]. Therefore, the relationship between COVID-19 disease and RBVs should be supported by large datasets.

Studies have sought how to determine whether patients who are likely to benefit from supportive care and early intervention are at risk and how to identify them [6,11]. While new tests are being developed for the diagnosis of COVID-19, Banerjee et al. [8] stated that these applications require specialized equipment and facilities. Estimating the diagnosis and prognosis of diseases without using advanced devices and methods can help with various problems, such as patient comfort, as well as health system and economic inefficiencies. For this purpose, Beck et al. [17] and Xu et al. [18] have reported that more economical and faster alternative methods are being developed to assist clinical procedures.

Uncertainties in the routine blood values of COVID-19 patients, in addition to difficulties in diagnosis and treatment have increased the interest in machine learning (ML) and artificial intelligence (AI) approaches. Artificial intelligence models have the power to reveal hidden relationship structures between features [19]. Artificial intelligence approaches are frequently used in real-time decision making to reduce drug costs, improve patient comfort, and improve the quality of healthcare services [5,19].

There are several artificial intelligence methods to predict the diagnosis and mortality of COVID-19 [4,17]. Most of these studies have relied on computed tomography (CT) [19], while far fewer studies relied on RBVs [4,5,20]. Imaging-based solutions are costly, time-consuming, and require specialized equipment [20]. Diagnosis based on RBV values can provide an effective, rapid, and cost-effective alternative for the early detection and prognosis of COVID-19 cases [5,20,21].

Previous AI studies did not use most of the RBV parameters and reported relatively poor classifier performance compared to the current study [2,3,5,6]. In addition, previous studies [8,19–25] have generally focused on the early diagnosis of COVID-19 disease and have addressed relatively smaller samples. Artificial intelligence studies on predicting the prognosis of the disease and detecting severely or mildly infected patients in the early period based on RBVs alone are insufficient. New studies could reduce the intensity of the ICU and help health services by detecting severe and mildly infected patients with COVID-19 early [2,5,19,20].

Most ML approaches involve the process of transforming the feature vector from the first multidimensional space to the second multidimensional space and detecting the vector by a linear classifier [26]. The differences between ML models generally lie in the transformation algorithms and their number and order. In addition, transformation algorithms can be in the form of reducing and increasing the space dimension. The popular machine learning classifier algorithms used for data analysis are: multilayer perceptron (feedforward neural network with several layers, linear classifier) [27], support vector machine [28], K-nearest neighbors method [29], XGBoost classifier [30], random forest method [31], logistic regression [32], and decision trees [33].

ML algorithms typically require a sufficiently large number of samples. However, in our case, the dataset has to be reduced to avoid dimensionality problems by finding a matrix that has fewer columns and is similar to the original matrix. Since the new matrix consists of fewer features, it can be used more efficiently than the original matrix. Dimensionality reduction is the process of finding matrices with fewer columns. Feature selection is one of the techniques used to reduce dimensionality, when irrelevant and redundant features are discarded [26,34]. In addition, the selection of appropriate features can reduce the measurement cost and provide a better understanding of the problem [26]. Feature selection methods can be classified as filters, embedded methods, and wrappers (forward selection, backward elimination, recursive feature elimination) [26,34]. Because feature selection is part of the training process in embedded methods, our method lies between filters and wrappers. Searching for the best subset of features is performed during training of the classifier, e.g., when optimizing weights in a neural network. Therefore, embedded methods present a lower computational cost than wrappers [26].

Most of the feature selection methods are filters, although we can find representative methods for all three categories [26]. The large number of available feature selection methods complicates the selection of the best method for a given problem [34]. The latest methods that have become popular among researchers are feature selection based on correlation (CFS) [35], filtering based on consistency [36], INTERACT [37], knowledge gain (InfoGain) [38], ReliefF [39], recursive feature elimination for support vector machines (SVM-RFE) [40], Lasso editing [41], and the minimum redundancy maximum relevance (mRMR) algorithm (developed specifically for dealing with microarray data) [26].

In [42], a classifier based on the LogNNet neural network was described using a handwriting recognition example from the MNIST database. Velichko [43] demonstrated the use of the LogNNet to calculate risk factors for the presence of a disease based on a set of medical health indicators. The LogNNet neural network is a feedforward network that improves classification accuracy by passing the feature vector through a special reservoir matrix and transforming it into a feature vector of different size [44]. Previous studies have shown that the higher the entropy of a chaotic mapping that fills a reservoir matrix, the better the classification accuracy [45]. Therefore, the procedure for optimizing chaotic map parameters plays an important role in the presented data analysis method using the LogNNet neural network. In addition, due to the characteristics of chaotic mapping, RAM usage by a neural network can be significantly reduced. In [43], the operation of the LogNNet algorithm on a device with 2 kB of RAM was presented. This result demonstrated that LogNNet can be used in Internet of Things (IoT) mobile devices.

In this study, we apply the LogNNet neural network for the diagnosis and prognosis of COVID-19 using the RBV values measured at the time of admission to the hospital. The wrapper-type backward feature elimination algorithm has been successfully adapted to LogNNet. The novelty of the presented method is the approach to the diagnosis and prognosis of COVID-19 using routine blood values.

The paper has the following structure. Section 2 describes the data collection procedure, the basic LogNNet architecture, and K-fold cross-validation technique. Section 3 presents examples of using the feature selection methodology for two datasets. In this section, the most important RBVs (features) effective in the diagnosis and prognosis of the disease were selected. Using various feature combinations, the performance of the LogNNet model in the diagnosis and prognosis of the disease was calculated. Section 4 discusses the results and compares them with known developments. In conclusion, a general description of the study and its scientific significance are given.

2. Materials and Methods

This study was conducted in accordance with the Declaration of Helsinki, 1989. Data were collected retrospectively from the information system of Erzincan Binali Yıldırım University Mengücek Gazi Training and Research Hospital (EBYU-MG) between April and December 2021. The study had three main stages: data collection, LogNNet training with selection of main features, and testing of feature combinations (Figure 1).

The RBV of the patients consisted of biochemical, hematological, and immunological tests. Patients admitted to the ICU were defined as severely infected, while patients who could not be admitted to the ICU (non-ICU, subjects in all wards) were defined as mildly infected. The dataset SARS-CoV-2-RBV1 included information on n = 2648 COVID-19 positive outpatients and n = 2648 COVID-19 negative (control group), for a total of 5296 patients. The dataset SARS-CoV-2-RBV2 contained information of n = 203 ICU and n = 3696 non-ICU COVID-19 patients. Raw data records included patients' diagnoses (COVID-19, heart disease, asthma, etc.), treatment units (ICU or non-ICU), age, and RBV data. The entire recording process took 20 h. In the raw data, RBV data were on a quantitative scale, diagnostic data were on a multinomial scale, and treatment units were on a binomial scale. In the data preprocessing stage, the string data were converted into numerical data. Categorical data were coded, repeated measurements were averaged, duplicates were removed, and quantitative data were normalized. The missing RBV data were complemented by the mean of the respective parameter distribution.

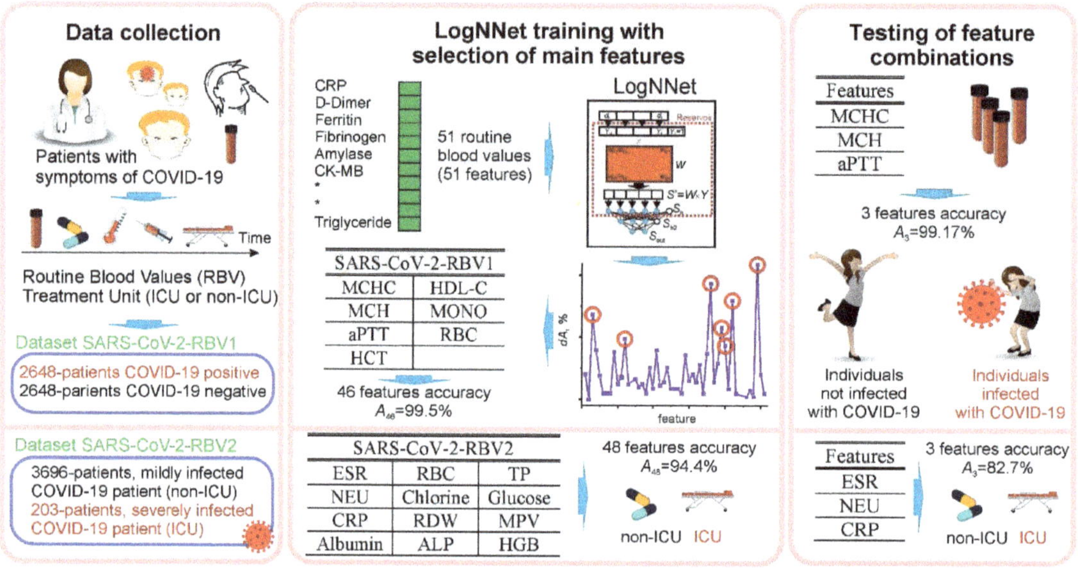

Figure 1. The main stages of the study for the diagnosis and prognosis of COVID-19 using the routine blood values: data collection, LogNNet training with the selection of main features, testing combinations of the most important features that influence the diagnosis and prognosis of the disease.

2.1. Characteristic of Participants, Workflow and Define Datasets

In the EBYU-MG hospital, only the cases that were detected as SARS-CoV-2 by real-time reverse transcriptase polymerase chain reaction (RT-PCR) in nasopharyngeal or oropharyngeal swabs during the dates covered by this study were diagnosed with COVID-19. The research only included individuals over the age of 18. In order to prevent various complications, RBV results at the first admission were recorded.

The first SARS-CoV-2-RBV dataset (SARS-CoV-2-RBV1) includes the information of 2648 patients diagnosed with COVID-19 and receiving outpatient treatment in hospital on the specified dates, and the same number of patients (control group) whose COVID-19 tests were negative. The control group was randomly selected from individuals over the age of 18 who had applied to the emergency COVID-19 service but had a negative RT-PCR test. With the feature selection procedure, the most important RBV features that are effective in the diagnosis of the disease were selected from the SARS-CoV-2-RBV1 dataset. The selected features were fed into LogNNet neural network to examine the method's performance in diagnosing COVID-19 disease.

The second SARS-CoV-2-RBV dataset (SARS-CoV-2-RBV2) includes the information of 3899 patients who were treated for COVID-19 in hospital on the specified dates. The treatment units of these patients at the first admission were examined. The SARS-CoV-2-RBV2 dataset contains n = 203 ICU and n = 3696 non-ICU COVID-19 patients. Then, with the feature selection procedure, the most influential RBV traits in the prognosis of the disease were selected from the SARS-CoV-2-RBV2 dataset. Selected features were fed into the LogNNet neural network to examine the performance of this method in determining the prognosis and severity of COVID-19 disease.

The SARS-CoV-2-RBV1 and SARS-CoV-2-RBV2 datasets are presented in Tables 1 and 2. SARS-CoV-2-RBV1 and SARS-CoV-2-RBV2 datasets include immunological, hematological, and biochemical RBV parameters and each dataset consists of 51 features. In the SARS-

CoV-2-RBV1 dataset, positive COVID-19 test results were coded as 1 and negative as 0 (COVID-19 = 1, non-COVID-19 = 0).

Table 1. Feature numbering for SARS-CoV-2-RBV1 datasets.

№	Feature	№	Feature	№	Feature	№	Feature	№	Feature
1	CRP	12	NEU	23	MPV	34	GGT	45	Sodium
2	D-Dimer	13	PLT	24	PDW	35	Glucose	46	T-Bil
3	Ferritin	14	WBC	25	RBC	36	HDL-C	47	TP
4	Fibrinogen	15	BASO	26	RDW	37	Calcium	48	Triglyceride
5	INR	16	EOS	27	ALT	38	Chlorine	49	eGFR
6	PT	17	HCT	28	AST	39	Cholesterol	50	Urea
7	PCT	18	HGB	29	Albumin	40	Creatinine	51	UA
8	ESR	19	MCH	30	ALP	41	CK		
9	Troponin	20	MCHC	31	Amylase	42	LDH		
10	aPTT	21	MCV	32	CK-MB	43	LDL		
11	LYM	22	MONO	33	D-Bil	44	Potassium		

CRP: C-reactive protein; INR: international normalized ratio; PT: prothrombin time; PCT: Procalcitonin; ESR: erythrocyte sedimentation rate; aPTT: activated partial prothrombin time; LYM: lymphocyte count; NEU: neutrophil count; PLT: platelet count; WBC: white blood cell count; BASO: basophil count; EOS: eosinophil count; HCT: hematocrit; HGB: hemoglobin; MCH: mean corpuscular hemoglobin; MCHC: mean corpuscular hemoglobin concentration; MCV: mean corpuscular volume; MONO: monocyte count; MPV: mean platelet volume; PDW: platelet distribution width; RBC: red blood cells; RDW: red cell distribution width; ALT: alanine aminotransaminase; AST: aspartate aminotransferase; ALP: alkaline phosphatase; CK-MB: creatine kinase myocardial band; D-Bil: direct bilirubin; GGT: gamma-glutamyl transferase; HDL-C: high-density lipoprotein-cholesterol; CK: creatine kinase; LDH: lactate dehydrogenase; LDL: low-density lipoprotein; T-Bil: total bilirubin; TP: total protein; eGFR: estimating glomerular filtration rate; UA: uric acid.

Table 2. Feature numbering for SARS-CoV-2-RBV2 datasets.

№	Feature	№	Feature	№	Feature	№	Feature	№	Feature
1	ALT	12	Chlorine	23	eGFR	34	MONO	45	Fibrinogen
2	AST	13	Cholesterol	24	Urea	35	MPV	46	INR
3	Albumin	14	Creatinine	25	UA	36	NEU	47	PT
4	ALP	15	CK	26	BASO	37	PDW	48	PCT
5	Amylase	16	LDH	27	EOS	38	PLT	49	ESR
6	CK-MB	17	LDL	28	HCT	39	RBC	50	Troponin
7	D-Bil	18	Potassium	29	HGB	40	RDW	51	aPTT
8	GGT	19	Sodium	30	LYM	41	WBC		
9	Glucose	20	T-Bil	31	MCH	42	CRP		
10	HDL-C	21	TP	32	MCHC	43	D-Dimer		
11	Calcium	22	Triglyceride	33	MCV	44	Ferritin		

ALT: alanine aminotransaminase; AST: aspartate aminotransferase; ALP: alkaline phosphatase; CK-MB: creatine kinase myocardial band; D-Bil: direct bilirubin; GGT: gamma-glutamyl transferase; HDL-C: high-density lipoprotein-cholesterol; CK: creatine kinase; LDH: lactate dehydrogenase; LDL: low-density lipoprotein; T-Bil: total bilirubin; TP: total protein; eGFR: estimating glomerular filtration rate; UA: uric acid; BASO: basophil count; EOS: eosinophil count; HCT: hematocrit; HGB: hemoglobin; LYM: lymphocyte count; MCH: mean corpuscular hemoglobin; MCHC: mean corpuscular hemoglobin concentration; MCV: mean corpuscular volume; MONO: monocyte count; MPV: mean platelet volume; NEU: neutrophil count; PDW: platelet distribution width; PLT: platelet count; RBC: red blood cells; RDW: red cell distribution width; WBC: white blood cell count; CRP: C-reactive protein; INR: international normalized ratio; PT: prothrombin time; PCT: procalcitonin; ESR: erythrocyte sedimentation rate; aPTT: activated partial prothrombin time.

In the SARS-CoV-2-RBV2 dataset, severely infected (ICU) COVID-19 patients were coded as 1, while mildly infected (non-ICU) COVID-19 patients were coded as 0. Datasets are available for download in the Supplementary Materials.

2.2. LogNNet Architecture

Figure 2 demonstrates the principle of operation of the neural network LogNNet [43].

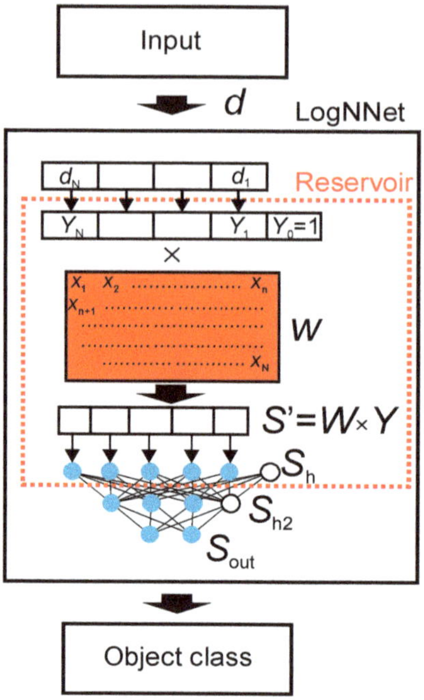

Figure 2. LogNNet architecture [43].

An object in the form of a feature vector, denoted as d, is inputted to LogNNet. The feature vector contains N coordinates (d_1, d_2, ... , d_N), where the number N is defined by the user. The classifier output determines the object class to which the input feature vector d belongs. The number of possible classes is denoted as M. LogNNet contains a reservoir with a special matrix, denoted as W. The matrix W was filled in a row-by-row pattern with numbers generated by the chaotic mapping x_n. We use chaotic mapping based on the congruential generator Equation (1) (see Table 3) and the algorithm of matrix W filling shown in Algorithm 1. Vector d is converted into a vector Y of dimension $N + 1$ with an additional coordinate $Y_0 = 1$, and each component is normalized by dividing by the maximum value of this component in the training base. The next step is a multiplication of a special matrix W with the dimension $(N + 1) \times P$ and a vector Y. The result is a vector S' with P coordinates, which is normalized [42] and converted into a vector S_h of dimension $P + 1$ with zero coordinate $S_h[0] = 1$, which plays the role of a bias element. In this way, the primary transformation of the feature vector d into the second $(P + 1)$-dimensional space is completed. Then, the vector S_h is fed to a two-layer linear classifier, with the number of neurons H in the hidden layer S_{h2}, and the number of outputs M in the output layer S_{out}. To indicate the parameters of the neural network, the following designation LogNNet N:P:H:M is used.

Table 3. Chaotic map equation and list of optimized parameters with limits.

Chaotic Map	List of Optimized Parameters (Limits)	Equation
Congruent generator	K (−100 to 100) D (−100 to 100) L (2 to 10,000) C (−100 to 100)	$\begin{cases} x_{n+1} = (D - K \cdot x_n) \bmod L \\ x_1 = C \end{cases}$ (1)

Algorithm 1. Algorithm of matrix *W* filling.

```
xn: = C;
for j: = 1 to P do
for i: = 0 to N do
begin
xn: = (D−K * xn) mod L; // Congruential generator formula
W [i,j]: = xn/L;
end;
```

The training of the linear classifier LogNNet was carried out using the backpropagation method [42].

2.3. *Optimization of Reservoir Parameters*

The optimal chaotic mapping parameters were selected using a special algorithm. The ranges of the parameters are indicated in Table 3. Before optimization, it is necessary to set the following values of the constant parameters of the model: the value $P + 1$, which determines the dimension of the vectors S_h and S_{h2}, the number of layers in the linear classifier, the number of epochs *Ep* for backpropagation training, and the number of neurons in the classifier's hidden layer, in the case of a two-layer classifier. The training of the LogNNet network is performed by two nested iterations [46]. The inner iteration trains the output LogNNet classifier by backpropagation of error on the training set, and the outer iteration optimizes the model parameters.

During the optimization process, the training and validation bases coincided and were equivalent to the initial datasets (SARS-CoV-2-RBV1 or SARS-CoV-2-RBV2). The outer iteration implements the particle swarm method with fitness function equal to classification accuracy. Outer iteration ends either when the desired values of the classification accuracy are reached, or when the specified number of iterations in the particle swarm method is completed. As a result, the optimized model parameters (chaotic mapping parameters) at the output allow us to obtain the highest classification accuracy on the validation set.

2.4. *Classification Accuracy, K-Fold Cross-Validation and Balancing Techniques*

The K-fold cross-validation technique was used to test LogNNet. This method is well suited for the medical databases, which are not split into test and training sets. The elements of the set (SARS-CoV-2-RBV1 or SARS-CoV-2-RBV2) are divided into *K* parts ($K = 5$). One of the parts is taken as the test sample, and the remaining *K*-1 parts are used for the training sample. Then, the average value of the metrics is calculated for all *K* cases when one of the *K* parts of the set becomes the test sample in turn. A distinctive feature of the method is that the separate test data are not needed for the training process. Applying the K-fold cross-validation technique, we calculate the classification metrics: classification accuracy, *A*, precision, recall, and F1-metric. Wherever we talk about the classification accuracy *A* in this article, we imply the value obtained by the K-fold cross-validation method.

To obtain a higher value of *A*, the training *K*-1 parts of the sets were balanced as in [43]. The balancing implies equalizing the number of objects for each class, supplementing the classes with copies of already existing objects, and sorting the training set in sequential order. The balancing process can be illustrated by the following example. The training set consists of 10 objects divided into 2 classes. Each object is assigned a feature vector dz_{m}, where z is the object number $z = 1, \ldots, 10$, m is the class number $m = 1, \ldots, 2$. For example, we have 7 objects of class 1 ($d1_1$, $d2_1$, $d4_1$, $d5_1$, $d6_1$, $d7_1$, $d10_1$) and three objects of class 2 ($d3_2$, $d8_2$, $d9_2$). We find the maximum number of objects (*MAX*) in the classes, and *MAX* equals 7 for class 1. We supplement the remaining groups with copies of the already existing objects (duplication) to equalize the number to *MAX*. Therefore, for class 2, we acquire the group ($d3_2$, $d8_2$, $d9_2$, $d3_2$, $d8_2$, $d9_2$, $d3_2$). Then, we compose a balanced training data set, choosing one object from each group in turn. As a result, we achieve the following training set: ($d1_1$,

$d3_2, d2_1, d8_2, d4_1, d9_2, d5_1, d3_2, d6_1, d8_2, d7_1, d9_2, d10_1, d3_2$), which consists of 14 vectors and has the same number of objects in every class.

2.5. Threshold Approach

The simplest approach for classifying by one feature in the presence of only two classes is based on determining the threshold value separating the classes *Vth*. For the SARS-CoV-2-RBV1 dataset, we introduce an additional designation of the type of threshold value Type 1 or Type 2 in accordance with the rule:

$$\begin{cases} \text{Type 1: if feature value } > Vth \text{ then ``COVID-19'' else ``non-COVID-19''} \\ \text{Type 2: if feature value } > Vth \text{ then ``non-COVID-19'' else ``COVID-19''} \end{cases} \quad (2)$$

The threshold type indicates which side of the threshold the sick and healthy classes are on.

For the SARS-CoV-2-RBV2 dataset (after balancing, see Section 2.4), we introduce a similar relation for the type of threshold value:

$$\begin{cases} \text{Type 1: if feature value } > Vth \text{ then ``ICU'' else ``non-ICU''} \\ \text{Type 2: if feature value } > Vth \text{ then ``non-ICU'' else ``ICU''} \end{cases} \quad (3)$$

Threshold accuracy after balancing datasets (see Section 2.4) is determined as

$$Ath = \frac{TP + TN}{TP + TN + FP + FN} \quad (4)$$

were *TP* denotes true positive, *TN* true negative, *FP* false positive, and *FN* false negative.

K-fold validation is not used when calculating *Ath*.

The threshold value *Vth* was determined by stepwise enumeration and finding the maximum value of *Ath*.

The threshold method reflects the dependence of one feature and COVID-19 and indicates the classification success (Equations (2)–(4)). In practical applications, the LogNNet is a more powerful classification tool than the simple threshold method, revealing more information between features and COVID-19.

2.6. Feature Selection Method

The feature selection method is based on a wrapper-type backward feature elimination algorithm and has two consecutive steps. First, redundant features and features that make training of the neural network difficult are removed. In backward elimination, the algorithm starts with all the features and removes the least significant feature at each iteration. The features are removed by zeroing the corresponding components of the input vectors *d*. The second stage includes sorting the remaining features according to their contribution to the classification metric.

Features selection for the dataset SARS-CoV-2-RBV2 illustrates this method. Let us suppose a reservoir optimization was carried out and an accuracy of A_{51} = 93.665% was obtained (using K-fold cross-validation), where the designation A_{NF} means the classification accuracy when using *NF* = 51 features. Let us introduce additional pointers, denote the set of removed features by *FR*, and denote the set of selected features by *FS*. For example, A_{49}(*FR* [3,33]) denotes accuracy at *NF* = 49 features with features *z* = 3 and *z* = 33 removed, and A_4(*FS* [1,22,33,41,55] denotes accuracy at *NF* = 4 features with the main features from the set *FS*, *z* = 1, 22, 33, 41, 55. Next, we plot the dependence of the value of dA_{51} on the number of the removed feature *z* (see Figure 3a), where

$$dA_{51}(z) = A_{51} - A_{50}(FR[z]) \quad (5)$$

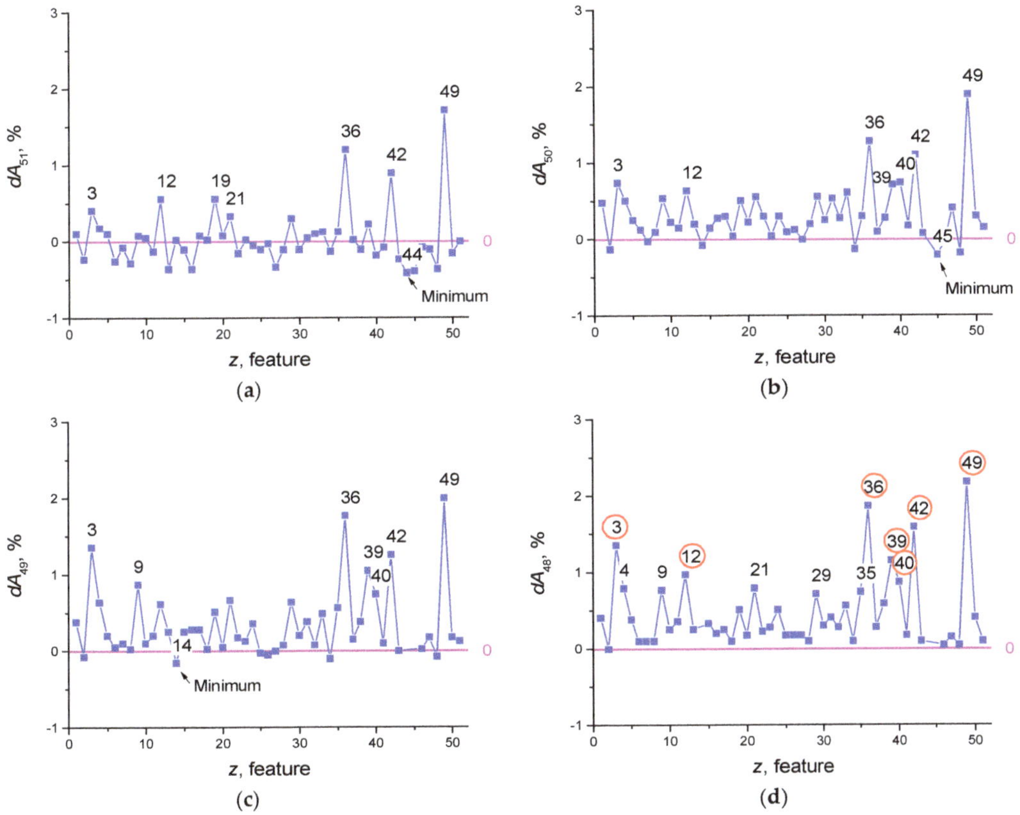

Figure 3. Function of the feature strength $dA_{51}(z)$ (**a**), $dA_{50}(z)$ (**b**), $dA_{49}(z)$ (**c**), $dA_{48}(z)$ (**d**).

Dependence $dA(z)$ is a function of the feature strength. The value $A_{50}(FR[z])$ characterizes the classification accuracy of the neural network using $NF = 50$ features, after deleting the feature with number z. Positive feature strength dA_{51} (Figure 3a and Equation (5)) means that the removal of the feature reduces the classification accuracy of the network and the feature is useful. Negative dA_{51} means that the feature interferes with learning (redundant) and its removal leads to an increase in the classification properties of the neural network. After the first selection iteration, the seven most useful features can be identified having numbers z = 49, 36, 42, 19, 12, 3, 21 (Figure 3a). The feature that makes learning the most difficult is number z = 44 (in Figure 3 it is indicated by the index 'Minimum'). Its removal makes $A_{50}(FR\ [44])$ = 94.075%, which exceeds the previous value A_{51} = 93.665%.

The next iteration involves calculating the dependence of $dA_{50}(z)$ (Figure 3b), where

$$dA_{50}(z) = A_{50}(FR[44]) - A_{49}(FR[44,z]) \tag{6}$$

Equation (6) implies the exclusion of the worst feature z = 44 and the exclusion of all other features in turn. As a result, the next feature to exclude will be the feature z = 45, and the best accuracy will be $A_{49}(FR\ [44,45])$ = 94.28%.

Iterations continue until all dA values are greater than or equal to zero. Figure 3c,d shows graphs for Equations (7) and (8)

$$dA_{49}(z) = A_{49}(FR[44,45]) - A_{48}(FR[44,45,z]) \tag{7}$$

$$dA_{48}(z) = A_{48}(FR[44,45,14]) - A_{47}(FR[44,45,14,z]) \tag{8}$$

The graph in Figure 3d reflects the dependence $dA_{48}(z)$ that has positive values. Thus, the best classification accuracy corresponds to $A_{48}(FR\ [14,44,45]) = 94.434\%$, after removing the features z = 44, 45, 14. During the selection, the set of the seven best features with highest feature strength dA also changed from the set [3,12,19,21,36,42,49] (Figure 3a) to [3,12,36,39,40,42,49] (Figure 3d, red circle).

The second stage arranges the features according to their strength in descending order of peak values dA. For the considered example, the sequence contains the following first 12 values [3,4,9,12,21,29,35,36,39,40,42,49] (Figure 3d).

3. Results

3.1. Dataset SARS-CoV-2-RBV1

LogNNet 51:50:20:2 architecture was used for SARS-CoV-2-RBV1 dataset. Reservoir optimization following the method from Section 2.3 with the number of epochs $Ep = 50$ led to the parameters of the congruential generator listed in Table 4.

Table 4. Optimal reservoir parameters.

Dataset SARS-CoV-2-RBV1				Dataset SARS-CoV-2-RBV2			
K	*D*	*L*	*C*	*K*	*D*	*L*	*C*
93	68	9276	73	47	99	8941	56

Feature selection was performed with the number of epochs $Ep = 100$. Prior to selection, the $dA_{51}(z)$ shape is plotted in Figure 4a. After feature selection, the redundant features have the numbers z = 21, 37, 42, 49, 40, and the $dA_{46}(z)$ plot is shown in Figure 4b. The influence of features with numbers z = 20, 19, 10, 17 has increased.

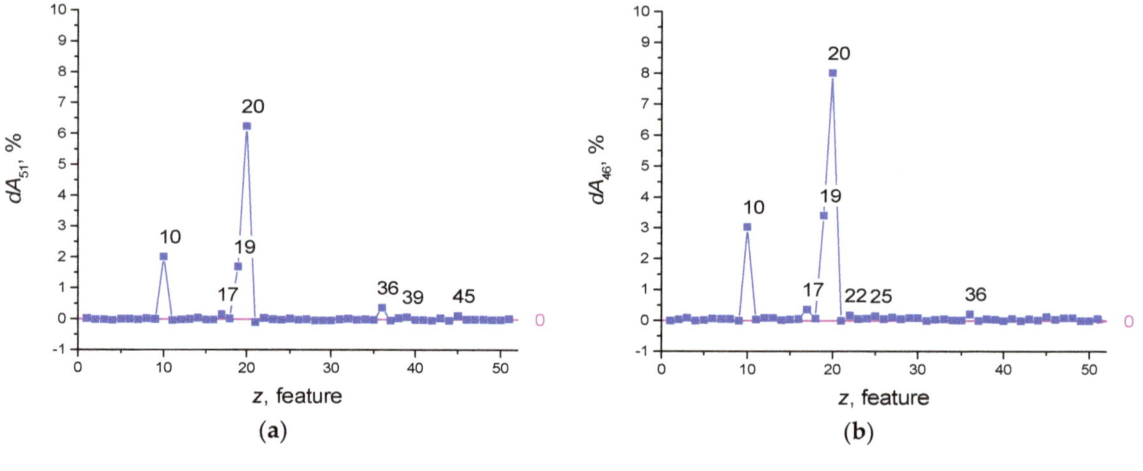

Figure 4. Function of the feature strength $dA_{51}(z)$ (**a**), $dA_{46}(z)$ (**b**).

The dependence of $A_{46}(FR\ [21,37,40,42,49])$ on the number of epochs is shown in Figure 5, and the values of other metrics are shown in Table 5.

$Ep = 100$ will be taken as the optimal value of the number of epochs. The RBV values found most important in the diagnosis of COVID-19 are the features listed in Table 6. The most important of these are MCHC, MCH, and aPTT. MCHC in a blood test allows to find out the average amount of hemoglobin in an erythrocyte.

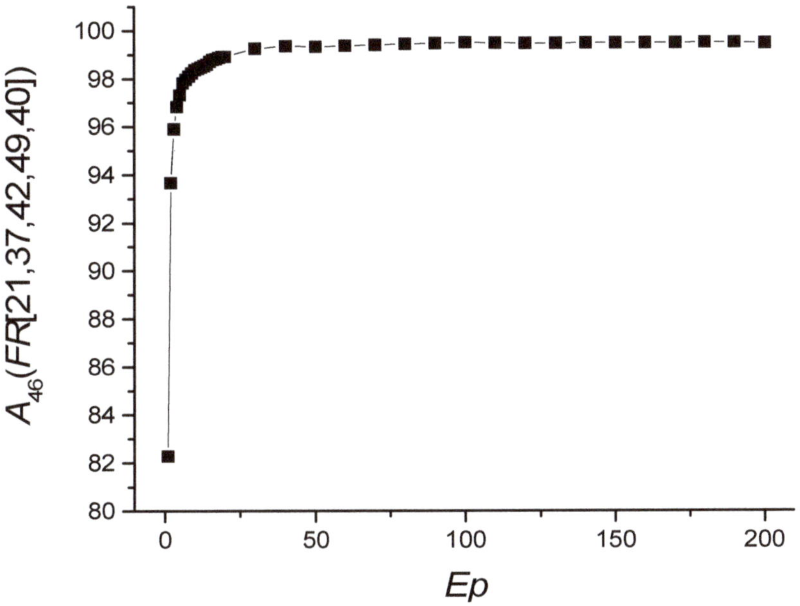

Figure 5. Dependence of A_{46}(*FR* [21,37,40,42,49]) on the number of epochs *Ep*.

Table 5. Classification metrics depending on the number of training epochs *Ep*.

Ep	A_{46}(FR [21,37,40,42,49])	Precision "Non-COVID-19"	Precision "COVID-19"	Recall "Non-COVID-19"	Recall "COVID-19"	F1 "Non-COVID-19"	F1 "COVID-19"
10	98.376	0.978	0.99	0.991	0.977	0.984	0.984
30	99.339	0.992	0.995	0.995	0.992	0.993	0.993
100	99.509	0.994	0.996	0.996	0.994	0.995	0.995
150	99.49	0.994	0.996	0.996	0.994	0.995	0.995
200	99.471	0.994	0.995	0.995	0.994	0.995	0.995

Table 6. The seven features found to be most important in the diagnosis of COVID-19.

Number	dA_{46}	Features
20	8.007	MCHC
19	3.399	MCH
10	3.022	aPTT
17	0.359	HCT
36	0.208	HDL-C
22	0.17	MONO
25	0.151	RBC

MCH: corpuscular hemoglobin; MCHC: corpuscular hemoglobin concentration; aPTT: activated partial prothrombin time; HCT: hematocrit; HDL-C: high-density lipoprotein-cholesterol; MONO: monocyte count; RBC: red blood cells.

The efficiency of LogNNet in determining the diagnosis of COVID-19 using only seven features and their combinations is shown in Table 7.

Using only one feature 20 (MCHC) or 36 (HDL-C) in determining the diagnosis of COVID-19 provides a high classification accuracy of A_1(*FS* [20]), A_1(*FS* [36]) ~94%. The combination of 2 features 20 (MCHC) and 19 (MCH) allows to reach accuracy A_2(*FS* [19,20]) ~99.15%.

The accuracy of the model in diagnosing the disease with seven features was almost equal to the accuracy rate in using all 46 features (A_7~99.4 vs. A_{46}~99.59) (Table 7).

Table 7. LogNNet efficiency for various combinations of features.

Combinations of Features	A	Precision "Non-COVID-19"	Precision "COVID-19"	Recall "Non-COVID-19"	Recall "COVID-19"	F1 "Non-COVID-19"	F1 "COVID-19"
$A_{46}(FR\ [21,37,40,42,49])$	99.509	0.994	0.996	0.996	0.994	0.995	0.995
$A_7(FS\ [10,17,19,20,22,25,36])$	99.358	0.991	0.996	0.996	0.991	0.994	0.994
$A_1(FS\ [>20])$	94.279	0.930	0.958	0.959	0.926	0.944	0.942
$A_1(FS\ [>19])$	52.418	0.526	0.524	0.500	0.548	0.509	0.532
$A_1(FS\ [10])$	52.398	0.516	0.947	0.972	0.075	0.672	0.100
$A_1(FS\ [36])$	94.429	0.935	0.955	0.956	0.932	0.945	0.943
$A_2(FS\ [19,20])$	99.150	0.989	0.994	0.994	0.989	0.992	0.991
$A_2(FS\ [20,36])$	97.583	0.973	0.979	0.979	0.972	0.976	0.976
$A_2(FS\ [19,36])$	94.373	0.934	0.955	0.957	0.931	0.945	0.943
$A_3(FS\ [10,19,20])$	99.169	0.989	0.995	0.995	0.989	0.992	0.992
$A_5(FS\ [10,17,19,22,25])$	51.699	0.526	0.546	0.784	0.250	0.604	0.277

Threshold Accuracy on One Feature

Table A1 in Appendix A contains threshold accuracy Ath, threshold values Vth, type, and change limits for all features. Values of threshold accuracy Ath are sorted in descending order. Case distribution histograms for features with the highest threshold accuracy (LDL, HDL-C, Cholesterol, MCHC, Triglyceride, Amylase) are shown in Figure 6. An LDL level lower than 116.1 mg/dL, HDL-C level lower than 43.1 mg/dL, Cholesterol level lower than 206.3 mg/dL, Triglyceride level lower than 163.3 mg/dL, MCHC level higher than 31.3 g/dL, and Amylase level higher than 76.3 u/L mg/dL are critical levels for the detection of sick individuals. Considering any of these critical levels, the patients and healthy individuals could be detected with accuracy between Ath = 85% and Ath = 94%.

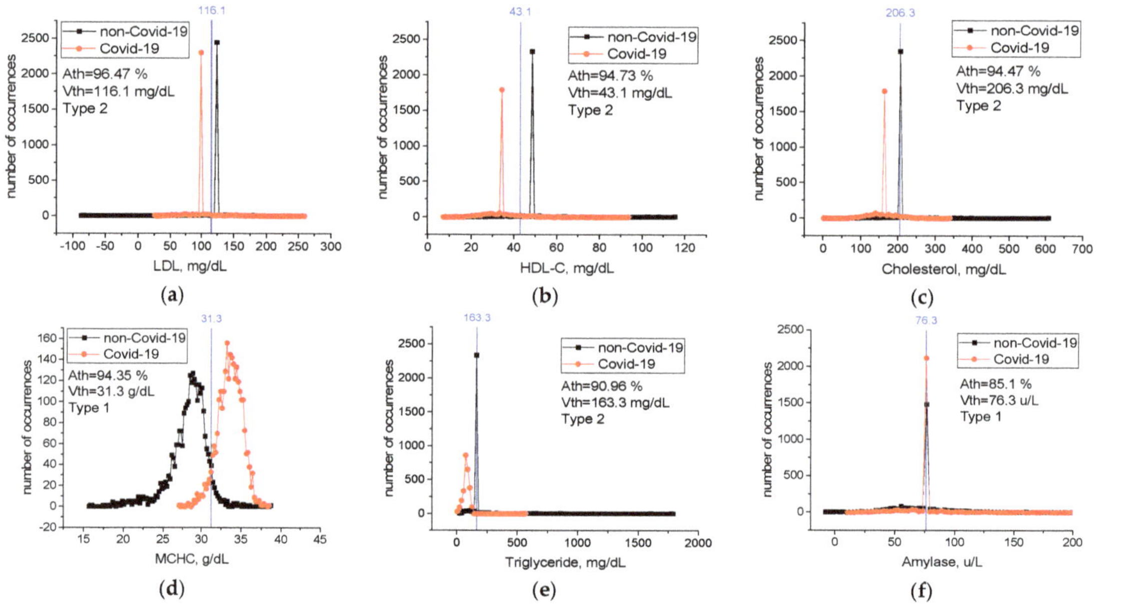

Figure 6. Case distribution histograms for LDL (**a**), HDL-C (**b**), Cholesterol (**c**), MCHC (**d**), Triglyceride (**e**), Amylase (**f**) from sick and healthy individuals and the threshold values Vth of these features (blue line) in the diagnosis of the disease. Histogram bin sizes are listed in Table A1.

For features from Table 6 not included in Figure 6, case distribution histograms (MCH, aPTT, HCT, MONO, RBC) are demonstrated in Figure 7. The success of these features alone in detecting sick and healthy individuals was less than 60% (Figure 7). However, the combination of MCHC with MCH and the combination of MCHC with HDL-C in detecting sick and healthy individuals is higher than their individual performance (Table 7). Revealed high-level mutual information among these variables helps LogNNet to diagnose COVID-19. The combinations of MCH, aPTT, HCT, MONO, and RBC features are not effective in the diagnosis of the disease (A_5(*FS* [10,17,19,22,25]), Table 7). We think that there is a low correlation between these features and COVID-19.

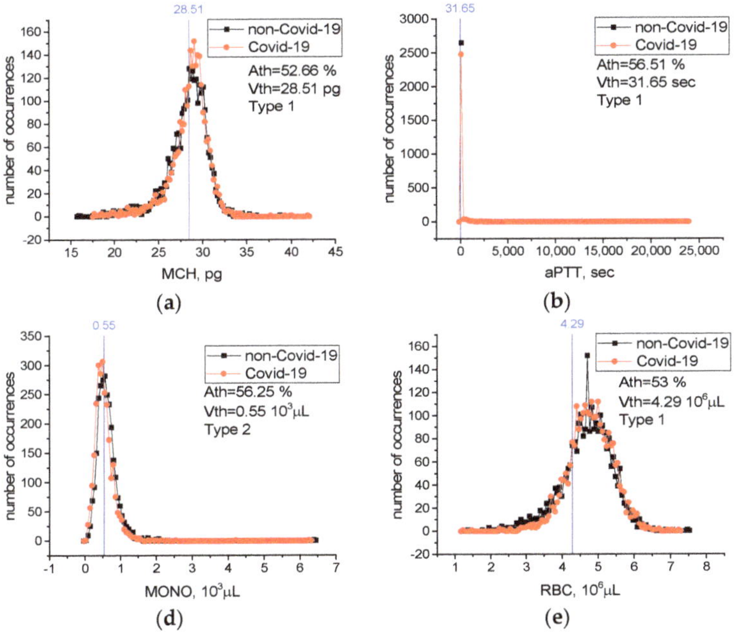

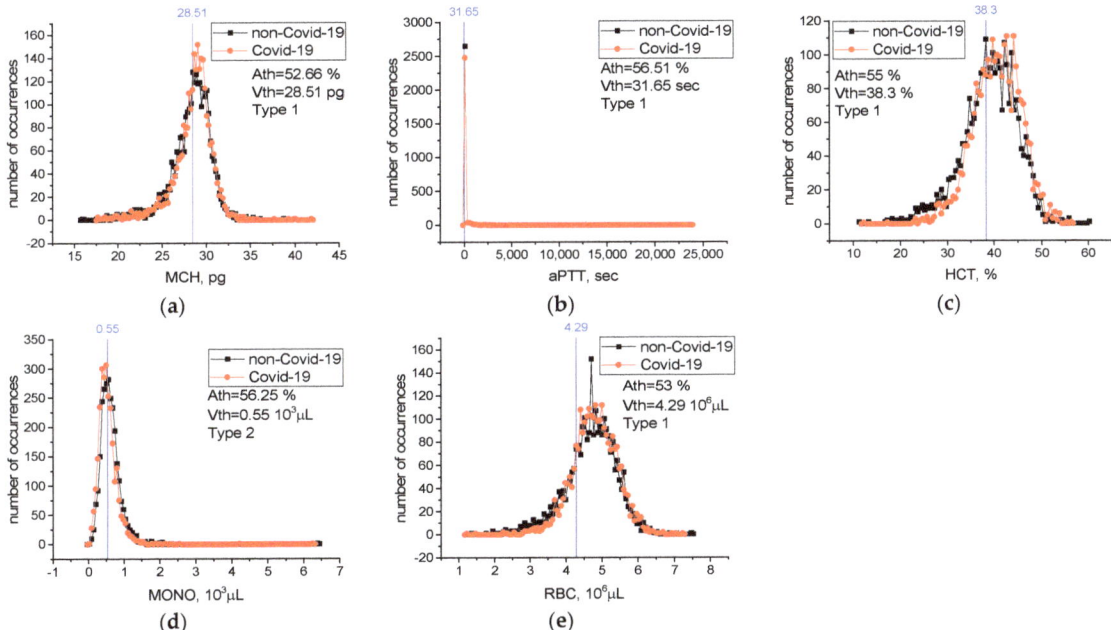

Figure 7. Case distribution histograms for MCH (**a**), aPTT (**b**), HCT (**c**), MONO (**d**), RBC (**e**) from sick and healthy individuals and the threshold values *Vth* of these features in the diagnosis of the disease. Histogram bin sizes are listed in Table A1.

3.2. Dataset SARS-CoV-2-RBV2

LogNNet 51:50:20:2 architecture was used for the SARS-CoV-2-RBV2 dataset. The result of reservoir optimization obtained following the method from Section 2.3 with the number of epochs $Ep = 50$ led to the parameters of the congruential generator indicated in Table 4. Feature selection was carried out with the number of epochs $Ep = 150$. Prior to selection, feature strength corresponded to $dA_{51}(z)$ (Figure 3a). After feature selection, the redundant features are with numbers z = 44, 45 and 14, and the $dA_{48}(z)$ graph is shown in Figure 3d.

The dependence of A_{48}(*FR* [14,44,45]) on the number of epochs is shown in Figure 8, and the values of other metrics are shown in Table 8.

$Ep = 150$ is be taken as the optimal value of the number of epochs. The metrics for the "ICU" case are significantly worse than for the "non-ICU" case because of limited data for the "ICU" case. The most important RBVs in identifying severely and mildly infected COVID-19 patients are the features listed in Table 9. The most important of these are ESR and NEU.

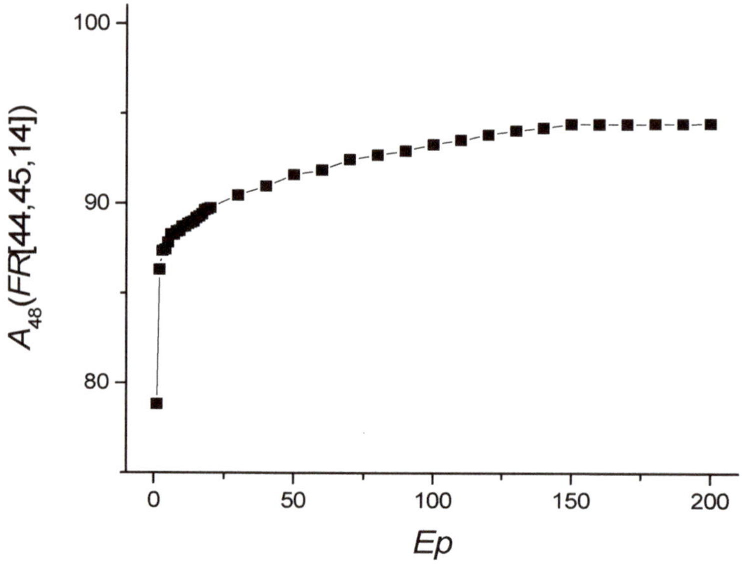

Figure 8. Dependence of A_{48}(*FR* [14,44,45]) on the number of epochs *Ep*.

Table 8. Classification metrics depending on the number of training epochs *Ep*.

Ep	A_{48}(FR [14,44,45])	Precision "Non-ICU"	Precision "ICU"	Recall "Non-ICU"	Recall "ICU"	F1 "Non-ICU"	F2 "ICU"
10	88.715	0.993	0.307	0.887	0.881	0.937	0.451
30	90.459	0.993	0.347	0.906	0.876	0.947	0.492
100	93.306	0.990	0.433	0.939	0.821	0.964	0.562
150	94.434	0.989	0.49	0.952	0.797	0.97	0.599
200	94.486	0.987	0.495	0.955	0.767	0.97	0.592

Table 9. The 12 features found to be most important in detecting severely (ICU) and mildly (non-ICU) infected COVID-19 patients.

Number	dA_{48}	Features
49	2.18	ESR
36	1.872	NEU
42	1.59	CRP
3	1.359	Albumin
39	1.154	RBC
12	0.974	Chlorine
40	0.872	RDW
4	0.795	ALP
21	0.795	TP
9	0.769	Glucose
35	0.744	MPV
29	0.718	HGB

ESR: erythrocyte sedimentation rate; NEU: neutrophil count; CRP: C-reactive protein; RBC: red blood cells; RDW: red cell distribution width; ALP: alkaline phosphatase; TP: total protein; MPV: mean platelet volume; HGB: hemoglobin.

The efficiency of LogNNet when using only the 12 features and their combinations to identify severely and mildly infected COVID-19 patients are shown in Table 10.

Table 10. LogNNet efficiency for various combinations of features.

Combinations of Features	A	Precision "Non-ICU"	Precision "ICU"	Recall "Non-ICU"	Recall "ICU"	F1 "Non-ICU"	F1 "ICU"
A_{48}(*FR* [14,44,45])	94.434	0.989	0.49	0.952	0.797	0.97	0.599
A_{12}(*FS* [3,4,9,12,21,29,35,36,39,40,42,49])	90.946	0.990	0.364	0.914	0.831	0.950	0.499
A_1(*FS* [49])	59.598	0.950	0.059	0.605	0.418	0.694	0.097
A_1(*FS* [49])	75.040	0.955	0.085	0.773	0.341	0.851	0.133
A_3(*FS* [36,42,49])	82.712	0.989	0.210	0.827	0.826	0.900	0.334
A_7(*FS* [3,12,36,39,40,42,49])	89.355	0.991	0.341	0.896	0.846	0.940	0.469

The recall value indicates what percentage of individuals diagnosed as mild or severe patients by the specialist could be recognized as mild or severe patients by our model. In other words, the recall value indicates the success of our model in distinguishing mild or severe patients. The precision value indicates the percentage of the individuals diagnosed as mild or severe patients by our model who were also defined as mild or severe patients by the specialist. In other words, the precision value shows the success of our model in diagnosing mild or severe patients.

The accuracy of the model run with 12 features to identify mildly and severely infected patients was close to the accuracy rate of the model run with 48 features (A_{12}~90.9 vs. A_{48}~94.94) (Table 10). The accuracy with the seven features model run was 89.3%, where the model success in diagnosing the mildly infected (precision value) was 99.1%, and success in recognizing mildly infected patients (recall value) was 89.6%. The metrics for the "ICU" case are significantly worse than for the "non-ICU" case. Here, our model decided in favor of the diagnosis of mildly infected (high precision for non-ICU, low precision for ICU) due to the sample number unbalance of our mildly infected and severely infected patients.

Threshold Accuracy on One Feature

Table A2 in Appendix A contains values of threshold accuracy *Ath*, threshold values *Vth*, as well as types and limits of change for all features. Rows in the table are sorted in descending order of threshold accuracy *Ath*. Case distribution histograms for features with the highest threshold accuracy (NEU, Albumin, WBC, CRP, Urea, Calcium) are shown in Figure 9.

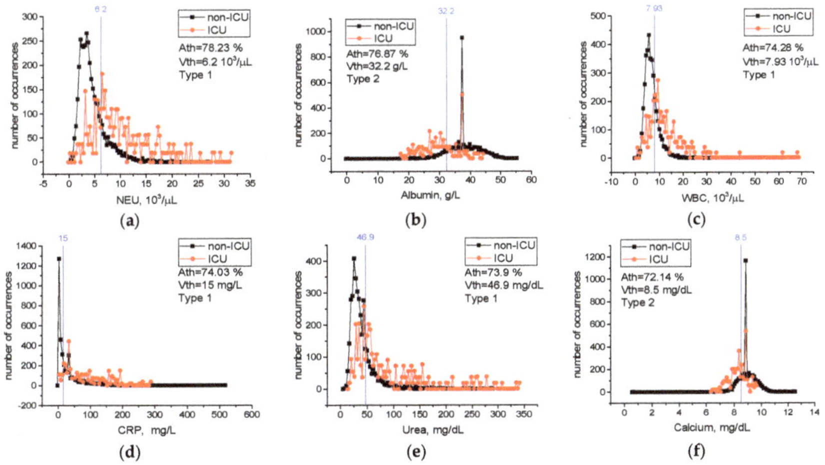

Figure 9. Case distribution histograms for NEU (**a**), Albumin (**b**), WBC (**c**), CRP (**d**), Urea (**e**), Calcium (**f**) from mildly and severely infected COVID-19 patients and the threshold values *Vth* of these features (blue line) in the prognosis of the disease. Histogram bin sizes are listed in Table A2.

Cases with an NEU level higher than $6.2 \times 10^3/\mu L$, WBC level higher than $7.93 \times 10^3/\mu L$, CRP level higher than 15 mg/dL, Urea level higher than 46.9 mg/dL, Albumin level lower than 32.2 g/L, and Calcium level lower than 8.5 mg/dL most likely require intensive care treatment (Figure 9). Considering any of these critical levels, patients requiring intensive care and patients not requiring intensive care could be correctly identified with the accuracy between Ath = 72% and Ath = 78%.

For features from Table 9 not included in Figure 9, case distribution histograms (ESR, RBC, Chlorine, RDW, ALP, TP, Glucose, MPV, HGB) are demonstrated in Figure 10. The success of these features alone in detecting mildly and severely infected patients varies between Ath = 54.3% and Ath = 71.5% (Figure 10). However, the performance of the combination of the ESR, NEU, and CRP features in detecting mild and severely infected patients was higher than their individual performance (Table 10). In addition, combinations of these properties with the Albumin, RBC, Chlorine, and RDW properties improved performance in detecting severely and mildly infected patients [A_3(FS [36,42,49] = 82.7% vs. A_7(FS [3,12,36,39,40,42,49] = 89.3% (Table 10). We think that there is a low level of correlation between the characteristics of ALP, TP, Glucose, MPV, and HGB and the severity of COVID-19 (A_7(FS [3,12,36,39,40,42,49])) = 89.4% vs. A_{12}(FS [3,4,9,12,21,29,35,36,39,40,42,49]) = 90.9% (Table 10). Therefore, the combination of the ESR, NEU, CRP, Albumin, RBC, Chlorine, and RDW blood values is an important source of variation in determining the severity of the disease, and high-level confidential information may be found among these variables. The combination of these features may have important effects in the prognosis of COVID-19 disease and in identifying patients in need of intensive care.

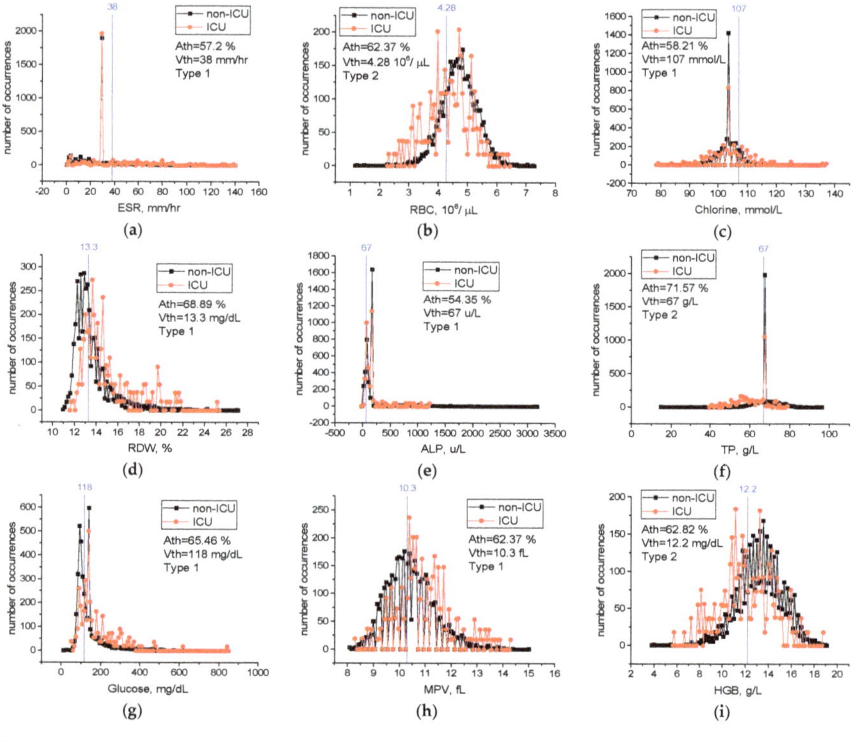

Figure 10. Case distribution histograms for ESR (**a**), RBC (**b**), Chlorine (**c**), RDW (**d**), ALP (**e**), TP (**f**), Glucose (**g**), MPV (**h**), HGB (**i**) from mildly and severely infected COVID-19 patients and the threshold values Vth of these features (blue line) in the prognosis of the disease. Histogram bin sizes are listed in Table A2.

4. Discussion

COVID-19 is a systemic multi-organ damage disease that causes severe acute respiratory syndrome, death, and continues to spread [3,47]. Despite the use of vaccines, the spread of the disease cannot be stopped, and important mutations have been detected in the structure of the virus [1]. It is likely that COVID-19 will continue to be present in our lives. Despite the large number of studies on COVID-19, some of these studies were contradictory and pathological aspects of the disease could not be fully determined [48]. Changes in many RBVs and hematological abnormalities were observed during the course of the disease [6,48]. The fact that most patients lost their lives in case of severe infection has led to a fight against the disease all over the world [10,49]. In addition, Brinati et al. [19] and Zhang et al. [49] pointed out that various complications may occur during the treatment process of COVID-19, and this makes it important to predict the prognosis of the disease in the early period. Similarly, Mertoğlu et al. [1] and Huyut and İlkbahar [3] stated that the early prediction of the diagnosis and prognosis of the disease are important in the first response to severely infected COVID-19 patients.

As with immunodiagnostic testing, RT-PCR testing may present difficulties in identifying true positive and negative individuals infected with COVID-19 [4,50]. Indeed, Teymouri et al. [50] and D'Cruz et al. [51] suggested that to increase the sensitivity of the RT-PCR test, the test should be repeated on multiple samples and the application methodology should be improved. However, these procedures represent a troublesome process for health personnel and patients. These difficulties in diagnosing COVID-19 have further increased the importance of RBVs methods [1,2]. In this context, it is possible to determine both the diagnosis and the prognosis of the disease with RBVs (biomarkers), which are easier to obtain, more economical, and faster to measure [1–6].

In an ML study for the diagnosis of COVID-19 based on RBVs, Brinati et al. [19] explained that AI models are based on clinical features and can be used for processes, such as disease diagnosis and prognosis. AI models that use the RBVs can be both an adjunct and an alternative method to rRT-PCR [20]. In addition, AI application results can provide information about the infection risk level and can be used in the rapid triage and quarantine of high-risk patients [20].

In this study, the most effective RBV biomarkers in the diagnosis and prognosis of COVID-19 were determined by a two-step feature selection procedure for use in peripheral IoT devices with low computing resources. Our LogNNet neural network model, fed with selected features, identified sick and healthy individuals, and especially mildly infected patients, with high accuracy.

In the first dataset used in this study, the RBVs of COVID-19 positive (n = 2648) patients and COVID-19 negative (n = 2648) individuals were recorded. In the second dataset, the RBVs of 3899 patients (n = 203 ICU and n = 3696 non-ICU) hospitalized with the diagnosis of COVID-19 were recorded. Hence, 51 features of all patients were identified (Tables 1 and 2). A two-stage feature selection procedure (see Section 2.5) was applied on the datasets and features were found for each dataset. The features selected for the first dataset were fed into the LogNNet neural network, and the accuracy of the method in the diagnosis of COVID-19 was calculated. Then, the selected features for the second dataset were fed into LogNNet neural network, and the performance of the method in identifying mildly and severely infected patients (determining the prognosis of the disease) was assessed.

Previous studies on the diagnosis and prognosis of COVID-19 have indicated the changes in most of the RBV parameters and biomarkers [1–3,5]. Mertoglu et al. [1] and Yang et al. [52] reported that the most effective RBV biomarkers in the diagnosis and prognosis of COVID-19 are CRP and LYM. However, other studies conducted for this purpose have reported blood values of CRP, procalcitonin, ferritin, ALT, aPTT, and ESR [3,4,6]. Banerjee et al. [8] used random forest, glmnet, generalized linear models, and ANN neural network models to determine the diagnosis of COVID-19 with 14 RBV values of 81 COVID-19 positive and 517 healthy individuals. Glmnet was found to be the most successful model in the diagnosis of the disease with 92% sensitivity and 91% accuracy [8]. Brinati et al. [19]

used various ML methods with 13 RBV values for diagnosis of the disease (102 COVID-19 negative, 177 positive) and noted that the models with the highest accuracy were random forest (82%) and logistic regression (78%). Similarly, Cabitza et al. [20] used various ML models to rapidly detect COVID-19 using many RBV parameters and found the models with the highest accuracy were random forest (88%), support vector machine (SVM) (88%), and k-nearest neighbor (86%). Joshi et al. [22] developed a trained logistic regression model using some RBVs on a dataset of 380 cases, reporting good sensitivity (93%) but low specificity (43%). Yang et al. [21] applied various ML models on 27 RBV parameters of a large patient population of 3356 individuals (42% COVID-19 positive), and found the gradient boost tree model to be the most successful model in the diagnosis of the disease with 76%-sensitivity and 80%-specificity value. In a COVID-19 study using chest computed tomography (CT) data and RBV parameters, Mei et al. [23] showed a model combining CNN and multilayer sensor and found the success of the model in diagnosing the disease with 84% sensitivity and 83% specificity. Soares [24] proposed a model combining SVM, ensembling, and SMOTE Boost models to diagnose COVID-19 using 15 RBV parameters in a population of 599 individuals, and found the success of the model in diagnosing the disease with 86% specificity and 70% sensitivity. Running various ML models to diagnose COVID-19 with the RBV parameters, Soltan et al. [25] found the XGBoost method to be the most successful model with 85% sensitivity and 90% precision. Huyut [53] used 28 routine blood values with age on a variety of supervised ML models to detect a large population of severely and mildly infected COVID-19 patients. The models with the highest AUC in identifying mildly infected patients were local weighted-learning (0.95%), Kstar (0.91%), Naïve bayes (0.85%), and K nearest neighbor (0.75%).

This study identified the seven most important biomarkers in the diagnosis of COVID-19 (Table 6). Among these features, the most important biomarkers were MCHC, MCH, and aPTT. The overall accuracy rate of the LogNNet model, which was run with seven features, was A_7(*FS* [10,17,19,20,22,25,36]) ~99.3%, and the precision rate of patient identification was 99.6%. In addition, the different combinations of features that are important in the diagnosis of patients were examined. The overall accuracy of the LogNNet model run only with MCHC and MCH features was A_2(*FS* [19,20]) ~99.1% and the precision rate of patient identification was 99.4%. The overall accuracy rate of our model using only the MCHC feature was 94.2%, while the overall accuracy rate of the model using only the HDL-C feature was 94.4%. According to the calculated critical levels of the main features, such as LDL, HDL-C, Cholesterol, Triglyceride, MCHC, and Amylase (Figure 6), the health and sickness status of individuals could be determined accurately. The fact that the performance of the combination of MCHC and MCH and the combination of MCHC and HDL-C in the detection of sick and healthy individuals was higher than the individual performances suggested that there is a high level of confidential information between these blood feature combinations and COVID-19. This information was revealed by the LogNNet neural network method. These combinations of features can be used by LognNNet in diagnosis of COVID-19 disease with high results.

Studies indicate that the ALT, AST, LDH, direct bilirubin, and aPTT RBVs are increased in severe COVID-19 patients, while the hemoglobin values are decreased significantly compared to mildly infected patients [6,23,54]. However, in other studies, the LYM, NEU, WBC, MCH, MPV, and RDW hematological RBVs were higher in severe COVID-19 patients, when compared to mildly infected patients [1–3,6]. Mousavi et al. [16], Zhang et al. [54], and Zheng et al. [55] determined that patients with severe COVID-19 had lower EOS, MONO, RBC, hematocrit, hemoglobin, and MCHC hematological values, when compared to mild patients. Huyut et al. [6], in a study of patients who died from COVID-19, showed that the ESR, INR, PT, CRP, D-dimer, and ferritin biomarkers are the most important biomarkers to detect the mortality of the disease. Luo et al. [56] proposed a multi-criteria decision making (MCDM) algorithm combining ideal the solution similarity sequencing technique (TOPSIS) and naive Bayes (NB) as a feature selection procedure to predict the severity of COVID-19 from initial RBV values. With the MCDM model, the WBC, LYM, NEU values, and age were the most effective features in determining the severity of the disease with 82% accuracy obtained by ROC analysis [56]. Similarly, Ma et al. [57] and Lai et al. [58] noted that the high WBC and NEU values are important manifestations of bacterial infection and indicate a serious disease state that complicates the clinical situation. Numerous studies have shown that other proinflammatory marker levels, including CRP, ferritin, and IL-6, are associated with worse outcomes [59–61]. Cheng et al. [62] reported that high levels of inflammatory markers, such as ESR, CRP, and procalcitonin, may indicate hyperinflammatory reactions in COVID-19 patients. Cavalcante-Silva et al. [63] stated that the neutrophil count was increased in severe COVID-19 patients and the neutrophils are the main effector cells in the development of COVID-19. The different neutrophil mechanisms, e.g., neutrophil enzymes and cytokines, are potential targets for treating particularly severe cases of COVID-19 [63].

This study identifies the twelve most important biomarkers to determine the prognosis of COVID-19 (detecting severely and mildly infected patients) (Table 9). The most important of them are ESR, NEU, CRP, albumin, and RBC biomarkers. The overall accuracy of the LogNNet model, which was run with twelve features, was 90.9%, the success rate in diagnosing mildly infected patients (precision rate) was 99.0%, and the success rate in diagnosing severely infected patients (precision rate) was 36.6% (Table 10). However, the success of the LogNNet model, which was run with twelve features, in distinguishing mild and severe patients according to their real conditions (recall value), was 91.4% and 83.1%, respectively (Table 10).

The calculated critical levels of NEU, WBC, CRP, Urea, Albumin, and Calcium features are important levels in determining the severity of infection of the patients (Figure 9). Moreover, the performance of the combination of the ESR, NEU, CRP, Albumin, RBC, Chlorine, and RDW features in detecting infected patients being higher than their individual performance indicates a high level of confidential information about COVID-19 among these blood features. This information was revealed by the LogNNet neural network. The combinations of features can be used as important biomarkers in the prognosis of the COVID-19 disease and in identifying patients in need of intensive care.

Our model decided in favor of the diagnosis of mildly infected patients (high precision for non-ICU, low precision for ICU) because of the unbalanced sample size of mildly infected and severely infected patients. However, our model showed a high recall value in identifying mildly and severely infected patients. The model run with only three features showed an average of 82.6% agreement with the expert opinion in distinguishing mildly or severely infected patients (Table 10). However, severe patient diagnosis of our model showed low agreement with expert opinion (low precision "ICU") (Table 10), and the success of our model in diagnosing severe patients is low. As a result, the LogNNet model, which is run with the features in Table 10, can be used safely with high sensitivity (recall) to confirm the expert opinion in recognizing mild and severely infected patients. In addition, our model can be an alternative tool for diagnosing mildly infected patients using the features in Table 10. Furthermore, the success of the LogNNet model using few features in distinguishing mild and severe patients and diagnosing mildly infected patients is high.

Other studies [19,64,65] confirming the association of RBV features with COVID-19 highlight the importance of the clinical research direction that our model takes. The poor performance of our model in diagnosing severe patients (low precision for the ICU) is an expected situation. Several studies have stated that severe COVID-19 patients experienced more changes in the RBV values than mildly infected patients, and that various complications could occur during the severe disease process [1–3,6]. There are many factors affecting the intensive care need of an individual with COVID-19 and difficulties in determining this process with only RBV values [1–6]. However, there are few studies on determining the severity of infection in patients with COVID-19 based on the RBV values alone.

Cabitza et al. [20], Soltan et al. [25], and Rabanser et al. [66] stated that the reported performance values are good enough, especially in terms of screening, considering the economic benefits and rapid results of the developed artificial intelligence models. Moreover, Brinati et al. [19] suggested the necessity of conducting studies on the predictability of arterial blood gas tests in addition to routine blood values for the diagnosis of COVID-19. In this context, we plan our next studies as follows. The first phase is to identify the diagnosis and prognosis of COVID-19 with LogNNet model using the arterial blood gases. The next phase is to determine the mortality of COVID-19 with the LogNNet model using the RBV values.

Velichko [43] reported a method for the estimation of the occupied RAM in the implementation of the LogNNet on Arduino microcontrollers. The LogNNet 51:50:20:2 model, discussed above, takes about 13.7 kB of RAM. As the matrix W occupies ~10.4 kB, this memory can be freed due to RAM saving algorithm, and the algorithm will use ~3.3 kB. Therefore, the model can be placed on microcontrollers with a RAM size of 16 kB, e.g., Arduino Nano.

With recent advancements in information and communication technologies due to the adoption of IoT technology, smart health monitoring and support systems have a higher development and acceptability margin to improve wellness [67,68]. The integration of medical technologies into IoT is called the Internet of Medical Things (IoMT) [69].

In this context, the availability of low-cost, single-chip microcontrollers and advances in wireless communication technology have encouraged researchers to design low-cost embedded systems for healthcare monitoring applications [67]. Doctors can use patients' data to remotely monitor their physiological health status and diagnose their disorders [68]. In a study designed for mobile health applications, Hu et al. [70] used various graphical biosensors to monitor conditions, such as heart attack, brain problems, and high blood pressure (seizures, mental disorder, etc.). In a study for a similar purpose, Vizbaras et al. [71] reported that the stretching and bending vibrations of various chemical bonds are molecule-specific. Therefore, certain infrared spectral ranges are of particular interest in biomedical sensing. In addition, this approach can be used to selectively detect important biomolecules, such as glucose, lactate, urea, ammonia, serum albumin, and so on. Clifton et al. [72] demonstrated the use of wearable sensors for routine healthcare in their study of the large-scale clinical adoption of "intelligent" predictive monitoring systems.

Mobile sensors for the measurement of routine blood parameters to be used in the real-time detection of various diseases are being developed rapidly with the advancements of technology [73–76]. The RBV values can be measured using a low-cost, mobile microscope, an ocular camera, and a smartphone [73]. Chan et al. [74] determined PT and INR blood values by monitoring the micro-mechanical movements of a copper particle with a proof-of-concept using the vibration motor and camera in smartphones. Farooqi et al. [75] followed the diabetic patients with telemonitoring and Bluetooth-enabled self-monitoring devices and produced new solutions for the glycemic control of the patients. Zhang et al. [76] determined various biochemical parameters by electrochemical controls.

In the feature, the data can be obtained in real time and used to provide immediate medical advice before the health problems of the patients occur and progress. The technique presented in this study can be used to create mobile health monitoring systems.

The output of the LogNNet model can be used in different scenarios. The presented feature selection method can be used in conjunction with molecular testing to obtain high sensitivity and certainty regarding suspected cases. In this way, more positive patients can be identified, isolated, and treated in a timely manner. Likewise, the outputs of our model can be used while the results of other tests are awaited. The results of this study demonstrated that the LogNNet neural network model can be used with high productivity for clinical decision support systems and mobile diagnostics.

Various independent biomarkers used in the study need to be tested in the diagnosis and prognosis of other infectious diseases. The low number of ICU patient groups compared to the non-ICU group was one of the limitations of this study.

5. Conclusions

Determining the mild or severe infection status of COVID-19 patients using various diagnostic tests and imaging results can be costly, time consuming, and is subject to different complications during the process. In this case, the patient's health may be at higher risk and health services may face tragic situations under intense pressure. This study provides a fast, reliable, and economic alternative mobile tool for the diagnosis and prognosis of COVID-19 based on the RBV values measured only at the time of admission to the hospital.

In this study, the most effective RBVs in the diagnosis and prognosis of COVID-19 were determined using a feature selection method for the LogNNet reservoir neural network. The most important RBVs in the diagnosis of the disease were MCHC, MCH, and aPTT. The most important RBVs in the prognosis of the disease were ESR, NEU, CRP, albumin, and RBC. The LogNNet deep neural network model accurately and precisely detected almost all COVID-19 patients using only a few RBV features.

The health and sickness status of individuals could be determined largely accurately using threshold levels of the LDL, HDL-C, Cholesterol, Triglyceride, MCHC, and Amylase features. In addition, the LogNNet neural network revealed that the performance of the combination of MCHC and MCH and the combination of MCHC and HDL-C in the detection of sick and healthy individuals was higher than the individual performances of these features.

Threshold levels of the NEU, WBC, CRP, Urea, Albumin, and Calcium main properties were found to be significant in the detection of severely and mildly infected patients. As revealed by the LogNNet network, the combination of ESR, NEU, CRP, Albumin, RBC, Chlorine, and RDW features is an important source of variation in the prognosis of COVID-19. We propose to use this combination of the features with LogNNet as important biomarkers in the prognosis of the disease and in identifying patients in need of intensive care.

The results of this study can be effectively used in medical peripheral devices of the IoT (IoTM) with low RAM resources, including clinical decision support systems, remote internet medicine, and telemedicine.

Supplementary Materials: The following supporting information can be downloaded at: https://data.mendeley.com/datasets/8hdnzv23x7, SARS-CoV-2-RBV1.sav, SARS-CoV-2-RBV2.sav, SARS-CoV-2-RBV3.sav.

Author Contributions: Conceptualization, M.T.H. and A.V.; methodology, M.T.H. and A.V.; software, A.V.; validation, M.T.H. and A.V.; formal analysis, M.T.H.; investigation, A.V.; resources, M.T.H.; data curation, M.T.H.; writing—original draft preparation, M.T.H. and A.V.; writing—review and editing, M.T.H. and A.V.; visualization, M.T.H. and A.V.; supervision, M.T.H.; project administration, M.T.H.; funding acquisition, A.V. All authors have read and agreed to the published version of the manuscript.

Funding: This research was supported by the Russian Science Foundation (grant no. 22-11-00055, https://rscf.ru/en/project/22-11-00055/ (accessed on 22 June 2022)).

Institutional Review Board Statement: The dataset used in this study was collected in order to be used in various studies in the estimation of the diagnosis, prognosis and mortality of COVID-19. The necessary permissions for the collected dataset were given by the Ministry of Health of the Republic of Turkey and the Ethics Committee of Erzincan Binali Yıldırım University. This study was conducted in accordance with the 1989 Declaration of Helsinki. Erzincan Binali Yıldırım University Human Research Health and Sports Sciences Ethics Committee Decision Number: 2021/02-07.

Informed Consent Statement: In this study, a dataset including only routine blood values, RT-PCR results (positive or negative) and treatment units of the patients was downloaded retrospectively from the information system of our hospital in digital environment. A new sample was not taken from the patients. There is no information in the dataset that includes identifying characteristics of individuals. It was stated that routine blood values would only be used in academic studies, and written consent was obtained from the institutions for this. In addition, therefore, written informed consent was not administered for every patient.

Data Availability Statement: The data used in this study can be shared with the parties, provided that the article is cited.

Acknowledgments: We thank the method of Erzincan Mengücek Gazi Training and Research Hospital for their support in reaching the material used in this study. Special thanks to the editors of the journal and to the anonymous reviewers for their constructive criticism and improvement suggestions.

Conflicts of Interest: The authors declare no conflict of interest.

Appendix A

Table A1. Threshold method parameters for SARS-CoV-2-RBV1 dataset and histogram bin sizes for Figures 6 and 7.

№	Feature	*Ath*, %	*Vth*	Units	Type	Min	Max	Bin Size
43	LDL	96.47	116.14	mg/dL	2	−83	258	3.4
36	HDL-C	94.73	43.09	mg/dL	2	8	115	1
39	Cholesterol	94.47	206.33	mg/dL	2	5	606	6
20	MCHC	94.35	31.31	g/dL	1	15.9	38.6	0.2
48	Triglyceride	90.96	163.35	mg/dL	2	34	1782	17
31	Amylase	85.1	76.35	u/L	1	0	1193	3
51	UA	81.12	5.39	mg/dL	1	0	14.3	
47	TP	79.68	68.05	g/L	2	15	96	
32	CK-MB	78.91	19.87	u/L	2	0	685.5	
42	LDH	74.98	258.40	u/L	1	0	2749	
29	Albumin	74.91	39.61	g/L	2	0	55.87	
37	Calcium	74.21	9.01	mg/dL	2	0	12.55	
30	ALP	74.13	154.35	u/L	1	0	3150	
38	Chlorine	72.62	103.47	mmol/L	2	79	345	
34	GGT	71.6	35.51	u/L	1	0	2732	
1	CRP	70.54	4.29	mg/L	1	1	1650	
41	CK	70.47	111.96	u/L	2	0	4665	
45	Sodium	69.24	139.02	mmol/L	1	108	175	
3	Ferritin	68.75	49.69	μg/L	1	0.2	1650	
46	T-Bil	68.52	0.58	mg/dL	2	−0.35	20.95	
33	D-Bil	66.09	0.16	mg/dL	2	−0.06	20	
11	LYM	66.01	1.50	10^3/μL	2	0.08	715	
40	Creatinine	64.03	1.01	mg/dL	1	0	202	
7	PCT	63.22	0.12	ng/mL	1	0.12	1500	
4	Fibrinogen	63.18	307.94	mg/dL	2	10.9	668.07	
35	Glucose	62.42	122.05	mg/dL	1	11	846	
49	eGFR	61.48	87.22	no unit	2	3.483	561.746	
27	ALT	61.35	29.54	u/L	1	0	2110	
28	AST	60.65	32.19	u/L	1	0	2927	
2	D-Dimer	60.37	385.41	μg/L	2	1.06	9610	
50	Urea	58.19	40.99	mg/dL	1	0	427	
14	WBC	58.08	5.71	10^3/μL	2	0.4	127	
13	PLT	57.46	200.26	10^3/μL	2	9	768	
8	ESR	57.38	14.07	mm/hr	1	2	124	
16	EOS	56.4	0	10^3/μL	1	0	4.41	
21	MCV	56.25	84.03	fL	1	56.7	122.1	
22	MONO	56.25	0.54	10^3/μL	2	0.03	6.4	0.06
44	Potassium	55.63	4.36	mmol/L	1	0	59	
26	RDW	55.49	13.21	%	2	0	30.8	
15	BASO	55.04	0.029	10^3/μL	2	0	0.38	
17	HCT	55	38.33	%	1	11.4	60.1	60
10	aPTT	56.51	31.06	Sec	1	12	23,843.7	238
12	NEU	54.8	2.60	10^3/μL	2	0.49	66.43	
18	HGB	54.12	12.31	g/L	1	3.7	19	
5	INR	53.15	0.735	no unit	2	0.12	88	
25	RBC	53	4.29	10^6/μL	1	1.24	7.48	0.06
19	MCH	52.66	28.51	pg	1	15.9	41.9	0.2
24	PDW	51.93	11.89	fL	1	0	25.3	
23	MPV	51.79	9.81	fL	1	0	15	
6	PT	51.79	13.09	Sec	1	2	181	
9	Troponin	50.19	25	ng/L	1	0.01	25,000	

Table A2. Threshold method parameters for SARS-CoV-2-RBV2 dataset and histogram bin sizes for Figures 9 and 10.

№	Feature	*Ath*, %	*Vth*	Units	Type	Min	Max	Bin Size
36	NEU	78.23	6.20	10^3/µL	1	0.1	31.26	0.3
3	Albumin	76.87	32.20	g/L	2	0.08	55	0.5
41	WBC	74.28	7.93	10^3/µL	1	0.4	68.3	0.6
42	CRP	74.03	15.051	mg/L	1	0.15	514	5
24	Urea	73.92	46.95	mg/dL	1	6	339	3
11	Calcium	72.14	8.50	mg/dL	2	0.6	12.43	0.1
21	TP	71.57	67.00	g/L	2	15	96	0.8
30	LYM	71.48	1.02	10^3/µL	2	0.08	58.87	
40	RDW	68.89	13.30	%	1	11	27	0.16
48	PCT	67.85	0.151	ng/mL	1	0.052	100	
2	AST	66.39	44.92	u/L	1	4	2927	
16	LDH	66.11	267.37	u/L	1	20	1547	
9	Glucose	65.46	118.13	mg/dL	1	17	846	8
7	D-Bil	65.04	0.209	mg/dL	1	0.01	20	
44	Ferritin	64.17	238.116	µg/L	1	2.4	2000	
15	CK	63.66	99.92	u/L	1	2	4665	
43	D-Dimer	63.61	1074	µg/L	1	1.06	37,000	
29	HGB	62.82	12.20	g/L	2	4	19	0.15
47	PT	62.78	14.30	Sec	1	9.4	129	
23	eGFR	62.55	80.47	no unit	2	4.724	561.746	
35	MPV	62.37	10.30	fL	1	8.1	15	0.07
39	RBC	62.37	4.28	10^6/µL	2	1.24	7.22	0.06
50	Troponin	61.86	10.19	ng/L	1	1	4600	
20	T-Bil	61.81	0.58	mg/dL	1	0.01	29	
8	GGT	61.41	57.36	u/L	1	1	1085	
19	Sodium	61.01	145	mmol/L	1	112	175	
37	PDW	60.86	11.51	fL	1	7.6	25.3	
32	MCHC	60.72	32.11	g/dL	2	3.6	39.2	
28	HCT	59.71	36.63	%	2	12	56.3	
1	ALT	59.02	39.80	u/L	1	0.7	1349	
33	MCV	58.79	85.93	fL	1	55.8	117.8	
6	CK-MB	58.72	19.38	u/L	1	1	575.4	
14	Creatinine	58.39	1.26	mg/dL	1	0.46	202	
12	Chlorine	58.21	107	mmol/L	1	79	137	0.58
45	Fibrinogen	57.22	334	mg/dL	1	70.56	681.88	
49	ESR	57.2	38.03	mm/hr	1	2	139	1.37
5	Amylase	56.46	75.7	10^3/µL	2	11	874	
46	INR	56.38	1.42	no unit	1	0.77	110	
51	aPTT	56.33	36.12	Sec	2	12	414	
25	UA	55.92	5.412	mg/dL	1	0.9	15	
38	PLT	55.61	160	%	2	5	1199	
34	MONO	55.22	0.474	sec	2	0.03	6.29	
18	Potassium	54.99	3.815	mmol/L	2	2.4	59	
27	EOS	54.72	0.111	10^3/Ml	2	0.01	4.41	
4	ALP	54.35	63.98	u/L	1	1	3150	31
22	Triglyceride	53.27	141.6	10^6/µL	1	32	1402	
31	MCH	53.11	28.22	pg	2	15.6	41.9	
13	Cholesterol	53.11	170	mg/dL	2	5	354	
10	HDL-C	53.02	34.69	mg/dL	2	8	93	
26	BASO	52.75	0.01	10^3/µL	1	0.01	0.38	
17	LDL	51.26	115.1	mg/dL	1	15	258	

References

1. Mertoglu, C.; Huyut, M.; Olmez, H.; Tosun, M.; Kantarci, M.; Coban, T. COVID-19 is more dangerous for older people and its severity is increasing: A case-control study. *Med. Gas Res.* **2022**, *12*, 51–54. [CrossRef] [PubMed]
2. Mertoglu, C.; Huyut, M.T.; Arslan, Y.; Ceylan, Y.; Coban, T.A. How do routine laboratory tests change in coronavirus disease 2019? *Scand. J. Clin. Lab. Investig.* **2021**, *81*, 24–33. [CrossRef]
3. Huyut, M.T.; İlkbahar, F. The effectiveness of blood routine parameters and some biomarkers as a potential diagnostic tool in the diagnosis and prognosis of Covid-19 disease. *Int. Immunopharmacol.* **2021**, *98*, 107838. [CrossRef] [PubMed]
4. Huyut, M.T.; Huyut, Z. Forecasting of Oxidant/Antioxidant levels of COVID-19 patients by using Expert models with biomarkers used in the Diagnosis/Prognosis of COVID-19. *Int. Immunopharmacol.* **2021**, *100*, 108127. [CrossRef]
5. Huyut, M.; Üstündağ, H. Prediction of diagnosis and prognosis of COVID-19 disease by blood gas parameters using decision trees machine learning model: A retrospective observational study. *Med. Gas Res.* **2022**, *12*, 60–66. [CrossRef]

6. Tahir Huyut, M.; Huyut, Z.; İlkbahar, F.; Mertoğlu, C. What is the impact and efficacy of routine immunological, biochemical and hematological biomarkers as predictors of COVID-19 mortality? *Int. Immunopharmacol.* **2022**, *105*, 108542. [CrossRef]
7. Guan, W.; Ni, Z.; Hu, Y.; Liang, W.; Ou, C.; He, J.; Liu, L.; Shan, H.; Lei, C.; Hui, D.S.C.; et al. Clinical Characteristics of Coronavirus Disease 2019 in China. *N. Engl. J. Med.* **2020**, *382*, 1708–1720. [CrossRef]
8. Banerjee, A.; Ray, S.; Vorselaars, B.; Kitson, J.; Mamalakis, M.; Weeks, S.; Baker, M.; Mackenzie, L.S. Use of Machine Learning and Artificial Intelligence to predict SARS-CoV-2 infection from Full Blood Counts in a population. *Int. Immunopharmacol.* **2020**, *86*, 106705. [CrossRef]
9. Huyut, M.T.; Soygüder, S. The Multi-Relationship Structure between Some Symptoms and Features Seen during the New Coronavirus 19 Infection and the Levels of Anxiety and Depression post-Covid. *East. J. Med.* **2022**, *27*, 1–10. [CrossRef]
10. Amgalan, A.; Othman, M. Hemostatic laboratory derangements in COVID-19 with a focus on platelet count. *Platelets* **2020**, *31*, 740–745. [CrossRef]
11. Li, X.; Wang, L.; Yan, S.; Yang, F.; Xiang, L.; Zhu, J.; Shen, B.; Gong, Z. Clinical characteristics of 25 death cases with COVID-19: A retrospective review of medical records in a single medical center, Wuhan, China. *Int. J. Infect. Dis.* **2020**, *94*, 128–132. [CrossRef] [PubMed]
12. Kukar, M.; Gunčar, G.; Vovko, T.; Podnar, S.; Černelč, P.; Brvar, M.; Zalaznik, M.; Notar, M.; Moškon, S.; Notar, M. COVID-19 diagnosis by routine blood tests using machine learning. *Sci. Rep.* **2021**, *11*, 10738. [CrossRef]
13. Jiang, S.Q.; Huang, Q.F.; Xie, W.M.; Lv, C.; Quan, X.Q. The association between severe COVID-19 and low platelet count: Evidence from 31 observational studies involving 7613 participants. *Br. J. Haematol.* **2020**, *190*, e29–e33. [CrossRef]
14. Zheng, Y.; Zhang, Y.; Chi, H.; Chen, S.; Peng, M.; Luo, L.; Chen, L.; Li, J.; Shen, B.; Wang, D. The hemocyte counts as a potential biomarker for predicting disease progression in COVID-19: A retrospective study. *Clin. Chem. Lab. Med.* **2020**, *58*, 1106–1115. [CrossRef] [PubMed]
15. Lippi, G.; Plebani, M.; Henry, B.M. Thrombocytopenia is associated with severe coronavirus disease 2019 (COVID-19) infections: A meta-analysis. *Clin. Chim. Acta* **2020**, *506*, 145–148. [CrossRef]
16. Mousavi, S.A.; Rad, S.; Rostami, T.; Rostami, M.; Mousavi, S.A.; Mirhoseini, S.A.; Kiumarsi, A. Hematologic predictors of mortality in hospitalized patients with COVID-19: A comparative study. *Hematology* **2020**, *25*, 383–388. [CrossRef]
17. Beck, B.R.; Shin, B.; Choi, Y.; Park, S.; Kang, K. Predicting commercially available antiviral drugs that may act on the novel coronavirus (SARS-CoV-2) through a drug-target interaction deep learning model. *Comput. Struct. Biotechnol. J.* **2020**, *18*, 784–790. [CrossRef]
18. Xu, X.; Jiang, X.; Ma, C.; Du, P.; Li, X.; Lv, S.; Yu, L.; Ni, Q.; Chen, Y.; Su, J.; et al. A Deep Learning System to Screen Novel Coronavirus Disease 2019 Pneumonia. *Engineering* **2020**, *6*, 1122–1129. [CrossRef]
19. Brinati, D.; Campagner, A.; Ferrari, D.; Locatelli, M.; Banfi, G.; Cabitza, F. Detection of COVID-19 Infection from Routine Blood Exams with Machine Learning: A Feasibility Study. *J. Med. Syst.* **2020**, *44*, 135. [CrossRef]
20. Cabitza, F.; Campagner, A.; Ferrari, D.; Di Resta, C.; Ceriotti, D.; Sabetta, E.; Colombini, A.; De Vecchi, E.; Banfi, G.; Locatelli, M.; et al. Development, evaluation, and validation of machine learning models for COVID-19 detection based on routine blood tests. *Clin. Chem. Lab. Med.* **2021**, *59*, 421–431. [CrossRef]
21. Yang, H.S.; Hou, Y.; Vasovic, L.V.; Steel, P.A.D.; Chadburn, A.; Racine-Brzostek, S.E.; Velu, P.; Cushing, M.M.; Loda, M.; Kaushal, R.; et al. Routine Laboratory Blood Tests Predict SARS-CoV-2 Infection Using Machine Learning. *Clin. Chem.* **2020**, *66*, 1396–1404. [CrossRef] [PubMed]
22. Joshi, R.P.; Pejaver, V.; Hammarlund, N.E.; Sung, H.; Kyu, S.; Lee, H.; Scott, G.; Gombar, S.; Shah, N.; Shen, S.; et al. Short communication A predictive tool for identi fi cation of SARS-CoV-2 PCR-negative emergency department patients using routine test results. *J. Clin. Virol.* **2020**, *129*, 104502. [CrossRef] [PubMed]
23. Mei, X.; Lee, H.C.; Diao, K.Y.; Huang, M.; Lin, B.; Liu, C.; Xie, Z.; Ma, Y.; Robson, P.M.; Chung, M.; et al. Artificial intelligence–enabled rapid diagnosis of patients with COVID-19. *Nat. Med.* **2020**, *26*, 1224–1228. [CrossRef]
24. Soares, F. A novel specific artificial intelligence-based method to identify COVID-19 cases using simple blood exams. *medRxiv* **2020**. [CrossRef]
25. Soltan, A.A.; Kouchaki, S.; Zhu, T.; Kiyasseh, D.; Taylor, T.; Hussain, Z.B.; Peto, T.; Brent, A.J.; Eyre, D.W.; Clifton, D. Artificial intelligence driven assessment of routinely collected healthcare data is an effective screening test for COVID-19 in patients presenting to hospital. *medRxiv* **2020**. [CrossRef]
26. Remeseiro, B.; Bolon-Canedo, V. A review of feature selection methods in medical applications. *Comput. Biol. Med.* **2019**, *112*, 103375. [CrossRef]
27. Bikku, T. Multi-layered deep learning perceptron approach for health risk prediction. *J. Big Data* **2020**, *7*, 50. [CrossRef]
28. Battineni, G.; Chintalapudi, N.; Amenta, F. Machine learning in medicine: Performance calculation of dementia prediction by support vector machines (SVM). *Inform. Med. Unlocked* **2019**, *16*, 100200. [CrossRef]
29. Xing, W.; Bei, Y. Medical Health Big Data Classification Based on KNN Classification Algorithm. *IEEE Access* **2020**, *8*, 28808–28819. [CrossRef]
30. Hoodbhoy, Z.; Noman, M.; Shafique, A.; Nasim, A.; Chowdhury, D.; Hasan, B. Use of machine learning algorithms for prediction of fetal risk using cardiotocographic data. *Int. J. Appl. Basic Med. Res.* **2019**, *9*, 226. [CrossRef]
31. Alam, M.Z.; Rahman, M.S.; Rahman, M.S. A Random Forest based predictor for medical data classification using feature ranking. *Inform. Med. Unlocked* **2019**, *15*, 100180. [CrossRef]

32. Schober, P.; Vetter, T.R. Logistic Regression in Medical Research. *Anesth. Analg.* **2021**, *132*, 365–366. [CrossRef] [PubMed]
33. Podgorelec, V.; Kokol, P.; Stiglic, B.; Rozman, I. Decision trees: An overview and their use in medicine. *J. Med. Syst.* **2002**, *26*, 445–463. [CrossRef]
34. Guyon, I.; Gunn, S.; Nikravesh, M.; Zadeh, L.A. *Feature Extraction: Foundations and Applications*; Studies in Fuzziness and Soft Computing; Springer: Berlin/Heidelberg, Germany, 2008; ISBN 9783540354888.
35. Hall, M.A. Correlation-based Feature Selection for Machine Learning. Ph.D. Thesis, Department of Computer Science, The University of Waikato, Hamilton, NewZealand, April 1999; pp. 51–69.
36. Dash, M.; Liu, H. Consistency-based search in feature selection. *Artif. Intell.* **2003**, *151*, 155–176. [CrossRef]
37. Zhao, Z.; Liu, H. Searching for interacting features. In Proceedings of the 20th International Joint Conference on Artificial Intelligence, Hyderabad, India, 6–12 January 2007; pp. 1156–1161.
38. Hall, M.A.; Smith, L.A. Practical feature subset selection for machine learning. In Proceedings of the Computer Science '98, 21st Australasian Computer Science Conference ACSC'98, Perth, Australia, 4–6 February 1998; Volume 20, pp. 181–191.
39. Kononenko, I. Estimating attributes: Analysis and extensions of RELIEF. In *European Conference on Machine Learning*; Springer: Berlin/Heidelberg, Germany, 1994; Volume 784, pp. 171–182. [CrossRef]
40. Le Thi, H.A.; Nguyen, V.V.; Ouchani, S. Gene selection for cancer classification using DCA. In *International Conference on Advanced Data Mining and Applications*; Springer: Berlin/Heidelberg, Germany, 2008; Volume 5139, pp. 62–72. [CrossRef]
41. Tibshirani, R. Regression Shrinkage and Selection via the Lasso. *J. R. Stat. Soc. Ser. B* **1996**, *58*, 267–288. [CrossRef]
42. Velichko, A. Neural network for low-memory IoT devices and MNIST image recognition using kernels based on logistic map. *Electronics* **2020**, *9*, 1432. [CrossRef]
43. Velichko, A. A method for medical data analysis using the lognnet for clinical decision support systems and edge computing in healthcare. *Sensors* **2021**, *21*, 6209. [CrossRef]
44. Velichko, A.; Heidari, H. A Method for Estimating the Entropy of Time Series Using Artificial Neural Networks. *Entropy* **2021**, *23*, 1432. [CrossRef]
45. Izotov, Y.A.; Velichko, A.A.; Boriskov, P.P. Method for fast classification of MNIST digits on Arduino UNO board using LogNNet and linear congruential generator. *J. Phys. Conf. Ser.* **2021**, *2094*, 32055. [CrossRef]
46. Heidari, H.; Velichko, A. An improved LogNNet classifier for IoT application. *J. Phys. Conf. Ser.* **2021**, *2094*, 032015. [CrossRef]
47. Mattiuzzi, C.; Lippi, G. Which lessons shall we learn from the 2019 novel coronavirus outbreak? *Ann. Transl. Med.* **2020**, *8*, 48. [CrossRef] [PubMed]
48. Kim, S.; Kim, D.-M.; Lee, B. Insufficient Sensitivity of RNA Dependent RNA Polymerase Gene of SARS-CoV-2 Viral Genome as Confirmatory Test using Korean COVID-19 Cases. *Preprints* **2020**, 1–4. [CrossRef]
49. Zhang, J.J.; Cao, Y.Y.; Tan, G.; Dong, X.; Wang, B.C.; Lin, J.; Yan, Y.Q.; Liu, G.H.; Akdis, M.; Akdis, C.A.; et al. Clinical, radiological, and laboratory characteristics and risk factors for severity and mortality of 289 hospitalized COVID-19 patients. *Allergy Eur. J. Allergy Clin. Immunol.* **2021**, *76*, 533–550. [CrossRef] [PubMed]
50. Teymouri, M.; Mollazadeh, S.; Mortazavi, H.; Naderi Ghale-noie, Z.; Keyvani, V.; Aghababaei, F.; Hamblin, M.R.; Abbaszadeh-Goudarzi, G.; Pourghadamyari, H.; Hashemian, S.M.R.; et al. Recent advances and challenges of RT-PCR tests for the diagnosis of COVID-19. *Pathol. Res. Pract.* **2021**, *221*, 153443. [CrossRef]
51. D'Cruz, R.J.; Currier, A.W.; Sampson, V.B. Laboratory Testing Methods for Novel Severe Acute Respiratory Syndrome-Coronavirus-2 (SARS-CoV-2). *Front. Cell Dev. Biol.* **2020**, *8*, 468. [CrossRef]
52. Yang, A.P.; Liu, J.P.; Tao, W.Q.; Li, H.M. The diagnostic and predictive role of NLR, d-NLR and PLR in COVID-19 patients. *Int. Immunopharmacol.* **2020**, *84*, 106504. [CrossRef]
53. Huyut, M.T. Automatic Detection of Severely and Mildly Infected COVID-19 Patients with Supervised Machine Learning Models. *IRBM* **2022**, *1*, 1–12. [CrossRef]
54. Zhang, C.; Shi, L.; Wang, F.S. Liver injury in COVID-19: Management and challenges. *Lancet Gastroenterol. Hepatol.* **2020**, *5*, 428–430. [CrossRef]
55. Zheng, M.; Gao, Y.; Wang, G.; Song, G.; Liu, S.; Sun, D.; Xu, Y.; Tian, Z. Functional exhaustion of antiviral lymphocytes in COVID-19 patients. *Cell. Mol. Immunol.* **2020**, *17*, 533–535. [CrossRef]
56. Luo, J.; Zhou, L.; Feng, Y.; Li, B.; Guo, S. The selection of indicators from initial blood routine test results to improve the accuracy of early prediction of COVID-19 severity. *PLoS ONE* **2021**, *16*, e0253329. [CrossRef]
57. Ma, Y.; Hou, L.; Yang, X.; Huang, Z.; Yang, X.; Zhao, N.; He, M.; Shi, Y.; Kang, Y.; Yue, J.; et al. The association between frailty and severe disease among COVID-19 patients aged over 60 years in China: A prospective cohort study. *BMC Med.* **2020**, *18*, 274. [CrossRef] [PubMed]
58. Lai, C.C.; Shih, T.P.; Ko, W.C.; Tang, H.J.; Hsueh, P.R. Severe acute respiratory syndrome coronavirus 2 (SARS-CoV-2) and coronavirus disease-2019 (COVID-19): The epidemic and the challenges. *Int. J. Antimicrob. Agents* **2020**, *55*, 105924. [CrossRef] [PubMed]
59. Feld, J.; Tremblay, D.; Thibaud, S.; Kessler, A.; Naymagon, L. Ferritin levels in patients with COVID-19: A poor predictor of mortality and hemophagocytic lymphohistiocytosis. *Int. J. Lab. Hematol.* **2020**, *42*, 773–779. [CrossRef]
60. Zhou, F.; Yu, T.; Du, R.; Fan, G.; Liu, Y.; Liu, Z.; Xiang, J.; Wang, Y.; Song, B.; Gu, X.; et al. Clinical course and risk factors for mortality of adult inpatients with COVID-19 in Wuhan, China: A retrospective cohort study. *Lancet* **2020**, *395*, 1054–1062. [CrossRef]

61. Chen, G.; Wu, D.; Guo, W.; Cao, Y.; Huang, D.; Wang, H.; Wang, T.; Zhang, X.; Chen, H.; Yu, H.; et al. Clinical and immunological features of severe and moderate coronavirus disease 2019. *J. Clin. Investig.* **2020**, *130*, 2620–2629. [CrossRef] [PubMed]
62. Cheng, L.; Li, H.; Li, L.; Liu, C.; Yan, S.; Chen, H.; Li, Y. Ferritin in the coronavirus disease 2019 (COVID-19): A systematic review and meta-analysis. *J. Clin. Lab. Anal.* **2020**, *34*, 1–18. [CrossRef]
63. Cavalcante-Silva, L.H.A.; Carvalho, D.C.M.; Lima, É.D.A.; Galvão, J.G.; da Silva, J.S.d.F.; de Sales-Neto, J.M.; Rodrigues-Mascarenhas, S. Neutrophils and COVID-19: The road so far. *Int. Immunopharmacol.* **2021**, *90*, 107233. [CrossRef]
64. Pan, F.; Ye, T.; Sun, P.; Gui, S.; Liang, B.; Li, L.; Zheng, D.; Wang, J.; Hesketh, R.L.; Yang, L.; et al. Time Course of Lung Changes on Chest CT During Recovery From 2019 Novel Coronavirus (COVID-19) Pneumonia. *Radiology* **2020**, *295*, 200370. [CrossRef]
65. Zhao, D.; Yao, F.; Wang, L.; Zheng, L.; Gao, Y.; Ye, J.; Guo, F.; Zhao, H.; Gao, R. A Comparative Study on the Clinical Features of Coronavirus 2019 (COVID-19) Pneumonia with Other Pneumonias. *Clin. Infect. Dis.* **2020**, *71*, 756–761. [CrossRef]
66. Rabanser, S.; Günnemann, S.; Lipton, Z.C. Failing loudly: An empirical study of methods for detecting dataset shift. *Adv. Neural Inf. Process. Syst.* **2019**, *32*. [CrossRef]
67. Al-Aubidy, K.M.; Derbas, A.M.; Al-Mutairi, A.W. Real-time patient health monitoring and alarming using wireless-sensor-network. In Proceedings of the 2016 13th International Multi-Conference on Systems, Signals & Devices (SSD), Leipzig, Germany, 21–24 March 2016; pp. 416–423. [CrossRef]
68. Taiwo, O.; Ezugwu, A.E. Smart healthcare support for remote patient monitoring during Covid-19 quarantine. *Inform. Med. Unlocked* **2020**, *20*, 100428. [CrossRef] [PubMed]
69. Lamonaca, F.; Balestrieri, E.; Tudosa, I.; Picariello, F.; Carnì, D.L.; Scuro, C.; Bonavolontà, F.; Spagnuolo, V.; Grimaldi, G.; Colaprico, A. An Overview on Internet of Medical Things in Blood Pressure Monitoring. In Proceedings of the 2019 IEEE International Symposium on Medical Measurements and Applications (MeMeA), Istanbul, Turkey, 26–28 June 2019; pp. 1–6.
70. Hu, F.; Xiao, Y.; Hao, Q. Congestion-aware, loss-resilient bio-monitoring sensor networking for mobile health applications. *IEEE J. Sel. Areas Commun.* **2009**, *27*, 450–465. [CrossRef]
71. Vizbaras, A.; Simonyte, I.; Droz, S.; Torcheboeuf, N.; Miasojedovas, A.; Trinkunas, A.; Buciunas, T.; Dambrauskas, Z.; Gulbinas, A.; Boiko, D.L.; et al. GaSb Swept-Wavelength Lasers for Biomedical Sensing Applications. *IEEE J. Sel. Top. Quantum Electron.* **2019**, *25*, 1–12. [CrossRef]
72. Clifton, L.; Clifton, D.A.; Pimentel, M.A.F.; Watkinson, P.J.; Tarassenko, L. Predictive monitoring of mobile patients by combining clinical observations with data from wearable sensors. *IEEE J. Biomed. Health Inform.* **2014**, *18*, 722–730. [CrossRef]
73. Pfeil, J.; Nechyporenko, A.; Frohme, M.; Hufert, F.T.; Schulze, K. Examination of blood samples using deep learning and mobile microscopy. *BMC Bioinform.* **2022**, *23*, 1–14. [CrossRef]
74. Chan, J.; Michaelsen, K.; Estergreen, J.K.; Sabath, D.E.; Gollakota, S. Micro-mechanical blood clot testing using smartphones. *Nat. Commun.* **2022**, *13*, 1–12. [CrossRef]
75. Farooqi, M.H.; Abdelmannan, D.K.; Mubarak, M.; Abdalla, M.; Hamed, A.; Xavier, M.; Joyce, T.; Cadiz, S.; Nawaz, F.A. The Impact of Telemonitoring on Improving Glycemic and Metabolic Control in Previously Lost-to-Follow-Up Patients with Type 2 Diabetes Mellitus: A Single-Center Interventional Study in the United Arab Emirates. *Int. J. Clin. Pract.* **2022**, *2022*, 6286574. [CrossRef]
76. Zhang, Y.; Zhang, Y.; Li, H.; Cao, Y.; Han, S.; Zhang, K.; He, W. Covalent Biosensing Polymer Chain Reaction Enabling Periphery Blood Testing to Predict Tumor Invasiveness with a Platelet Procancerous Protein. *Anal. Chem.* **2022**, *94*, 1983–1989. [CrossRef]

sensors

MDPI

Article

Deep Learning and 5G and Beyond for Child Drowning Prevention in Swimming Pools

Juan Carlos Cepeda-Pacheco and Mari Carmen Domingo *

Department of Network Engineering, BarcelonaTech (UPC) University, 08860 Castelldefels, Spain
* Correspondence: cdomingo@entel.upc.edu

Abstract: Drowning is a major health issue worldwide. The World Health Organization's global report on drowning states that the highest rates of drowning deaths occur among children aged 1–4 years, followed by children aged 5–9 years. Young children can drown silently in as little as 25 s, even in the shallow end or in a baby pool. The report also identifies that the main risk factor for children drowning is the lack of or inadequate supervision. Therefore, in this paper, we propose a novel 5G and beyond child drowning prevention system based on deep learning that detects and classifies distractions of inattentive parents or caregivers and alerts them to focus on active child supervision in swimming pools. In this proposal, we have generated our own dataset, which consists of images of parents/caregivers watching the children or being distracted. The proposed model can successfully perform a seven-class classification with very high accuracies (98%, 94%, and 90% for each model, respectively). ResNet-50, compared with the other models, performs better classifications for most classes.

Keywords: deep learning; 5G and beyond; child drowning prevention; network slicing architecture

Citation: Cepeda-Pacheco, J.C.; Domingo, M.C. Deep Learning and 5G and Beyond for Child Drowning Prevention in Swimming Pools. *Sensors* **2022**, *22*, 7684. https://doi.org/10.3390/s22197684

Academic Editors: Andrei Velichko, Dmitry Korzun and Alexander Meigal

Received: 25 July 2022
Accepted: 6 October 2022
Published: 10 October 2022

1. Introduction

Drowning is a major health problem worldwide. According to the World Health Organization (WHO, Geneva, Switzerland), in 2015, around 360,000 people died from drowning [1]. More than half of these deaths are of people younger than 25.

The WHO Global report on drowning [2] states that the highest rates of drowning deaths occur among children aged 1–4, followed by children aged 5–9 years. In fact, in countries like Australia, drowning is the leading cause of unintentional injury death in children aged 1–3 years, and in the USA, drowning is responsible for more deaths among children aged 1–4 years than any other cause (except birth defects) [3]. Furthermore, drowning is the third leading cause of death worldwide for those aged from 5 to 14. In the Western Pacific Region, children aged 5–14 years die more frequently from drowning than from any other cause.

Drowning happens quickly and quietly and its signs often go unnoticed. Young children can drown silently in as little as 25 s, even in the shallow end or in a baby pool [4]. For all of these reasons, it is important for parents and caregivers to actively supervise their children around water, even if lifeguards are present.

The same report identifies the absence of or inadequate supervision as key risk factors for the drowning of children [1]. Another report [5] from the Royal Life Saving Society Australia (RSLA, Sydney, Australia) linked distracted parents to 77.8% of drownings in children aged 5–9 years in public and commercial pools between 1 July 2005 and 30 June 2015. In the cases of drowning without supervision, the parent or caregiver of the child was missing, or physically near the child but distracted (talking to another adult or attending to another child in his/her care). Furthermore, the German Lifeguard Association (DLRG, Bad Nenndorf, Germany) (the biggest organization of its kind in the world) reported that more than 300 people died in Germany during 2018 (from the beginning of the year through the summer) and associated the growing number of children drowning to their parents' obsession with mobile phones [6]. In addition, Royal Life Saving Australia reported that, between 2002 and 2017, 447 children under the age of four drowned. Roughly 5% of those deaths were a direct result of a failure to supervise owing to the use of electronic devices (smartphone, tablet, laptop, and so on) [7].

In order to solve the problem of inadequate child supervision, in this paper, we propose a novel 5G and beyond child drowning prevention system based on deep learning that detects and classifies distractions of inattentive parents or caregivers. It can be deployed in indoor swimming pools or outdoor locations such as beaches or aquatic recreation locations aided by unmanned aerial vehicle (UAV) (drones). The system detects distracted parents/caregivers in charge of a minor and alerts them to concentrate on the supervision task. A 5G network slicing architecture for child drowning prevention has also been introduced. To the best of our knowledge, this is the first paper that aims to avoid child drowning by detecting and classifying distractions of parents in charge of a minor in aquatic recreational spaces; it is also the first paper to use digital technologies such as artificial intelligence and modern communication technologies (such as 5G and beyond) to detect and alert distracted parents or caregivers. The main contributions of this study are as follows:

- The proposal of a real-time distraction detection system that takes place in an aquatic recreational environment (swimming pools).
- The collection of our own distracted parent/caregiver image dataset by harvesting images of real people at a swimming pool being distracted or supervising children.
- The implementation and evaluation of three types of well-known convolutional neural networks (CNNs) for the classification and detection system to determine the most suitable architecture for distraction detection.
- The development of a voice alert system, pager, or wearable device that reminds the parent or caregiver to focus on the task of child supervision.

The experimental results prove the feasibility of the child drowning prevention system. The proposed model can successfully perform a seven-class classification with very high accuracies (98%, 94%, and 90% for each model, respectively).

The paper is structured as follows. In Section 2, we introduce our proposed 5G-enabled child drowning prevention system. In Section 3, we identify the most relevant key performance indicators (KPIs). In Section 4, we explain the 5G-service-based architecture. In Section 5, we discuss the proposed 5G network slicing architecture for child drowning prevention from a technical perspective. In Section 6, we briefly describe the convolutional neural network architectures used in this research. The experiments and results are presented in Section 7. Finally, Section 8 concludes the paper and highlights some future research directions.

Related Work

Monitoring and supervision at swimming pools or aquatic recreation locations has drawn the attention of the research community [8], particularly for drowning prevention and early detection of possible drowning [9,10].

Some proposed drowning detection systems [11–13] employ underwater cameras to detect motionless drowned victims sunk at the bottom of the pool using techniques such as background extraction [13], which consists of detecting the moving objects by identifying the difference between the current frame and a reference frame, often called a 'background image' or 'background model'; however, these systems are limited to the victims that have sunk to the bottom of the pool, thus wasting precious time, as they are unable to detect the victims prior to them drowning.

Other proposed methods consist of overhead cameras mounted around the pool (such as our proposed system) [14–16]; these systems consist of two main parts: a vision component that can detect and track swimmers and an event-inference (water crisis) module that analyzes swimmer observation sequences for possible drowning behavior signals. Several studies have been carried out regarding the detection of swimmers based on overhead cameras [17,18]. This task is still challenging owing to disturbances at the water's surface (e.g., water exhibits random homogeneous blob movements, which could be easily misidentified as foreground objects) [19,20]. In addition, lightning and color variations over time due to ambient brightness even further complicate automated monitoring based on video surveillance. Several works apply background subtraction to solve the swimmer detection problem [13,19,20]. Currently, the development of wearable devices has become a very common practice. It has allowed researchers to develop sensor systems to monitor the physiological signals of high-performance swimming athletes [21,22], to detect pre-drowning symptoms and alert rescue staff [23], and to supervise children. Wearable sensor systems for infants can perceive external threats such as falls or drowning; the methods and techniques applied in wearable sensor systems are analyzed and discussed in [24]. In [20], a real-time detection method for constant monitoring of swimmers at an outdoor swimming pool is presented. A background subtraction scheme is introduced, where the background has been modeled as a composition of homogeneous region processes. Furthermore, to solve the foreground (swimmer) detection problem, a devised thresholding scheme has been proposed to attain a good trade-off between maximizing target detection while minimizing background noises. In addition, to enhance the visibility of the foreground (swimmer), a pre-processing filtering scheme able to classify each pixel of a current frame into different pixel types has been proposed; this way, appropriate filtering actions such as color compensation can be applied when necessary. In [19], a background subtraction scheme based on motion and intensity information has been developed to identify swimmers in each video frame. Image pixels are classified according to motion as random/stationary, ripple, and swimming. A motion map is developed through the computation of dense optical flow that characterizes the motion contents of image pixels over a short sequence of video frames rather than a single image. Intensity information has been modeled using a block-based mixture of Gaussians (MoG). However, these systems ([19,20]) only specify how to detect a swimmer; they do not specify how to detect if he/she is drowning.

Current improvements in computing power have enabled the use of deep learning algorithms for human detection and other computer-vision-related problems. Most state-of-the-art object detectors use deep learning algorithms to extract features from input images (or videos) and perform classification and localization, respectively [25]. In [26], a method to detect swimmers in low-quality video using two convolutional neural networks (YOLOv2 and Tiny-YOLO) has been proposed. Our proposed 5G and beyond child drowning prevention system is also based on deep learning (convolutional neural networks), but focuses on the detection of distracted parents/caregivers, not swimmer detection (as in [26]). In [27], a real-time vision system to detect drowning incidents using overhead cameras at an outdoor swimming pool is presented. The system uses a model comprising data fusion and hidden Markov modeling to learn of drowning events early. They focus on (1) foreground swimmer silhouette extraction and (2) behavioral recognition. The foreground detection module has already been reported in [20]. The system has analyzed water crisis episodes consisting of victims that suffer distress incidents (victims exhibit involuntary movements such as active struggling or waving [28]) and drowning incidents understood as suffocation. The detection of distress and early drowning episodes is based on visual indicators (instinctive response with repetitive arm movements of extending out and pressing down, perpendicular body (vertical up) in water with small movements in horizontal and diagonal directions). The experiments try to differentiate between three events (water crisis, treading, and normal swimming); the best testing errors obtained are 15.15% and 15.57%, with support vector machine (SVM) and reduced model (RM) classifier, respectively. Furthermore, the false alarm rate is at about one to five cases for each camera in a day. In addition, one challenge of their proposed system is that a drowning incident may happen in a way that is different from the learned instinctive drowning response model. In this case, it must be determined how the system will react to an event for which it is not trained [27]. Furthermore, specialists emphasize that drowning happens quickly and quietly, and its signs often go unnoticed (see Section 1). For this reason, in our current paper, we propose a novel technique to detect child drowning episodes that focuses on the caregivers of the children. To improve swimming pool safety, we use deep learning to detect a distracted caregiver of a child in a swimming pool, similarly to the detection of drivers' distractions on the road. The behavior of a driver is essential for traffic safety. On-road distractions deteriorate the driver's performance and may lead to the loss of vehicular control and traffic accidents. A distraction is anything that diverts the driver's attention from the primary task of navigating the vehicle and responding to critical events. The authors in [29–31] use deep learning to detect distracted driver behaviors such as texting, operating the radio, drinking, fixing hair and makeup, talking on the phone, and so on.

2. The Proposed 5G and Beyond Child Drowning Prevention System

In the proposed scenario, families need to register when they arrive at the swimming pool. A facial image of each family member is acquired to recognize them. The swimming pool database registers the age of each child and links the photos of the children with their parents and/or other family member/s. The family decides who is going to be the primary caregiver that is going to watch the children and be responsible for their safety inside the swimming pool and a pager is given to him/her. This task can be shared between the parents (or other family members 18 years or older) simultaneously, which means that none of them should be distracted. It is also possible that there is only one primary caregiver during a certain time slot and another during the next time slot (e.g., the father is the primary caregiver from 15:00 to 17:00 and the mother from 17:00 to 19:00).

After all of these decisions are made using the swimming pool app, the family can access the swimming pool area. The proposed 5G and beyond child drowning prevention system is shown in Figure 1.

If the primary caregiver decides to supervise the children outside of the pool, a specific seat will be assigned to him/her close to the swimming pool. This guarantees that he/she will have a good sight of the swimming pool to supervise the children. In addition, a video camera will be directly facing him/her to detect distractions. The cameras are strategically located at an optimal distance in a way not to obstruct people. In the case of multiple primary caregivers, the same or multiple video cameras can be facing them. Real-time video will be transmitted to the command center. Distractions of primary caregivers will be detected using a deep learning algorithm.

If the primary caregiver decides to supervise the child inside the pool, different video cameras mounted surrounding the pool will detect him/her using computer vision. For this purpose, a high-quality monitoring system is required that consists of video cameras with multiple high-end lenses that can zoom and steer around to detect critical details. The video cameras need to coordinate with each other to be able to track the primary caregivers at any time to detect possible distractions. The video cameras will identify the primary caregiver from different perspectives inside the pool. Automated analysis of the video footage will be carried out. A caregiver can be considered as 'distracted' if the convolutional neural network analyzes the images from all of the video cameras that are simultaneously capturing his/her behavior and he/she is characterized as being 'distracted' by most of them. That is, the images of the parents/caregivers are not combined, but the images from each camera are classified into a category. It is decided if the parent/caregiver is distracted or not by analyzing which category is repeated the most.

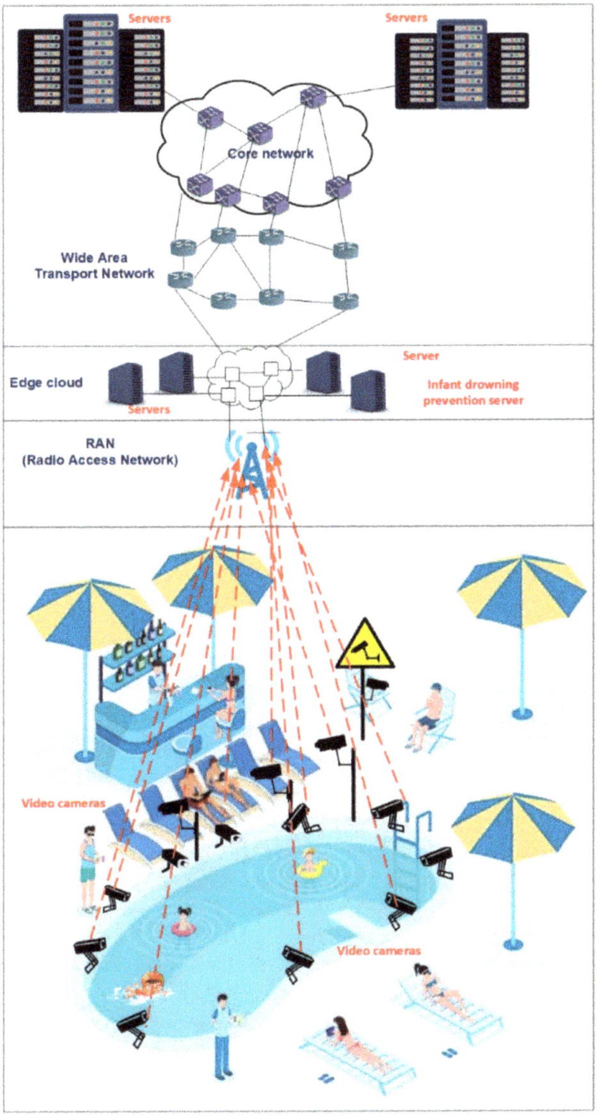

Figure 1. Proposed 5G-enabled child drowning prevention system.

When a distraction event is detected, an alert will warn the primary caregiver so that he/she focuses on active child supervision. We assume that alerts will be sent immediately if the kids to supervise are 5 years old or under. For kids that can swim (usually older than 5 years), parents will be alerted if the convolutional neural network detects a continuous distracted behavior for more than 10 s, because drowning accidents happen very quickly. Alert messages can be sent to a pager. The pager lights up or vibrates in case the caregiver is distracted. Alert messages can also be heard through the swimming pool speakers located in the closest vicinity of the caregiver. Furthermore, lifeguards will also get these notification messages and act accordingly. This information will be, for example, useful if certain caregivers are notified several times; in this case, lifeguards can supervise the associated children much closer and talk to the parents/caregivers or take other necessary steps if no change in their attitude is observed.

3. Related Key Performance Indicators

The proposed 5G-enabled child drowning prevention system can be identified as a mission critical communications (MCC) service because it requires real-time and reliable communications for a large number of users, as well as strong security and pre-emption handling [32]. Table 1 summarizes the major key performance indicators (KPIs) for child drowning prevention. The end-to-end latency can be measured as the time interval required to send the packages from a source to a destination, measured at the application level.

Table 1. Main KPIs for child drowning prevention.

	End-to-End Latency	Data Rate (Uplink/Downlink)	Reliability
5G-enabled child drowning prevention system	20 ms	40 Mbit/s for one video camera/1 Mbps for remote control	99.999%

Mission critical: A quality or characteristic of a communication activity, application, service, or device that requires low setup and transfer latency, high availability and reliability, the ability to handle large numbers of users and devices, strong security, and priority and pre-emption handling.

It would be possible for our use case to connect to the nearest edge server via Wi-Fi 7 (802.11be), because this standard will support a maximum throughput of at least 30 Gbps. Features operating at both the MAC (medium access control) layer and the physical layer (PHY) such as multi-access point coordinated beamforming, time-sensitive networking, and multi-link operation will bring Wi-Fi 7 latency performance into the sub-10 ms realm. These characteristics would be enough to support our high-throughput low-latency child drowning prevention use case. However, the IEEE task group announced draft 2.0 of 802.11be, and the final version will be released in 2024.

IEEE 802.11ax (Wi-Fi 6) received final approval from the IEEE Standards Board on 1 February 2021. This standard offers a theoretical speed of up to 9.6 Gbps and 10 ms latency. Wi-Fi 6 does not perform well in large-scale outdoor coverage scenarios and cannot meet the ultra-low latency requirements (<10 ms).

It has been shown in [33] that Wi-Fi 6 can achieve ultra-reliable low latency performance (i.e., <1 ms packet latency at 99.999% reliability) only when optimized and operating in a low load up to 0.16 bps/Hz that is not appropriate for our use case.

On the other hand, 5G can reach up to 10 Gbps (only slightly higher than Wi-Fi 6), but this technology has been designed to address the requirements of ultra reliable and low-latency communications (URLLC). URLLC has stringent requirements for capabilities such as latency, reliability, and availability. Some use cases include wireless control of industrial manufacturing or production processes, remote medical surgery, and transportation safety. It has been demonstrated in [33] that 5G NR (new radio)-FDD (frequency division duplex) has superior URLLC performance and meets the sub-ms delay requirement at >5× higher load than Wi-Fi 6.

Therefore, 5G is the appropriate technology for our use case thanks to its better latencies. The proposed system requires that real-time video is backhauled from the video cameras to the command center for remote control and analysis. The number of video cameras will vary depending on the size of the swimming pool. Moreover, 5G can be deployed in indoor swimming pools or even in outdoor locations such as beaches or aquatic recreation locations that extend several kilometers. In these cases where so many video images need to be processed as quickly and efficiently as possible, a 5G network is required to provide sufficiently high uplink data throughput and transmission reliability as well as sufficiently low latency. The short end-to-end latency will enable alert messages to be sent as fast as possible if necessary as drowning happens quickly. Reliability is critical to detect incidents, which means that performance should not be compromised irrespective of the channel conditions.

4. 5G Service-Based Architecture

Next, the 5G system architecture of the non-roaming case is illustrated in Figure 2 [34]. The user plane (UP) and control plane (CP) are decoupled to obtain scalable and flexible deployments. Whereas the CP is used for network signaling, the UP carries only user traffic.

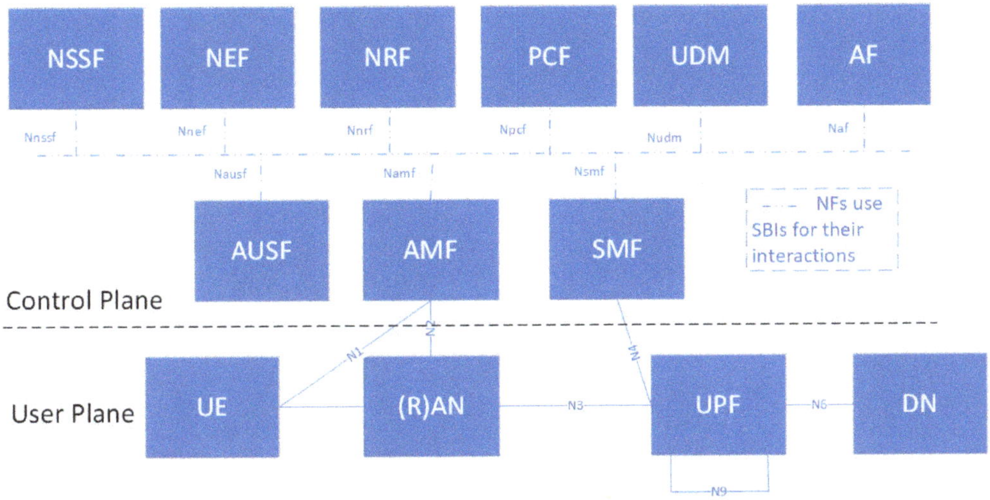

Figure 2. Service-based representation of the 5G non-roaming system architecture [34].

The user equipment (UE) in the user plane is connected to either the radio access network (RAN) or a non-3GPP access network (e.g., wireless local area network, WLAN) as well as to the access and mobility management function (AMF).

Next, we explain the network functions (NFs) of the 5G core network (see the upper part of the figure):

- Access and mobility management function (AMF): it is responsible for UE registration, reachability and mobility.
- Session management function (SMF): it offers UE IP address allocation and management, policy enforcement and quality of service, user plane function (UPF) selection, and control.
- User plane function (UPF): it is the anchor point for intra and inter radio access technology (RAT) mobility, packet routing, and forwarding.
- Policy control function (PCF): it integrates a policy framework for network slicing.
- Application function (AF): it is responsible for different services provided after the interaction with the core network.
- User data management (UDM): it is responsible for subscriptions and many services related to users.
- Authentication server function (AUSF): it performs the UE authentication service.
- Network slice selection function (NSSF): it offers an optimal selection of network instances serving the users.
- Network exposure function (NEF): it collects, stores, and exposes the services and capabilities provided by 3GPP NFs in a secure manner.
- NF repository function (NFR): it maintains and provides the deployed NF instances; it also supports the service discovery function.

5. A 5G Network Slicing Architecture for Child Drowning Prevention

Network slicing refers to the division of a physical network into multiple logical networks (network slices), so that each logical network can provide specific network characteristics for a particular use case. Network slicing provides services across multiple network segments and different administrative domains. A 5G slice can combine resources that belong to different infrastructure providers [35]. Network slicing is the best way for network operators to build and manage a network that meets the requirements from a wide range of users. Network slicing provides service flexibility and the ability to deliver services faster with high security, isolation, and according to the quality of service (QoS) requirements of the different applications. This way, network operators can manage their network resources efficiently and provide differentiated and scalable services.

Slices are isolated from each other, which means that faults or errors in one slice do not affect the proper functioning of another slice.

Next, we introduce the main design elements of our proposed 5G network slicing architecture for child drowning prevention (see Figure 3).

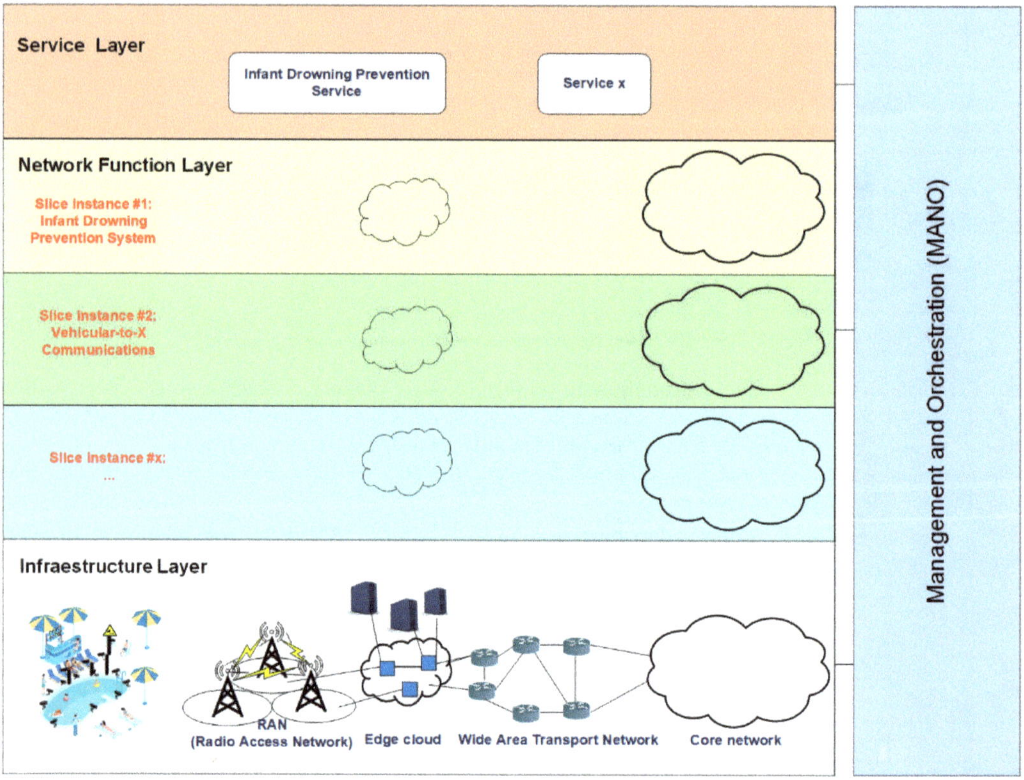

Figure 3. Network slicing architecture for child drowning prevention.

It is divided into three layers plus an additional management and orchestration layer, whose basic functionalities are summarized as follows:

Infrastructure layer: It refers to all of the parts of the physical network, because slices should be end-to-end. This layer includes the IoT networks, telecommunication networks, satellites, edge computing technologies, and the cloud. It provides the allocation of virtual or physical resources such as computing, storage, network, or radio.

We assume that all network devices are software defined networking (SDN)-enabled switches managed by SDN controllers that are able to program their routing tables.

The 5G core is generally divided into 'core—user plane' in charge of bearer delivery and 'core—control plane (CP)' in charge of control functions. Core—control plane will stay in the central cloud (network function virtualization, (NFV)), but 'core—user plane (UP)' will be distributed to its tens of edge nodes nationwide and be installed in edge clouds (NFV). Security, reliability, and latency will be critical for a 5G slice supporting the child drowning prevention case. For such a slice, all of the necessary (and potentially dedicated) network functions should be instantiated at the edge node. We consider that all the 5G core functions/units (UP) should be in the edge cloud close to the users. Multi-access edge computing (MEC) drastically reduces the latency between network nodes and remote servers in the cloud [36] because video processing servers are placed right where the core functions/units are located. This way, we can minimize the transmission delay to match the requirements of our delay-critical slice for such an MCC application. Furthermore, machine learning is crucial in supporting MCC by enabling a local decision making process at the edge servers [37].

Network function layer: It encapsulates all of the operations related to the configuration and life cycle management of the network functions that offer an end-to-end service. Network function virtualization (NFV) [38] and SDN (software-defined networking) [39] are two fundamental technologies to configure the virtual network resources. NFV decouples specific network functions from dedicated and expensive hardware platforms. This technology can provide software building blocks named VNFs (virtualized network functions) for the data plane that can be connected and chained according to the service type. SDN technology enables the separation of the control plane from the data plane to offer a flexible resource management.

Service layer: This layer provides a unified vision of the service requirements. Each service is represented by a service instance, which embeds all of the network characteristics that satisfy the SLA (service level agreement) requirements such as throughput or latency. A network slice instance (NSI) is a managed entity created by an operator's network with a lifecycle independent of the lifecycle of the service instance(s) [40]. An NSI provides the network characteristics required by a service instance. It is also possible that an NSI is shared across multiple service instances of a network operator.

Based on the main KPIs (see Section 3) and functional requirements of our use case, child drowning prevention, we propose that the drowning prevention slice has ultra-reliable and low-latency communications (URLLC) requirements. URLLC use cases (such as mission-critical applications) have stringent latency, reliability, and availability requirements.

Management and Orchestration (MANO): It is the framework for the management and orchestration of all network resources (computing, networking, storage, and virtual machine) in the cloud. It comprises three functional blocks: NFV orchestrator (NFVO), VNF manager (VNFM), and virtualized infrastructure manager (VIM). NFVO performs on-boarding of new network service and VNF packages, network service lifecycle management, and resource management. VNFM manages the lifecycle of VNF instances. VIM controls and manages the lifecycle of virtual resources as requested by the NFVO in an NFV infrastructure (NFVI) domain.

6. Convolutional Network Models

Convolutional neural networks (CNNs): They were created out of the need to be able to process images effectively and efficiently; nowadays, they are also used for speech recognition. However, their strength is in image processing. Next, we describe the CNNs used in our research.

VGG model: This architecture was proposed by Karen Simonyan and Andrew Zisserman [41]; it was the winner of the ImageNet Large-Scale Visual Recognition Challenge 2012 (ILSVRC12). It was designed with 16 hidden layers in VGG-16 and 19 hidden layers in VGG-19 versions. The architecture processes input images of size 224 × 224 pixels with three channels for color images (RGB). The image is passed through five convolutional blocks (Figure 4). In VGG-19, the first two blocks incorporate two convolutional layers and the remainders incoporate four convolutional layers. Each convolutional layer uses 3 × 3 filters and rectified linear unit (ReLU) as an activation function; the convolutional blocks also incorporate maxpooling layers to reduce image size and prevent overfitting problems; the upper layers are composed of two full-connected layers with 4096 neurons each, at the top, one output layer for image classification into 1000 different categories.

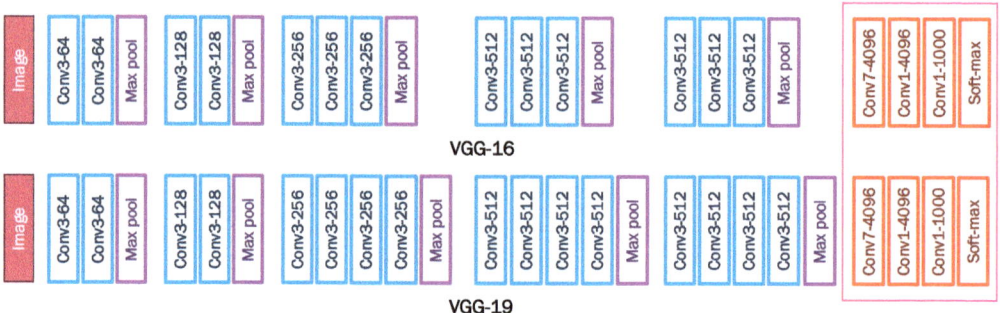

Figure 4. VGG-16 and VGG-19 architecture.

ResNet model: It is a type of advanced convolutional neural network; this model was proposed by Kaiming He in his 2016 document [42]. The ResNet-50 version consists of 50 layers. This model is based on the idea of residual and identity blocks that use skip connections (shortcut) (Figure 5), where the input is passed to a deeper layer. In other words, the simple deep convolutional neural network is inspired by VGG with 3 × 3 filters and a ReLU activation function, which is modified to become a residual network by adding skip connections to define residual blocks. On the top, the architecture contains a fully connected output layer with a softmax activation function for classification. Figure 6 shows the general configuration of the residual network architecture, including ResNet-50, ResNet-101, and ResNet-152.

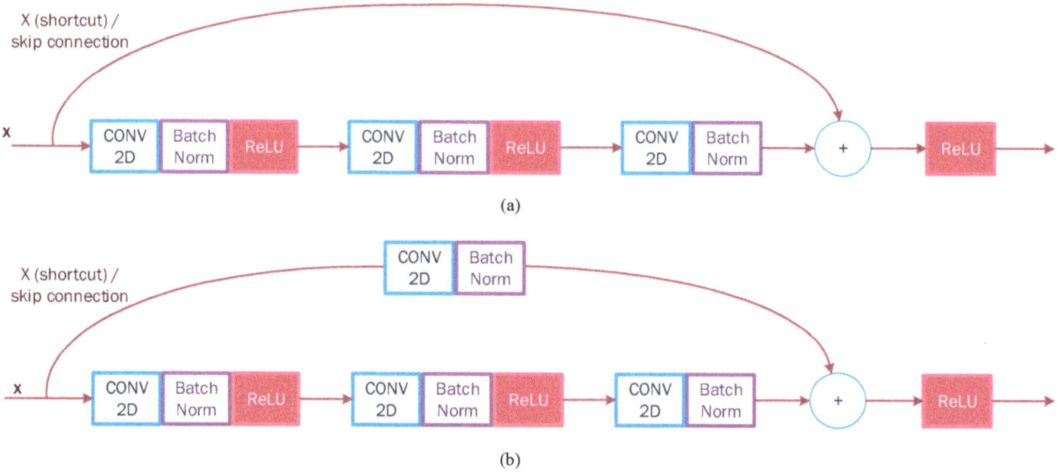

Figure 5. (**a**) ResNet identity block and (**b**) ResNet convolutional block.

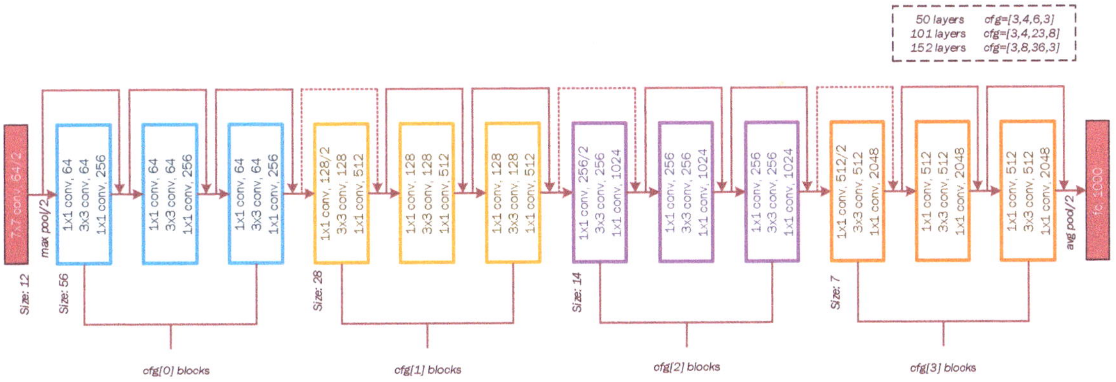

Figure 6. Configuration of residual network architecture, including ResNet-50, ResNet-101, and ResNet-152.

Inception-v3 model: This convolutional neural network was developed by Google. The first version of inception, called "GoogLeNet", was presented in the ImageNet Large-Scale Visual Recognition Challenge 2014 (ILSVRC14) [43]. This first version of the architecture is made up of 22 layers including convolutional, pooling, and a characteristic layer called inception; the latter is a type of convolutional layer, but it is characterized using only 1×1, 3×3, and 5×5 filters simultaneously (Inception blocks) (Figure 7); this way, the number of parameters to calculate is greatly reduced. This was achieved with what Google called bottlenecks, which were convolutional layers with 1×1 filters to reduce the complexity of the network. Google also includes auxiliary classifiers, intending to facilitate the propagation of the gradients backward and to reduce the cost involved Therefore, reducing the number of parameters and complexity resulted in a more powerful network.

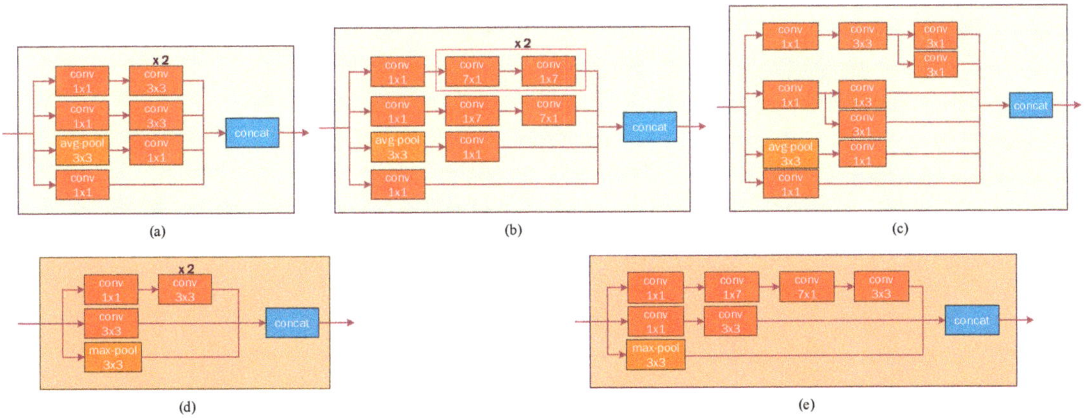

Figure 7. (**a**) Inception-A block, (**b**) inception-B block, (**c**) inception-C block, (**d**) reduction-A block, and (**e**) reduction-B.

Figure 8 shows the inception and reduction blocks that were set for the third version of this architecture.

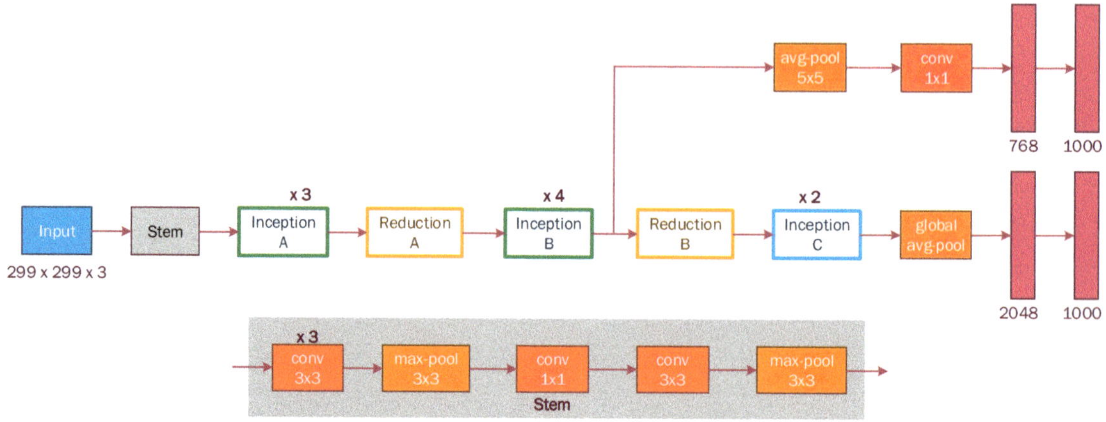

Figure 8. Inception-v3 architecture.

7. Experiments and Results

7.1. Dataset

The dataset is a collection of 38,000 images generated by us in the summer of 2019. The location of the video recording was the facilities of the Fontsanta swimming pool, located at Carrer del Marquès de Monistrol, 30, 08970 in Sant Joan Despí, Barcelona—Spain. Five primary caregivers (people in charge of the children) were involved in the development of these experiments. They were recorded on video, doing different activities (one video for each action related to each of the different categories) both inside and outside the water. The images captured from each video correspond to a specific category so that the images have been identified and labelled manually for each category. The capture was made taking into account that only the participants appear in the video to protect the privacy and confidentiality of other people who are at the swimming pool. The videos were recorded with high-resolution smart mobile devices (1920 × 1880), although the images are preprocessed according to the input data requirements of each model (224 × 224). The images were finally collected and classified into seven (7) categories:

- *I_distracted:* In the water distracted.
- *I_watching:* In the water watching the children.
- *O_distracted:* Out of the water distracted.
- *O_talk_cell:* Out of the water talking on a cell phone.
- *O_reading:* Out of the water reading a book.
- *O_chatting:* Out of the water chatting on a cell phone.
- *O_watching:* Out of the water watching the children.

To achieve a great performance during the training process with our own dataset, the videos were not shot from a single angle. Instead, they were shot from different angles, covering all potential perspectives of a caregiver. Furthermore, because the swimming pool is located outdoors, the varying lighting conditions throughout the day provide a richer dataset.

7.2. Experimental Settings

The dataset consists of approximately 38,000 images; it was split into two parts, keeping a ratio of 8:2, i.e., around 30,000 images for training and 8000 for testing. In addition, data augmentation was used to expand the training set and obtain better generalization. Data augmentation is a technique that expands our original training dataset virtually, through a random series of transformations from the original image, resulting in new plausible-looking images, in order to obtain a larger number of images for training. In computer vision, this technique became a standard for regularization, as well as to improve accuracy, generalization, and control of overfitting in CNNs. For this research, the techniques chosen are as follows: rescale = 1./255, rotation_range = 2, shear_range = 0.2, zoom_range = 0.2, and horizontal_flip = True.

We have selected the images from a different subject for testing purposes in order not to contaminate the testing set. Figures 9 and 10 show a set of images of each category with their training and testing labels.

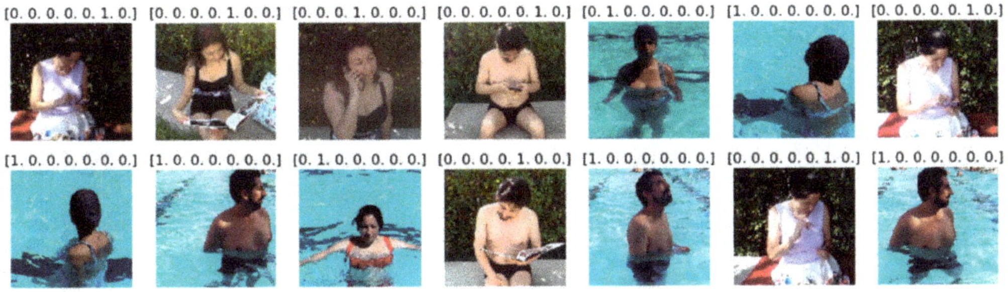

Figure 9. Image set of each category with their respective training labels.

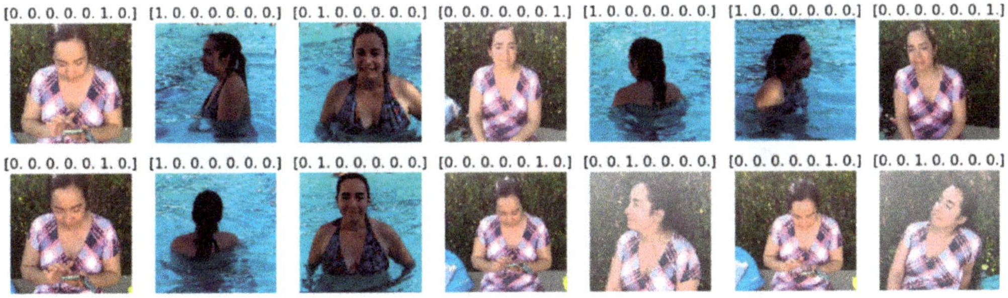

Figure 10. Image set of each category with their respective testing labels.

The algorithms were implemented in several Jupyter Notebooks in version 6.0.3 installed with anaconda programs suite, developed in Python. The experiments were carried out on a Lenovo computer 2.9 GHz Intel (R) Xeon (R) processor with 72 GB RAM, without GPU.

We implemented three different algorithms using the preset models from the python Keras library; each one was specifically adapted to obtain optimal results after each training. The transfer learning technique was used (further details will be provided in Section 7.4) to take advantage of the pre-trained weights. Early stopping and dropout were implemented as techniques to avoid overfitting to achieve an improvement of the generalization capacity. Accuracy was selected during the training process as a metric to evaluate the performance of each algorithm.

The setup of each model to be used is detailed below.

7.3. Convolutional Neural Network Architectures

In this paper, experiments were performed to evaluate the proposed approach with three different CNN architectures: VGG-19, ResNet-50, and Inception-v3. Table 2 presents a summary of the configuration for each model. For all experiments, we used an image size of $224 \times 224 \times 3$ and a batch size of 64.

Table 2. Architectures of the three CNN models.

Input	VGG-19 Image	ResNet-50 Image	Inception-v3 Image
Convolutional part	conv3-64 conv3-64 max pooling layer conv3-128 conv3-128 max pooling layer conv3-256 conv3-256 conv3-256 conv3-256 max-pooling layer conv3-512 conv3-512 conv3-512 conv3-512 max-pooling layer conv3-512 conv3-512 conv3-512 conv3-512 max-pooling layer	conv7-64, s = 2 max pooling layer [conv1-64; conv3-64; conv1-256]–[conv1-64] 2 blocks of [conv1-64; conv3-64; conv1-256] [conv3-128, s = 2; conv1-128; conv1-512]–[conv3-128, s = 2] 3 blocks of [conv1-128; conv3-128; conv1-512] [conv1-256, s = 2; conv3-256 conv1-1024]–[conv1-256, s = 2] 5 blocks of [conv1-256 conv3-256 conv1-1024] [conv1-512, s = 2; conv3-512; conv1-2048]–[conv1-512, s = 2] 2 blocks of [conv1-512 conv3-512 conv1-2048] global_average-pooling layer	Conv3-32, s = 2 Conv3-32 Conv3-64 max pooling layer Conv3-80 Conv3-192, s = 2 max pooling layer Inception A-256 Inception A-288 Inception A-288 Reduction A-768 Inception B-768 Inception B-768 Inception B-768 Inception B-768 Reduction B-1280 Inception C-2048 Inception C-2048 global_average-pooling layer
MLP classifier	FC layer-4096 FC layer-4096 FC layer-07	FC layer-2048 FC layer-2048 FC layer-07	FC layer-2048 FC layer-2048 FC layer-07

7.3.1. VGG-19

We implemented the VGG-19 version because it has a greater number of layers (deeper network) compared with the VGG-16 version mentioned above. It is made up of a 224 × 224 × 3 input layer, five convolutional blocks with kernel 3 × 3, ReLU activation function, without padding, and a maxpooling layer after each block followed by a flattened layer and two additional blocks; each additional block consists of a fully connected dense layer with 4092 neurons, a BatchNormalization layer, and a dropout layer. The last layer is a dense layer with a softmax activation function that contains seven neurons to classify our categories.

7.3.2. ResNet-50

This model contains an input layer of 224 × 224 × 3, fifty convolutional blocks with their respective skip connections, followed by a global average pooling layer. At the top of the model, we have added two additional blocks; each block consists of a fully connected dense layer with 2048 neurons, a BatchNormalization layer, and a dropout layer. The last layer is a dense layer with a softmax activation function that contains seven neurons for our classification.

7.3.3. Inception-v3

This model is composed of a 224 × 224 × 3 input layer, two convolutional blocks of three and two layers, followed by a maxpooling layer after each block. In the central part, it consists of several types of inception and reduction blocks, along with a global_average-pooling layer. At the top of the model, we added two additional blocks; each block consists of a dense layer fully connected with 2048 neurons, a BatchNormalization layer, and a dropout layer. The last layer is a dense layer with a softmax activation function that contains seven neurons for our classification.

7.4. Training

The dataset consists of approximately 38,000 images (N records); it was split into two parts, keeping a ratio of 8:2, i.e., around 30,000 images for the training set (n records) and 8000 for the testing set (N−n records). For the training, we applied cross-validation.

Cross-validation is a technique commonly used to validate machine learning models and estimate the performance of the model trained on unseen data. The most robust and widely used method of cross-validation is K iterations or K-fold cross-validation. This method consists of splitting the training dataset into K subsets (see Figure 11). During iterations, each of the subsets are used as validation data or testing folds and the rest (K−1) as training data or training folds. The cross-validation process is performed repeatedly for K iterations, with each of the subsets of validation data. The arithmetic average of the results of each iteration is finally performed to obtain a single result. This method is highly efficient as we evaluate it from K combinations of training and validation data, but it still has a disadvantage, that is, computationally, it is slow. However, the choice of the number of iterations depends on how large the dataset is. Cross-validation is most commonly used with K values ranging from 5 to 10. If the model (estimator) is a classifier and the target variable (y) is binary or multiclass (as in this research), the StratifiedKfold technique is used by default. This approach introduces stratified folds, i.e., by keeping the proportion of samples from each class in all folds. Therefore, the data from the training and testing folds are distributed equally. It is useful when unbalanced datasets are used. To evaluate the results, we used several metrics that are very common in machine learning applications for classification problems.

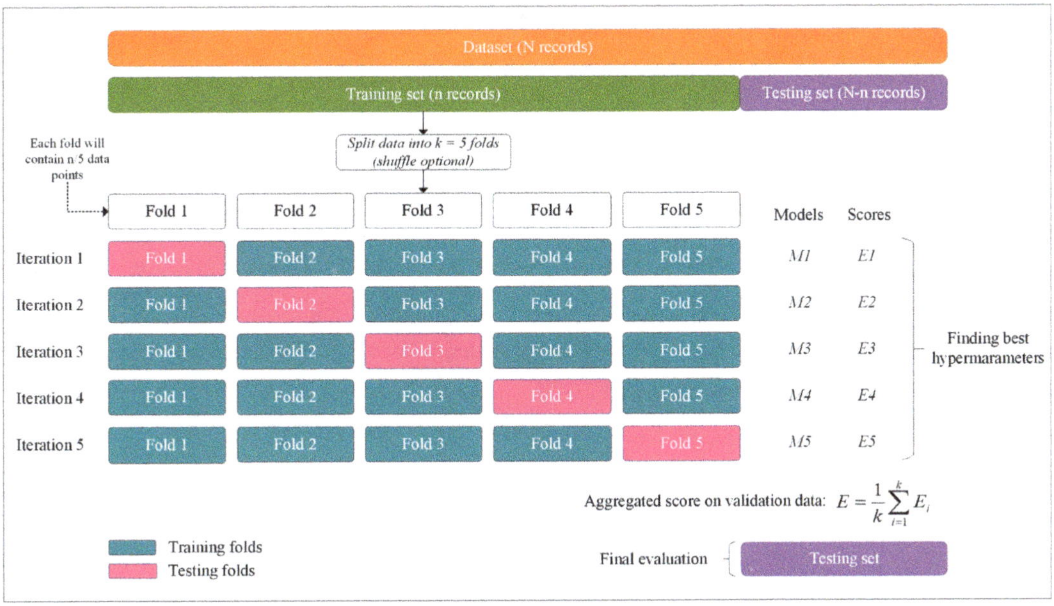

Figure 11. Use of each fold in the cross-validation process (fivefold representation).

7.4.1. Loss or Cost Function

A loss function is employed to optimize a machine learning algorithm. Several different cost functions can be used. Each of them penalizes errors differently. The loss function most commonly used in deep neural networks for classification problems is cross-entropy. In this research, we employed categorical cross-entropy. Categorical cross-entropy is a loss function that is used in multi-class classification tasks, where a sample can be considered to belong only to a specific category with a probability of 1 and to other categories with a probability of 0, and the model must decide which category each one belongs to.

7.4.2. Transfer Learning and Early Stopping

A model can be trained from scratch when it is not very large or when the necessary computational capacity for its execution is available. On the other hand, it is possible to take advantage of the benefits of pre-established models and use them in new models. This technique is known as transfer learning; this means that it allows us to transfer learning from a pre-trained model such as VGG-19, ResNet-50, Inception-v3, and so on (pre-trained models for 1000 objects' classification) and apply it to new classification algorithms. Furthermore, it is possible to unfreeze some pre-trained layers by adapting the model (fine-tuning) to re-train them along with the new fully connected layers; this method implies increasing the training time to avoid overfitting problems and to obtain optimal performance from the algorithm.

A popular technique to overcome overfitting is early stopping. For this purpose, at each iteration, the training set is divided into training and validation folds. The training folds are used to train the model and the validation folds are used as validation data at each iteration. In each training of the model, the validation folds help us to verify the accuracy of the model at the end of each epoch. Therefore, as soon as the test error starts to increase, the training is stopped.

7.5. Evaluation Metrics

To evaluate the results, we used several metrics that are very common in machine learning applications for classification problems.

7.5.1. Accuracy

It is defined as the number of predictions made correctly by the model of the total number of records.

$$accuracy = \frac{TP + TN}{TP + FP + FN + TN} \tag{1}$$

where TP represents true positives, TN represents true negatives, FP represents false positives, and FN represents false negatives.

7.5.2. Precision

We evaluate our data for its performance of "positive" predictions.

$$precision = \frac{TP}{TP + FP} \tag{2}$$

7.5.3. Recall (Sensitivity) (True Positive Rate)

It is calculated as the number of correct positive predictions divided by the total number of positives.

$$recall = \frac{TP}{TP + FN} \tag{3}$$

7.5.4. Specificity (True Negative Rate)

It is calculated as the number of correct negative predictions divided by the total number of negatives.

$$specificity = \frac{TN}{TN + FP} \tag{4}$$

7.5.5. F1 Score

It is the weighted average of precision and sensitivity. Therefore, this score takes into account both false positives and false negatives.

$$F1\ score = 2 \times \frac{(precision \times recall)}{(precision + recall)} \tag{5}$$

7.5.6. Loss

Loss is the value that reflects the sum of errors in our model. It indicates whether the model is performing well (high value) or not (low value); on the other hand, the accuracy can be defined as the number of correct predictions divided by the number of total predictions.

Therefore, if we analyze these two metrics together (loss and accuracy) (see Table 3), we can deduce more information about the model performance. If loss and accuracy are low, it implies that the model makes small errors in most of the data. However, if both are high, it makes large errors in some of the data. Low accuracy but high loss would mean that the model makes large errors in most of the data. However, if the accuracy is high and the loss is low, then the model makes small errors in only some of the data, which would be the ideal case.

Table 3. Analysis of both loss and accuracy metrics together.

	Low Loss	**High Loss**
Low Accuracy	A lot of small errors	A lot of big errors
High Accuracy	A few small errors	A few big errors

7.6. *Experimental Results*

After training with different configurations in the upper layers of each model, the following results were obtained.

7.6.1. Loss and Accuracy

For training, cross validation was performed; therefore, the early stopping technique was used to avoid overfitting (as mentioned above); thus, training is stopped once it has reached the maximum accuracy value. Furthermore, the checkpoint was used to save the weights of the trained model when a new maximum value arises and we can load it in the future. Table 4 shows a summary of the accuracy and loss for the training and testing of each model. We can see that, for training, all models achieve an accuracy above 99% and ResNet-50 achieves a higher loss value compared with the other two models. Furthermore, for testing, ResNet-50 achieves the highest accuracy, but also the largest loss of 98% and 0.3203, respectively. VGG-19 achieves an accuracy of 94% and the lowest loss of 0.0039 and, finally, Inception-v3 achieves an accuracy of 90% and a loss of 0.0364. Based on the accuracy, ResNet-50 has developed much better performance compared with the other trained models.

Table 4. Accuracy and loss for VGG-19, ResNet-50, and Inception-v3 model.

Models	**Training**		**Testing**	
	Accuracy	**Loss**	**Accuracy**	**Loss**
VGG-19	0.9987	0.0056	0.9445	0.0039
ResNet-50	0.9973	0.0110	0.9803	0.3203
Inception-v3	0.9993	0.0019	0.9044	0.0364

Table 5 shows the accuracy achieved by each model with each of the classification categories (seven), evidencing the performance in more detail. VGG-19 achieves an accuracy of 100% for I_watching and O_reading categories, an average accuracy of 97.42% for the remaining categories, and a lower value of 72.73% for the O_chatting category. Similarly, ResNet-50 achieves an accuracy of 100% for the I_watching and O_talk_cell categories and the worst result for the O_distracted category, with an accuracy of 95.4%. On the other hand, Inception-v3 achieves a high accuracy of 98.68% for the I_distracted category and a lower accuracy of 66.6% for the O_talk_cell category.

Table 5. Accuracy of each model with each category.

Parent Status	VGG-19 Accuracy (%)	ResNet-50 Accuracy (%)	Inception-v3 Accuracy (%)	Total Samples
I_distracted	98.99	97.75	98.68	1291
I_watching	100	100	96.83	883
O_distracted	92.32	95.4	95.2	1458
O_talk_cell	98.75	100	66.6	1036
O_reading	100	97.85	94.29	1069
O_chatting	72.73	97.97	90.91	935
O_watching	99.61	99.61	84.42	507

As this research work focuses on parental distraction detection for child drowning prevention, the "In the water watching the children" (I_watching) and "Out of the water watching the children" (O_watching) categories are the most relevant ones to detect if parents/caregivers are really supervising their children. All of the other categories just represent that the caregivers are distracted and should be warned. For I_watching, the VGG-19 and ResNet-50 models achieve an accuracy of 100% and Inception-v3 achieves an accuracy of 96.83%. Likewise, for O_watching, the VGG-19 and ResNet-50 models achieve an accuracy of 99.61% and Inception-v3 achieves an accuracy of 84.42% (Table 4).

7.6.2. Precision, Recall, and F1-Score

Accuracy should not be considered as a single metric for measuring model performance when using an unbalanced data set, as it counts the number of correct predictions regardless of the type of category, leaning towards the majority categories. In other words, from a dataset of 100 cases where 95 belong to the category "a" and five to category "b", if only all the cases in the first category are correctly predicted, an accuracy of 95% would be obtained. This value is misleading because 95% refers only to the correctly predicted values of one category (50% of the total predictions).

Because our data are unbalanced, we also consider other metrics such as recall, precision, specificity, and F1-score to evaluate our results. Table 6 shows the values obtained in every category based on the above-mentioned metrics for VGG-19. F1-score is the harmonic mean of precision and recall and it takes into account both false positives and false negatives. The VGG-19 model performs well because it achieves an accuracy between 96% and 99% for most categories and a smaller accuracy of 84% for the *O_reading* category. We can also observe that, for the most relevant categories (I_watching and O_watching), this model reaches an F1-score of 98%, demonstrating good performance in training.

Table 6. Evaluation metrics of the VGG-19 model.

Category	Precision	Recall	F1-Score	Total Samples
I_distracted	0.99	0.99	0.99	1291
I_watching	0.98	1.00	0.98	883
O_distracted	0.96	0.92	0.96	1458
O_talk_cell	0.99	0.99	0.99	1036
O_reading	0.87	1.00	0.87	1069
O_chatting	0.84	0.73	0.84	935
O_watching	0.98	1.00	0.98	507

Table 7 shows a summary of the already mentioned metrics in every category for the ResNet-50 model. It achieves an F1-score between 97% and 99% for all categories. It should be pointed out that this model reaches an F1-score of 98% and 99% for the most relevant categories (I_watching and O_watching), which is the best performance of the three models.

Table 7. Evaluation metrics of the ResNet-50 model.

Category	Precision	Recall	F1-Score	Total Samples
I_distracted	1.00	0.98	0.99	1291
I_watching	0.97	1.00	0.98	883
O_distracted	0.99	0.95	0.97	1458
O_talk_cell	0.95	1.00	0.98	1036
O_reading	1.00	0.98	0.99	1069
O_chatting	0.96	0.98	0.97	935
O_watching	0.98	1.00	0.99	507

Finally, Table 8 shows a summary of the already mentioned metrics in every category for the Inception-v3 model. This model achieves an F1-score between 91% and 98% for most categories, and a minimum F1-score of 79% for the O_talk_cell category. In this case, the Inception-v3 model achieves an F1-score of 98% for the I_watching category, but the lowest F1-score of 84% for the O_watching category (most relevant categories).

Table 8. Evaluation metrics of the Inception-v3 model.

Category	Precision	Recall	F1-Score	Total Samples
I_distracted	0.98	0.99	0.98	1291
I_watching	0.98	0.97	0.98	883
O_distracted	0.75	0.95	0.84	1458
O_talk_cell	0.98	0.67	0.79	1036
O_reading	0.98	0.94	0.96	1069
O_chatting	0.92	0.91	0.91	935
O_watching	0.84	0.84	0.84	507

According to this, we conclude that the ResNet-50 model shows excellent performance for this classification problem, reaching F1-scores of 98% and 99% in the I_watching and O_watching categories, respectively (see Table 7). However, the VGG-19 model with a value of 98% in the mentioned categories shows a solid performance as well (see Table 6).

7.6.3. Confusion Matrix, False Positive Rate, and False Negative Rate

Figures 12–14 show the confusion matrices for each model. The main diagonal shows the number of matches found for each category between the true labels (columns) and the predicted labels (rows).

All categories are well predicted. Considering the most relevant categories "In the water watching the children" (I_watching) and "Out of the water watching the children" (O_watching) mentioned above, it is possible to have some wrong predictions, which means that, in some cases, certain distractions have not been detected. The three models sometimes classify distracted behaviors of caregivers as 'watching the children' (false positives). These cases represent a risk for children's safety, but fortunately, do not occur often compared with the true positive values for these categories. Inception-v3 obtains less false positives for I_watching, with 14 versus 27 and 29 cases for VGG-19 and ResNet-50, respectively. ResNet-50 obtains less false positives for O_watching, with 8 versus 21 and 79 cases for VGG-19 and Inception-v3, respectively. We define the false positive rate as subtracting 1 from the specificity or as dividing false positives by the sum of false positives and true negatives. The false-positive rate for I_watching and the three models VGG-19, ResNet-50, and Inception-v3 is 0.43%, 0.46%, and 0.22%, respectively. The false-positive rate for O_watching and the three models (VGG-19, ResNet-50, and Inception-v3) is 0.31%, 0.12%, and 1.18%, respectively. In terms of the false-positive rate, we observe that the obtained values are always very small; VGG-19 and ResNet-50 perform a little worse than Inception-v3 for I_watching. ResNet-50 shows clearly the best results for O_watching.

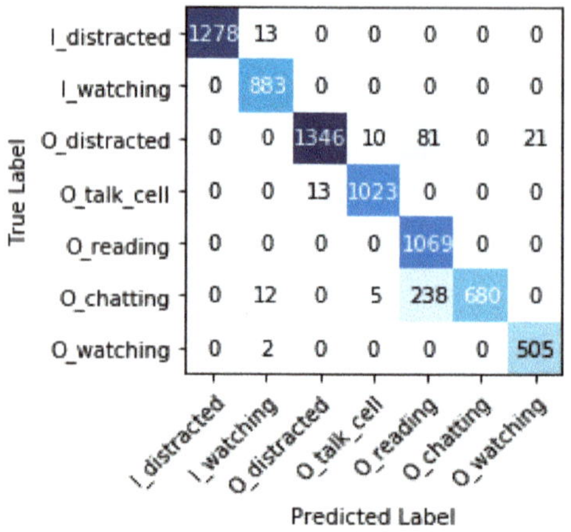

Figure 12. Confusion matrix VGG-19.

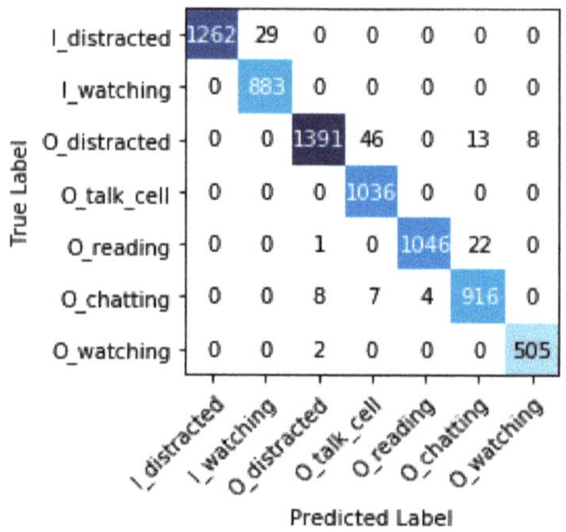

Figure 13. Confusion matrix ResNet-50.

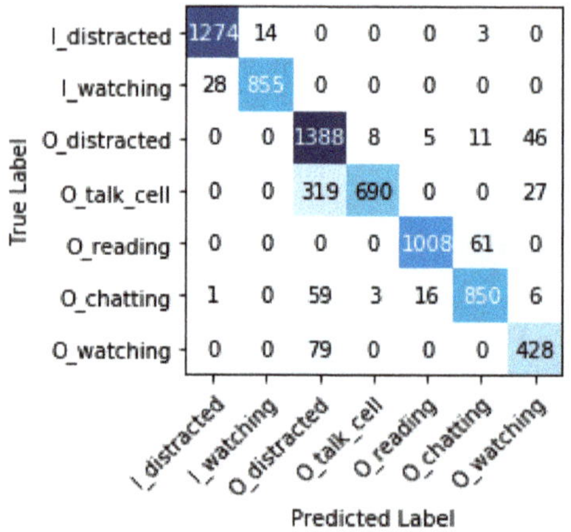

Figure 14. Confusion matrix Inception-v3.

Furthermore, the three models sometimes classify "watching the children" as distracted behaviors (false negatives). These cases do not pose any risk, but could be annoying for caregivers who are warned to supervise the children when they actually were doing so. ResNet-50 and VGG-19 do not obtain any false negatives for I_watching versus 28 cases for Inception-v3. ResNet-50 and VGG-19 obtain less false negatives for O_watching, with 2 cases each, versus 79 cases for Inception-v3. If we also consider the false-negative rate for the most relevant categories (we define the false-negative rate as subtracting one from recall), we can see that, for I_watching and the two models VGG-19 and ResNet-50, it is 0% and, for Inception-v3, it is 3.17%. The false-negative rate for O_watching and the two models VGG-19 and ResNet-50 is 0.39% and, for Inception-v3, it is 15.58%. The false-negative rates obtained are very small (with the exception of the O_watching category for Inception-v3). These results show that, for VGG-19 and ResNet-50, the child drowning prevention system works correctly with a minimal error rate versus Inception-v3.

8. Conclusions and Future Work

In this paper, a novel 5G and beyond child drowning prevention system that detects distracted parents or caregivers and alerts them to focus on active child supervision in swimming pools was developed. For this purpose, we evaluated and implemented three well-known CNN models: ResNet-50, VGG-19, and Inception-v3, to process and classify images. The proposed deep CNN models have revealed that they can be used to automatically detect (based on images) possible distractions of a caregiver who is supervising a child and generate alerts to warn them.

The proposed child drowning prevention system can successfully perform a seven-class classification with very high accuracies of 98% for ResNet-50, 94% for VGG-19, and 90% for Inception-v3. VGG-19 and ResNet-50 achieve the same high performance in the most relevant categories I_watching and O_watching, with accuracies of 100% and 99.61%, respectively. For I_watching, the three models achieve an F1-score of 98%. For O_watching, they reach a F1-score of 98%, 99%, and 84% for VGG-19, ResNet-50, and Inception-V3, respectively. In terms of false-positive rate, the obtained values are always very small; VGG-19 and ResNet-50 perform a little worse than Inception-v3 for I_watching. ResNet-50 shows the best results for O_watching. The false-negative rates obtained are also very small (with exception of the O_watching category for Inception-v3). VGG-19 and ResNet-50 models perform quite well with a minimal false-negative rate versus Inception-v3 for I_watching and O_watching of 0% and 0.39%, respectively. ResNet-50, compared with the other models performs a better classification for most categories. According to the results reached in this research, the proposed system was tested in a swimming pool, but we think it could also be implemented even in swimming lakes or beaches to avoid possible child drowning.

On the other hand, special attention must be paid to security/privacy. Although there is no doubt that distracted parent detection can save lives, associated privacy and security issues need to be analyzed to make our child drowning system socially acceptable. These issues include access rights to data (video images), storage of data, security of data transfer, data analysis rights, and the governing policies. The proposed child drowning prevention system may be vulnerable to a variety of active and passive security attacks (such as eavesdropping) with disastrous consequences (especially if unauthorized parties access underage images). For this reason, security and privacy risks should be minimized by applying existing technical solutions such as encryption, authentication mechanisms, and cryptographic access control during data collection and transmission, encryption message digests, and hashing to assure the integrity of data during data storage and processing. In addition, further works are also required to maintain the security and confidentiality of data by introducing advanced encryption-based techniques. All of these security and privacy challenges must be addressed so that the proposed child drowning prevention system comes out as a promising way to increase swimming pool safety.

We can define the total reaction time as the time elapsing from an observation (image), its transmission to the edge server, the image processing for activity recognition, and the transmission of an alert (if necessary) based on the observation ($D = D_{UE} + D_{Uplink} + D_{processing} + D_{Downlink}$). As future work, we would like to run the entire system (processing of the images with the neural network and transmission using 5G) in real time. The expected response time for our child drowning prevention system would be around twenty milliseconds (see Table 1). Neural networks have an infinitesimal response time once the weights and the topology have been defined [44]. Further, 5G has been designed to address the requirements of ultra reliable and low-latency communications (URLLC). URLLC has stringent requirements for capabilities such as latency, reliability, and availability. Some use cases include wireless control of industrial manufacturing or production processes, remote medical surgery, and transportation safety. Therefore, 5G is the appropriate technology for our use case.

Author Contributions: Conceptualization, J.C.C.-P. and M.C.D.; formal analysis, J.C.C.-P. and M.C.D.; investigation, J.C.C.-P.; methodology, J.C.C.-P.; software, J.C.C.-P.; supervision, M.C.D.; validation, J.C.C.-P.; writing—original draft, J.C.C.-P.; writing—review & editing, J.C.C.-P. and M.C.D. All authors have read and agreed to the published version of the manuscript.

Funding: This work was supported by the Agencia Estatal de Investigación of Ministerio de Ciencia e Innovación of Spain under project PID2019-108713RB-C51 MCIN/AEI/10.13039/501100011033.

Institutional Review Board Statement: Not applicable.

Informed Consent Statement: Not applicable.

Data Availability Statement: Not applicable.

Conflicts of Interest: The authors declare that they have no known competing financial interest or personal relationships that could have appeared to influence the work reported in this paper.

References

1. Meddings, D.; Altieri, E.; Bierens, J.; Cassell, E.; Gissing, A.; Guevarra, J. Preventing Drowning: An Implementation Guide. Available online: http://apps.who.int/iris/bitstream/10665/255196/1/9789241511933-eng.pdf?ua=1 (accessed on 15 February 2021).
2. World Health Organization Global Report on Drowning: Preventing a Leading Killer. Available online: http://apps.who.int/iris/bitstream/10665/143893/1/9789241564786_eng.pdf?ua=1&ua=1 (accessed on 5 April 2021).
3. Centers for Disease Control and Prevention. *N.C. for I.P. and C. WISQARS (Web-Based Injury Statistics Query and Reporting System)*. Available online: http://www.cdc.gov/injury/wisqars (accessed on 9 May 2021).
4. Lawler, K. More Than 600 Children Drown Every Year. Available online: http://search.ebscohost.com/login.aspx?direct=true&db=rzh&AN=116135707&site=ehost-live (accessed on 13 June 2021).
5. Royal Life Saving, Exploring Risk at Communal, Public and Commercial Swimming Pools A 10 Year Analysis of Drowning in Aquatic Facilities. 2018, pp. 1–48. Available online: https://www.royallifesaving.com.au/__data/assets/pdf_file/0009/37557/RLS_PublicPools_10YearReport.pdf (accessed on 20 June 2021).
6. Connolly, K. Child Drownings in Germany Linked to Parents' Phone "Fixation". Available online: https://www.theguardian.com/lifeandstyle/2018/aug/15/parents-fixated-by-phones-linked-to-child-drownings-in-germany (accessed on 17 August 2021).
7. Dunne, J. Kids Are Drowning Because Their Parents Are Distracted by Devices. Available online: https://10daily.com.au/news/australia/a180816zwp/kids-are-drowning-because-their-parents-are-distracted-by-devices-20180816 (accessed on 17 August 2021).
8. Alotaibi, A. Automated and Intelligent System for Monitoring Swimming Pool Safety Based on the IoT and Transfer Learning. *Electronics* **2020**, *9*, 2082. [CrossRef]
9. Jalalifar, S.; Kashizadeh, A.; Mahmood, I.; Belford, A.; Drake, N.; Razmjou, A.; Asadnia, M. A Smart Multi-Sensor Device to Detect Distress in Swimmers. *Sensors* **2022**, *22*, 1059. [CrossRef]
10. Burnay, C.; Anderson, D.I.; Button, C.; Cordovil, R.; Peden, A.E. Infant Drowning Prevention: Insights from a New Ecological Psychology Approach. *Int. J. Environ. Res. Public Health* **2022**, *19*, 4567. [CrossRef] [PubMed]
11. Meniere, J. System for Monitoring a Swimming Pool to Prevent Drowning Accidents 2000. U.S. Patent 6,133,838, 17 October 2000.
12. Menoud, E. Alarm and Monitoring Device for the Presumption of Bodies in Danger in a Swimming Pool. U.S. Patent 5,886,630, 23 March 1999.
13. Zhang, C.; Li, X.; Lei, F. *A Novel Camera-Based Drowning Detection Algorithm*; Springer: Berlin/Heidelberg, Germany, 2015; pp. 224–233. [CrossRef]
14. Lu, W.; Tan, Y.P. A camera-based system for early detection of drowning incidents. In Proceedings of the International Conference on Image Processing, Rochester, NY, USA, 22–25 September 2002; Volume 3, pp. 445–448. [CrossRef]

15. Lu, W.; Tan, Y.P. A Vision-Based Approach to Early Detection of Drowning Incidents in Swimming Pools. *IEEE Trans. Circuits Syst. Video Technol.* **2004**, *14*, 159–178. [CrossRef]
16. Kam, A.H.; Lu, W.; Yau, W.Y. A video-based drowning detection system. In Proceedings of the European Conference on Computer Vision, Copenhagen, Denmark, 28–31 May 2002; Volume 2353, pp. 297–311. [CrossRef]
17. Victor, B.; He, Z.; Morgan, S.; Miniutti, D. Continuous video to simple signals for swimming stroke detection with convolutional neural networks. In Proceedings of the IEEE Conference on Computer Vision and Pattern Recognition Workshops, Honolulu, HI, USA, 21–26 July 2017; pp. 122–131. [CrossRef]
18. Eng, H.L.; Toh, K.A.; Kam, A.H.; Wang, J.; Yau, W.Y. An automatic drowning detection surveillance system for challenging outdoor pool environments. In Proceedings of the Computer Vision, IEEE International Conference on, Nice, France, 13–16 October 2003; Volume 1, pp. 532–539. [CrossRef]
19. Chan, K.L. Detection of Swimmer Using Dense Optical Flow Motion Map and Intensity Information. *Mach. Vis. Appl.* **2013**, *24*, 75–101. [CrossRef]
20. Eng, H.L.; Wang, J.; Siew Wah, A.H.K.; Yau, W.Y. Robust Human Detection within a Highly Dynamic Aquatic Environment in Real Time. *IEEE Trans. Image Process.* **2006**, *15*, 1583–1600. [CrossRef]
21. Cosoli, G.; Antognoli, L.; Veroli, V.; Scalise, L. Accuracy and Precision of Wearable Devices for Real-Time Monitoring of Swimming Athletes. *Sensors* **2022**, *22*, 4726. [CrossRef]
22. Costa, J.; Silva, C.; Santos, M.; Fernandes, T.; Faria, S. Framework for Intelligent Swimming Analytics with Wearable Sensors for Stroke Classification. *Sensors* **2021**, *21*, 5162. [CrossRef]
23. Kałamajska, E.; Misiurewicz, J.; Weremczuk, J. Wearable Pulse Oximeter for Swimming Pool Safety. *Sensors* **2022**, *22*, 3823. [CrossRef]
24. Zhu, Z.; Liu, T.; Li, G.; Li, T.; Inoue, Y. Wearable Sensor Systems for Infants. *Sensors* **2015**, *15*, 3721–3749. [CrossRef]
25. Jiao, L.; Zhang, F.; Liu, F.; Yang, S.; Li, L.; Feng, Z.; Qu, R. A Survey of Deep Learning-Based Object Detection. *IEEE Access* **2019**, *7*, 128837–128868. [CrossRef]
26. Jensen, M.B.; Gade, R.; Moeslund, T.B. Swimming pool occupancy analysis using deep learning on low quality video. In Proceedings of the MMSports 2018—Proceedings of the 1st International Workshop on Multimedia Content Analysis in Sports, Co-Located with MM 2018, Seoul, Korea, 26 October 2018; pp. 67–73.
27. Eng, H.L.; Toh, K.A.; Yau, W.Y.; Wang, J. DEWS: A Live Visual Surveillance System for Early Drowning Detection at Pool. *IEEE Trans. Circuits Syst. Video Technol.* **2008**, *18*, 196–210. [CrossRef]
28. Carballo-Fazanes, A.; Bierens, J.J.L.M. The Visible Behaviour of Drowning Persons: A Pilot Observational Study Using Analytic Software and a Nominal Group Technique. *Int. J. Environ. Res. Public Health* **2020**, *17*, 6930. [CrossRef] [PubMed]
29. Alotaibi, M.; Alotaibi, B. Distracted Driver Classification Using Deep Learning. *Signal Image Video Process.* **2020**, *14*, 617–624. [CrossRef]
30. Tran, D.; Do, H.M.; Sheng, W.; Bai, H.; Chowdhary, G. Real-Time Detection of Distracted Driving Based on Deep Learning. *IET Intell. Transp. Syst.* **2018**, *12*, 1210–1219. [CrossRef]
31. Eraqi, H.M.; Abouelnaga, Y.; Saad, M.H.; Moustafa, M.N. Driver Distraction Identification with an Ensemble of Convolutional Neural Networks. *J. Adv. Transp.* **2019**, *2019*, 4125865. [CrossRef]
32. *TS 122 280-V15.3.0-LTE*; Mission Critical Services Common Requirements (3GPP TS 22.280 Version 15.3.0 Release 15). ETSI: Sophia Antipolis, France, 2018.
33. Maldonado, R.; Karstensen, A.; Pocovi, G.; Esswie, A.A.; Rosa, C.; Alanen, O.; Kasslin, M.; Kolding, T. Comparing Wi-Fi 6 and 5G Downlink Performance for Industrial IoT. *IEEE Access* **2021**, *9*, 86928–86937. [CrossRef]
34. ETSI. ETSI 5G; System Architecture for the 5G System (3GPP TS 23.501 Version 15.2.0 Release 15). *Eur. Telecommun. Stand. Inst. Tech. Rep. V15.2.0* **2018**, *15*, 4–220.
35. NGMN Alliance. *Next Generation Mobile Networks Alliance 5G Initiative 5G White Paper*; NGMN Alliance: Frankfurt am Main, Germany, 2015; p. 124. [CrossRef]
36. Shi, W.; Cao, J.; Zhang, Q.; Li, Y.; Xu, L. Edge Computing: Vision and Challenges. *IEEE Internet Things J.* **2016**, *3*, 637–646. [CrossRef]
37. Elbamby, M.S.; Perfecto, C.; Liu, C.F.; Park, J.; Samarakoon, S.; Chen, X.; Bennis, M. Wireless Edge Computing with Latency and Reliability Guarantees. *Proc. IEEE* **2019**, *107*, 1717–1737. [CrossRef]
38. Mijumbi, R.; Serrat, J.; Gorricho, J.L.; Bouten, N.; De Turck, F.; Boutaba, R. Network Function Virtualization: State-of-the-Art and Research Challenges. *IEEE Commun. Surv. Tutor.* **2016**, *18*, 236–262. [CrossRef]
39. Kreutz, D.; Ramos, F.M.V.; Veríssimo, P.E.; Rothenberg, C.E.; Azodolmolky, S.; Uhlig, S. Software-Defined Networking: A Comprehensive Survey. *Proc. IEEE* **2015**, *103*, 14–76. [CrossRef]
40. NGMN Alliance. *NGMN Alliance Description of Network Slicing Concept by NGMN Alliance*; Ngmn 5G P; NGMN Alliance: Frankfurt am Main, Germany, 2016; Volume 1, p. 19.
41. Simonyan, K.; Zisserman, A. Very deep convolutional networks for large-scale image recognition. In Proceedings of the 3rd International Conference on Learning Representations, ICLR 2015—Conference Track Proceedings, San Diego, CA, USA, 7–9 May 2015; pp. 1–14.
42. He, K.; Zhang, X.; Ren, S.; Sun, J. Deep Residual Learning for Image Recognition. In Proceedings of the IEEE Computer Society Conference on Computer Vision and Pattern Recognition, Las Vegas, NV, USA, 27–30 June 2016; pp. 770–778.

43. Szegedy, C.; Vanhoucke, V.; Ioffe, S.; Shlens, J.; Wojna, Z. Rethinking the inception architecture for computer vision. In Proceedings of the IEEE Computer Society Conference on Computer Vision and Pattern Recognition, Las Vegas, NV, USA, 27–30 June 2016; pp. 2818–2826.
44. Tango, F.; Botta, M. Real-Time Detection System of Driver Distraction Using Machine Learning. *IEEE Trans. Intell. Transp. Syst.* **2013**, *14*, 894–905. [CrossRef]

sensors

MDPI

Article

Machine Learning Sensors for Diagnosis of COVID-19 Disease Using Routine Blood Values for Internet of Things Application

Andrei Velichko [1,*], Mehmet Tahir Huyut [2,*], Maksim Belyaev [1], Yuriy Izotov [1] and Dmitry Korzun [3]

1 Institute of Physics and Technology, Petrozavodsk State University, 33 Lenin Ave., 185910 Petrozavodsk, Russia
2 Department of Biostatistics and Medical Informatics, Faculty of Medicine, Erzincan Binali Yıldırım University, 24000 Erzincan, Türkiye
3 Department of Computer Science, Institute of Mathematics and Information Technology, Petrozavodsk State University, 33 Lenin Ave., 185910 Petrozavodsk, Russia
* Correspondence: velichko@petrsu.ru (A.V.); tahir.huyut@erzincan.edu.tr (M.T.H.)

Abstract: Healthcare digitalization requires effective applications of human sensors, when various parameters of the human body are instantly monitored in everyday life due to the Internet of Things (IoT). In particular, machine learning (ML) sensors for the prompt diagnosis of COVID-19 are an important option for IoT application in healthcare and ambient assisted living (AAL). Determining a COVID-19 infected status with various diagnostic tests and imaging results is costly and time-consuming. This study provides a fast, reliable and cost-effective alternative tool for the diagnosis of COVID-19 based on the routine blood values (RBVs) measured at admission. The dataset of the study consists of a total of 5296 patients with the same number of negative and positive COVID-19 test results and 51 routine blood values. In this study, 13 popular classifier machine learning models and the LogNNet neural network model were exanimated. The most successful classifier model in terms of time and accuracy in the detection of the disease was the histogram-based gradient boosting (HGB) (accuracy: 100%, time: 6.39 sec). The HGB classifier identified the 11 most important features (LDL, cholesterol, HDL-C, MCHC, triglyceride, amylase, UA, LDH, CK-MB, ALP and MCH) to detect the disease with 100% accuracy. In addition, the importance of single, double and triple combinations of these features in the diagnosis of the disease was discussed. We propose to use these 11 features and their binary combinations as important biomarkers for ML sensors in the diagnosis of the disease, supporting edge computing on Arduino and cloud IoT service.

Keywords: COVID-19; biochemical and hematological biomarkers; routine blood values; feature selection method; LogNNet neural network; machine learning sensors; Internet of Medical Things; IoT

Citation: Velichko, A.; Huyut, M.T.; Belyaev, M.; Izotov, Y.; Korzun, D. Machine Learning Sensors for Diagnosis of COVID-19 Disease Using Routine Blood Values for Internet of Things Application. *Sensors* **2022**, *22*, 7886. https://doi.org/10.3390/s22207886

Academic Editor: Joel J. P. C. Rodrigues

Received: 15 September 2022
Accepted: 14 October 2022
Published: 17 October 2022

1. Introduction

Identified in 2019, COVID-19 is an infectious disease caused by the novel severe acute respiratory syndrome coronavirus (SARS-CoV-2) [1,2]. Since the World Health Organization (WHO) declared the SARS-CoV-2 infection as a pandemic, the epidemic still maintains its severity to this day [3,4]. The early diagnosis of patients is extremely important to manage this unprecedented emergency [5,6]. The preferred gold standard method for detecting SARS-CoV-2 infections is the reverse polymerase chain reaction (PCR) or reverse transcriptase-PCR (RT-PCR) technique [7]. However, the execution of the test is time consuming (not less than 4–5 h under optimum conditions) and many favorable conditions must be met, such as the use of special equipment and reagents, the collection of samples and the necessity of trained personnel [8]. Machine learning (ML) and artificial intelligence (AI) models provide a powerful motivation to uncover insights from patients' data in tragic events such as the COVID-19 pandemic or in situations wherein guidelines have not yet been created [9]. ML and AI methods select the relevant biomarkers, revealing their predictive importance and consistently detecting their interactions with each other. Moreover, the diagnostic performance of these methods has the ability to be improved [9–11]. AI studies for the early detection, diagnosis and prognosis of COVID-19 relied on computed tomography (CT) and RBVs. However, imaging-based solutions are costly and require specialized equipment. Machine learning (ML) and AI studies based on RBVs features are a more economical and rapid alternative method for the early detection, diagnosis and prognosis of COVID-19 [7,11,12]. Previous studies have indicated that this disease can accompany multi-organ dysfunction and cause a variety of symptoms [3,13–15]. COVID-19 can cause severe pneumonia and severe ARDS due to inflammatory cytokine storms [5,14]. The excessive and uncontrolled release of proinflammatory cytokines was considered the most important primary cause of death, similar to other infections caused by pathogenic coronaviruses [16].

The pathogen may require special attention in intensive care units (ICUs) and cause a serious respiratory disorder, in some cases leading to death [14,16]. Moreover, it is difficult to distinguish symptoms of COVID-19 from known infections in the majority of patients [14,17,18]. This predictive analytics is especially required in medical information systems (MISs) to support clinical or managerial decisions.

COVID-19 may be part of a broader spectrum of hyperinflammatory syndromes characterized by the cytokine release syndrome (CRS), such as secondary hemophagocytic lymphohistiocytosis (sHLH) [19–21]. The activation of the monocyte–macrophage system just before the disease leads to pneumonia [22,23]. During this period, changes in many routine laboratory parameters such as D-dimer and fibrinogen have been reported in COVID-19 patients [1,2,4,5,14,22,24]. High ferritin, D-dimer, lactate dehydrogenase and IL-6 levels are indicators of poor prognosis and risk of death in patients [25–27]. In addition, Winata and Kurniawan [28] reported increased D-dimer and fibrinogen degradation product (FDP) in all patients in the late stage of COVID-19. This indicates that D-Dimer and FDP levels are elevated due to increased hypoxia in severe COVID-19 conditions and are significantly associated with coagulation. Kurniawan et al. [29] reported that hyperinflammation, coagulation cascade, multi-organ failure, which play a role in the etiopathogenesis of COVID-19, and biomarkers associated with these conditions, such as CRP, D-Dimer, LDH and albumin, may be useful in predicting the outcome of COVID-19.

The previous studies detected the clinical significance of changes in the routine blood values (RBVs) in the diagnosis and prognosis of infectious diseases [1,2,4,5,30,31]. However, Jiang et al. [32], Zheng et al. [33] and Huyut [11] noted that information on early predictive RBVs should be supplemented with large samples, especially for severe and fatal cases of COVID-19.

The uncontrolled spread of the disease in pandemics distresses health systems. The early detection of patients in pandemics is an important but clinically difficult process in terms of morbidity and mortality [14,24]. The diagnosis and prognosis of COVID-19 with the use of advanced devices can provide support in improving patient comfort, health system and tackling economic inadequacies [6,11,12]. In this context, studies are carried out to diagnose and determine the severity of the disease in the early period by using ML and AI-based methods as well as RBVs data [7,11,12]. The basic element in ML approaches is to determine the feature vector with a linear classifier [30]. Since ML algorithms require a sufficiently large number of samples, the problem of dimensionality in these methods is inevitable. To minimize this problem, the dataset should be reduced by finding a less dimensional attribute matrix. The dimensionality problem can be minimized by discarding irrelevant features with the feature selection procedure [30,31].

Feature selection methods can be summarized under three main headings: embedded methods, filters and wrappers (backward elimination, forward selection, recursive feature elimination) [30,31]. Feature selection in embedded methods is part of the training process and, therefore, this method lies between filters and wrappers. In the embedded methods, the determination of the best subset of features is performed during the training of the classifier (for example, when optimizing weights in a neural network). In terms of computational cost, embedded methods are more economical than wrappers [30].

Although we can find many case studies for all three feature selection methods, most feature selection methods are filters [30]. The existence of a large number of available feature selection methods complicates the selection of the best method for a particular problem [31]. The popular feature selection methods include correlation-based feature selection (CFS) [34], consistency-based filtering [35], INTERACT [36], information gain [37], ReliefF [38], recursive feature elimination for support vector machines (SVM-RFE) [39], Lasso editing [40] and minimum redundancy maximum relevance (mRMR) algorithm (developed specifically for dealing with microarray data) [30].

We examined the SARS-CoV-2-RBV1 database using the LogNNet neural network [12]. LogNNet can be defined as a feed forward network that increases the classification accuracy by chaotic mapping that fills a reservoir matrix. It is important to optimize the chaotic map parameters in data analysis by applying the LogNNet neural network. In addition, by taking advantage of chaotic mapping, it is possible to significantly reduce the RAM usage by a neural network. These results show that LogNNet can be used effectively in Internet of Things (IoT) mobile devices.

The main point for many digital health solutions during the pandemic process is the production of effective, fast and inexpensive alternative methods for the early diagnosis and treatment of COVID-19 patients. However, even the most knowledgeable and experienced physicians can interpret little of the information contained in routine blood laboratory results, and it is extremely difficult to determine the severity of COVID-19 patients based on RBVs findings alone [41]. In this context, ML classification models run with RBV-based data to determine the preliminary diagnosis of COVID-19 can be an effective tool in clinical decision support systems with an accuracy of over 95%. In this study, 13 ML models and LogNNet neural networks were applied in the diagnosis of suspected cases with an alternative device, based on LogNNet and Andrunio solutions, as only RBV-based, and the most important features were determined. We made a clinical interpretation of the relationship between these features and their various combinations with the disease. We achieved the performance of all models in detecting the diagnosis of the disease and reached up to 99.8% accuracy. ML sensors (Sensors 1.0 type) for the diagnosis of the COVID-19 disease have been successfully tested in the IoT environment, and the diagnosis of the disease has been implemented in offline and online modes. In offline mode, ML sensors were run on an Arduino board with a LogNNet neural network with a total RAM consumption of ~4 kB. Obtaining the findings in this study over a large sample is an important advantage in terms of the validity of the study. We believe that this study will help to identify suspected patients with a high probability of being infected with COVID-19 at the time of admission to the hospital with a fast and economical method, which will make important contributions to the detection of the disease before it progresses.

The paper has the following structure. Section 2 present the related studies, Section 3 describes the data collection procedure, correlation analysis of features, machine learning methods and the implementation of LogNNet on an Arduino board. Section 4 presents the results from the correlation analysis of dataset, classification results, one, double, triple and 11 feature combinations in the detection of sick and healthy individuals, and the ML sensor concept for IoT. Section 5 discusses the results and compares them with known developments. Section 6 presents the limitations of the study. In conclusion, a general description of the study and its scientific significance are given.

2. Related Studies

The prompt diagnosis of COVID-19 seems to be a promising advancement for applying at-home health care and AAL [42]. The digitalization of healthcare calls for effective applications of human body sensors [43] and human sensing [44], including ML sensors, to continuously monitor various parameters of the human body in everyday life with the help of the IoT [45]. Everyday human body sensors testify to the growing number of applications in IoT-enabled ambient intelligence (AmI) systems [46]. The paradigms of ML sensors [47] and artificial intelligence (AI) sensors [48,49] are similar in meaning. The ML sensor paradigm was further developed by Warden et al. [47] and Matthew Stewart [50], wherein the authors introduced the terms Sensors 1.0 and Sensors 2.0 devices. Sensors 2.0 devices are a combination of both a physical sensor and a machine learning module in one package. Sensors 2.0 devices process data internally, ensuring data security, while in Sensors 1.0 devices, these modules are physically separated. In addition, the authors proposed the concept of creating a datasheet of ML sensors. Therefore, the development of technology for creating ML sensors for the diagnosis of the COVID-19 disease is an urgent problem.

In previous studies, the RBVs of people who lived and died from COVID-19, or patients with COVID-19 and healthy individuals, were statistically compared [1,3,14,22–24,26,51]. In addition, differences in many RBVs characteristics are known between mild and severe COVID-19 patient groups according to statistical methods. However, this study demonstrates that ML models using only one or two features can detect COVID-19 patients from a large group of patients with high accuracy. Therefore, this study will be an alternative approach with extremely high sensitivity for the diagnosis of COVID-19. ML algorithms allow for an easy interpretation of complex association structures in data by simultaneously evaluating the cumulative effects of numerous biomarkers to discover higher-order interactions [4,6,9]. With this benefit, the strengths of using ML in clinical medicine are considered as an opportunity. Although various clinical studies [7,52,53] have highlighted how blood test-based diagnosis can provide an effective and low-cost alternative for the early detection of COVID-19 cases, relatively few ML models have been applied to blood parameters [7,54].

An evaluation of lung CT images to predict lung cancer using deep learning with an improved abundant clustering technique and instant trained neural networks approach was performed in [55]. The authors achieved an accuracy of up to 98.42% in cancer diagnosis with a minimum classification error of 0.038. Cui et al. [56] examined the distribution of pixels in the images with the fuzzy Markov random field segmentation approach using positron emission tomography (PET) and computed tomography (CT) images of the affected area associated with lung tumor. The developed method provided an accuracy of 0.85 in recognizing the lung tumor region. Tomita et al. [57] ran a logistic regression (LR) analysis, support vector machine (SVM) and deep neural network (DNN) models with biochemical findings, lung function tests and bronchial challenge test features to predict the initial diagnosis of adult asthma. In the pre-diagnosis of adult asthma, the DNN model showed 0.98%-ACC, the SVM model 0.82%-ACC and the LR model 0.94%-ACC. Ryu et al. [58] used various ML models and a deep neural network model for the pre-diagnosis of diabetes mellitus using various physical and routine blood values features. The deep neural network has been the most successful model with a value of 0.80-AUC in diabetes mellitus. Kolachalama et al. [59] used a six-convolutional deep learning architecture (CNN) with histological images, biopsy results and some clinical phenotypes to classify kidney disease severity. The CNN model was found to be more successful with AUC values of 0.878, 0.875 and 0.904, respectively, than the pathologist-predicted fibrosis score (0.811, 0.800 and 0.786 AUC, respectively) for assessing 1-, 3- and 5-year renal survival. In a study conducted to identify patients at risk of early diagnosis of fatty liver disease, Wu et al. [60] used an artificial neural network model with three ML models. The most successful model in the diagnosis of risky patients was the random forest with 87.48-ACC and 0.92-AUC values. Oguntimilehin et al. [61] used an ML technique on a set of labeled typhoid fever contingent variables for the diagnosis of typhoid fever and to establish explicable rules. The labeled database is divided into five different levels of typhoid fever severity, with classification accuracies on both the training set and the test set of 95% and 96%, respectively. The application was implemented using Visual Basic as the front-end and MySQL as the back-end. Kouchaki et al. [62] used various ML methods to predict the resistance to MTB in Mycobacterium tuberculosis (MTB) patients given a specific drug in a timely manner and to identify resistance markers. Compared to the traditional molecular diagnostic test, the AUC values of the best ML classifiers were higher for all drugs. Logistic regression and gradient tree reinforcement methods performed better than other techniques. Taylor et al. [63] ran six machine learning algorithms with 10 features consisting of patient demographics, RBVs results and drug information for the diagnosis of and treatment decisions for urinary tract infection. The best performing model, XGBoost, diagnosed the presence of a urinary tract infection with a high AUC value (0.826–0.904 confidence interval).

Yang et al. [64] ran four ML models on 3356 patients (42% COVID-19 positive) using 27 features covering both blood count and biochemical parameters. A gradient boosted decision tree model was the most successful model in the diagnosis of the disease with a value of 0.85-AUC. Booth et al. [9] operated 26 RBVs data elements with a support vector machine to detect COVID-19 patients at high mortality risk and determined prognostic biomarkers with a value of 0.93-AUC. Huyut [11] classified severely and mildly infected patients from a large population of COVID-19 patients using 12 supervised ML models and 28 routine blood values. The models with the highest AUC for identifying mildly infected patients were found to be local weighted learning at 0.95%, Kstar at 0.91%, Naive bayes at 0.85% and K nearest neighbor at 0.75%. Brinati et al. [65] ran 13 RBVs with various ML methods to detect COVID-19 patients (102 negative and 177 COVID-19 positive). They noted that the models with the highest accuracy in the diagnosis of the disease were random forest (82%) and logistic regression (78%). Huyut and Velichko [12] determined the diagnosis and prognosis of the COVID-19 disease by running the LogNNet neural network model on 51 RBVs features. The model achieved an accuracy of 99% in the diagnosis of the disease and 84% in its prognosis. Zhang et al. [66] used a variety of demographic indicators and 21 RBVs using a Lasso-based neural network model to detect predictors of mortality from COVID-19. The success of the model in determining the clinical status of the patients was 98%-AUC. Alle et al. [67] applied the XGboost and logistic regression model on a dataset of various clinical and laboratory tests to predict COVID-19 mortality and found accuracy rates of 83% and 92%, respectively. Gao et al. [68] applied an ensemble model derived from support vector machine (SVM), gradient augmented decision tree (GBDT) and neural network (NN) algorithms using 28 immune/inflammatory features to detect COVID-19. The developed model reached 0.99 AUC in detecting infected patients. Vaishnav et al. [69] used various machine learning models to predict mortality from COVID-19, and the decision tree regression model produced a 70% accuracy and the random forest regression model a 76% accuracy. Huyut and İlkbahar [5] used various biomarkers with the CHAID decision tree to detect the diagnosis and prognosis of COVID-19. The model produced an 81.6% accuracy in recognizing the disease and a 93.5% accuracy in determining the prognosis of the disease. Huyut and Üstündağ [6] used 23 blood gas parameters with the CHAID decision tree to predict the diagnosis and prognosis of COVID-19. The model produced a 68.2% accuracy in recognizing the disease and a 65.0% accuracy in determining the prognosis of the disease. Kukar et al. [70] constructed a machine learning model based on 35 RBVs to diagnose 5333 negative and 160 positive COVID-19 patients with various bacterial and viral infections. The model showed an 81.9% sensitivity and a 97.9% specificity in detecting patients. Mei et al. [71] developed a model combining CNN and multilayer sensor to detect COVID-19 using computed tomography (CT), various clinical information elements and some RBVs data. The model reached an 84% sensitivity and an 83% specificity in recognizing the disease.

AI studies on the risk of poor outcome for COVID-19 patients need further validation with larger samples [11,25,72]. Furthermore, previous AI studies using RBVs for COVID-19 diagnosis and prognosis which covered the early stages of the outbreak included less blood values and reported poorer performance. Therefore, to detect the disease in the later stages of the epidemic, it is necessary to study ML models on a larger sample, which can achieve higher accuracy and use most RBVs.

3. Data and Methods

The data used in this study were collected retrospectively from the information system of Erzincan Binali Yıldırım University Mengücek Gazi Training and Research Hospital (EBYU-MG) between April and December 2021. The data used in this study are shared as open access under the name of "SARS-CoV-2-RBV1" in [12].

During the dates covered by this study, a diagnosis of SARS-CoV-2 was made by real-time reverse transcriptase polymerase chain reaction (RT-PCR) on nasopharyngeal or oropharyngeal swabs at the EBYU-MG hospital. RBVs results at first admission were recorded to prevent various complications.

3.1. Characteristic of Participants, Workflow and Datasets

Between the specified dates, the digital system of our hospital was scanned and patients diagnosed with COVID-19 (n = 2648) were selected from a large patient population (a dataset of approximately 80 thousand patients was scanned). The routine laboratory information of these patients was examined. The parameters (features) that were measured from at least 80% of the patients were used. Missing data were completed with the mean of the distribution and normalized. A total of 51 routine blood values calibrated from approximately 70 parameters were recorded. In addition, a group (control group) with the same number of negative COVID-19 tests (n = 2648) was identified and 51 characteristics of these individuals were recorded. Our control group arrived at the hospital only with the suspicion of COVID-19. Chronic disease information of the patients could not be reached. Only data of individuals over the age of 18 were recorded.

These two datasets were combined and named "SARS-CoV-2-RBV1" dataset. The SARS-CoV-2-RBV1 dataset includes immunological, hematological and biochemical RBVs parameters and consists of 51 features (Table 1). In the SARS-CoV-2-RBV1 dataset, positive COVID-19 test results were coded as 1 and negative test results as 0 (COVID-19 = 1, non-COVID-19 = 0).

Table 1. Feature numbering for SARS-CoV-2-RBV1 dataset [12].

№	Feature	№	Feature	№	Feature	№	Feature	№	Feature
1	CRP	12	NEU	23	MPV	34	GGT	45	Sodium
2	D-Dimer	13	PLT	24	PDW	35	Glucose	46	T-Bil
3	Ferritin	14	WBC	25	RBC	36	HDL-C	47	TP
4	Fibrinogen	15	BASO	26	RDW	37	Calcium	48	Triglyceride
5	INR	16	EOS	27	ALT	38	Chlorine	49	eGFR
6	PT	17	HCT	28	AST	39	Cholesterol	50	Urea
7	PCT	18	HGB	29	Albumin	40	Creatinine	51	UA
8	ESR	19	MCH	30	ALP	41	CK		
9	Troponin	20	MCHC	31	Amylase	42	LDH		
10	aPTT	21	MCV	32	CK-MB	43	LDL		
11	LYM	22	MONO	33	D-Bil	44	Potassium		

CRP: C-reactive protein; INR: international normalized ratio; PT: prothrombin time; PCT: procalcitonin; ESR: erythrocyte sedimentation rate; aPTT: activated partial prothrombin time; LYM: lymphocyte count; NEU: neutrophil count; PLT: platelet count; WBC: white blood cell count; BASO: basophil count; EOS: eosinophil count; HCT: hematocrit; HGB: hemoglobin; MCH: mean corpuscular hemoglobin; MCHC: mean corpuscular hemoglobin concentration; MCV: mean corpuscular volume; MONO: monocyte count; MPV: mean platelet volume; PDW: platelet distribution width; RBC: red blood cells; RDW: red cell distribution width; ALT: alanine aminotransaminase; AST: aspartate aminotransferase; ALP: alkaline phosphatase; CK-MB: creatine kinase myocardial band; D-Bil: direct bilirubin; GGT: gamma-glutamyl transferase; HDL-C: high-density lipoprotein cholesterol; CK: creatine kinase; LDH: lactate dehydrogenase; LDL: low-density lipoprotein; T-Bil: total bilirubin; TP: total protein; eGFR: estimating glomerular filtration rate; UA: uric acid.

The features in this dataset are calibrated and contain almost all of the routine blood values that are the subject of studies on COVID-19 in the literature. Therefore, we believe that the bias of our study using this dataset was minimized in comparison to the literature. In addition, the use of our dataset, which we share as open access, is important in terms of showing the reproducibility and auditability of the results.

3.2. Correlation Analysis of Features

To determine the level of correlation between diagnosis and biochemical blood parameters, the original dataset was analyzed using the point-biserial correlation test [73]. Pearson correlation coefficient was calculated for each feature–feature pair, and a correlation matrix was compiled. The correlation matrix makes it possible to judge the strength and structure (positive or negative) of the linear relationship between diagnosis–feature and feature–feature pairs. The correlation matrix was created using the pandas software package [74].

3.3. Machine Learning Methods, Hyperparameters, Accuracy Estimation

Machine learning algorithms can be applied to a wide range of problems such as classification, clustering, regression analysis, time series forecasting, etc. [75]. The SARS-CoV-2-RBV1 dataset under study has an output parameter divided into two classes (positive or negative diagnosis for COVID-19), so the task of the machine learning algorithm is reduced to binary classification based on 51 features. This study compared the accuracy of the most popular binary classification algorithms: multinomial naive Bayes (MNB), Gaussian naive Bayes (GNB), Bernoulli naive Bayes (BNB), linear discriminant analysis (LDA), K-nearest neighbors (KNN), support vector machine classifier with linear kernel (LSVM), support vector machine classifier with non-linear kernel (NLSVM), passive-aggressive (PA), multilayer perceptron (MLP), decision tree (DT), extra trees (ETs) classifier, random forest (RF), histogram-based gradient boosting (HGB).

Each classifier model has hyperparameters, for which optimization is necessary to obtain the most accurate models. For optimization, the software package "auto-sklearn" [76] was used.

Before training the models, the initial data were subjected to preprocessing, which makes it possible to speed up the training of the models and improve the accuracy of the classification. Preprocessing includes two stages: (1) normalization of numerical values of the input data, (2) generation of additional features. Normalization is a procedure consisting of bringing numerical data to a single format, which has the following options: quantile transformer (QT)—transforms feature values so that they correspond to a uniform or normal distribution; robust scaler (RS)—subtracts the median values for each feature and scales according to the interquartile range; MinMax (MM)—scales feature values so that they are all in the range from the minimum to the maximum value. The procedure for generating additional features transforms the original set of features into a set of features with a different dimension. This helps to select the most important features, compose additional features from them or present the input data in a special format for the ML algorithm. The following methods for generating additional features were used: polynomial (PN)—creates features that are polynomial combinations of the original features; random trees embedding (RTE)—creates a multidimensional sparse feature representation, in which the data in each new feature are represented by binary values; extra trees preprocessor (ETP)—selects a part of the most important features that are evaluated using the extra trees algorithm; linear SVM preprocessor (LSVMP)—selects some of the most important features that are evaluated using the support vector machine algorithm; independent component analysis (ICA)—selects a set of statistically independent features from the entire original set; Nystroem sampler (NS)—transforms a set of initial features using a low-rank matrix approximation by the Nystroem method.

The accuracy of models A_{NF} was assessed by the K-fold cross-validation method (K = 5) encapsulated in software packages, wherein the designation A_{NF} refers to the classification accuracy when using *NF* features. K-fold cross-validation method splits the original dataset into *K* parts and sequentially trains the model. One of the *K* parts of the dataset is used as a test sample, and the other parts as a training sample. Then, the obtained values of the classification accuracy on the test samples are averaged. The division of the base into parts is performed using stratification. Such approach makes it possible to reliably estimate the accuracy of models.

In this study, we used a less common ML algorithm based on the LogNNet neural network. The LogNNet 51:50:20:2 configuration was used, and a detailed configuration description is given in [75]. The LogNNet architecture is IoT-oriented and can run on devices with low computing resources (Section 3.4).

Each algorithm was given the same amount of time (1 h) to optimize the hyperparameters. A computer with an AMD Ryzen 9 3950X processor and 64 GB DDR-4 RAM was used to train the models.

3.4. Implementing LogNNet on an Arduino Board

The Arduino Nano 33 IoT board was chosen as a prototype IoT edge device with limited computing resources. It is based on a 32-bit Microchip ATSAMD21G18 microcontroller with an ARM Cortex-M0+ computing core, a clock frequency of 48 MHz, 256 KB of flash memory and 32 KB of RAM. The neural network LogNNet 51:50:20:2 from [12] was programmed on the Arduino board and tested. Arduino Nano 33 IoT test circuit, LogNNet architecture and board are presented in Figure 1.

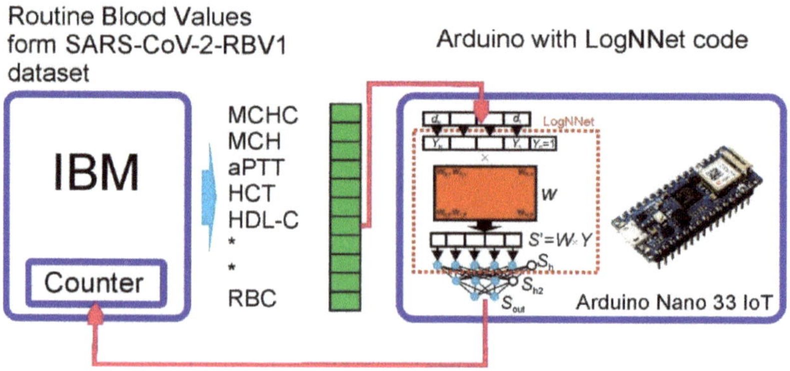

Figure 1. Arduino Nano 33 IoT test circuit and LogNNet architecture.

3.4.1. LogNNet Program for Arduino Board

LogNNet transforms the input feature vector *d* into a normalized vector *Y*, which is multiplied with the reservoir matrix *W* filled with a chaotic mapping. We used the mapping congruent generator (1) with the parameters indicated in Table 2 and the data [12]. Then, the transformed vector passes the output classifier (two-layer feed-forward neural network with two hidden layers).

Table 2. Chaotic map equation and list of parameters with limits.

Chaotic Map	List of Parameters	Equation
Congruent generator	$K = 93$ $D = 68$ $L = 9276$ $C = 73$	$\begin{cases} x_{n+1} = (D - K \cdot x_n) \bmod L \\ x_1 = C \end{cases}$ (1)

Let us denote the matrix of weight coefficients between the layers S_h and S_{h2} as W_1, and the matrix between the layers S_{h2} and S_{out} as W_2. At the output, there are two neurons for two classes (COVID-19 and non-COVID-19). Matrices of weight coefficients and values of normalization coefficients were calculated on a computer with high performance and saved in a separate library file. In addition, the library file (supplementary materials) contains the values of K, D, L and C required for calculating the W matrix, as well as data on configuration of the LogNNet 51:50:20:2 neural network.

When LogNNet is running, the values of the elements of the matrix W (2550 values) are sequentially calculated using the congruent generator method (1) each time a feature vector is input. This approach does not store the matrix W in the RAM memory of the controller, and it leads to memory saving; however, it slows down the calculations of the neural network.

The Arduino IDE development environment was used to implement the algorithm. The library file with the matrices W_1 and W_2 and other coefficients necessary for the operation of the neural network were loaded at the beginning of the program. The complete code of the program is presented in Appendix A, Algorithm A1. The algorithm is divided into functions and procedures:

- Function "Fun_activ"—activation function, lines 10–12;
- Procedure "Reservoir"—calculation of coefficients of reservoir matrix W by congruent generator formula, multiplication of arrays and calculation of neurons in layer Sh, lines 14–28;
- Procedure "Hidden_Layer"—calculation of neurons in the hidden layer Sh2, lines 30–39;
- Function "Output_Layer_Layer"—calculation of the output layer Sout, lines 41–54;
- The "void loop" block is an executable loop, lines 61–77;
- "void setup" block—initialization block, lines 61–77.

The scaling factor "scale_factor = 1000" makes it possible to convert data from a floating point type to an integer (and vice versa), by multiplying (dividing) by a factor and rounding. In the Arduino, a float variable takes 4 bytes of RAM, and an integer variable takes 2 bytes of RAM. Therefore, storing matrices W_1, W_2 and other data in integer format are more efficient, and during library initialization, the data takes 2 times less RAM memory.

3.4.2. Test Scheme

Neural network testing is the serial sending of SARS-CoV-2-RBV1 data to the Arduino board and counting the correct network responses. The data is generated on an external computer (Figure 1). For sending data, a protocol was implemented that separates the elements of the feature vector Y using the symbol "T" to avoid data gluing. At the end of the vector Y, special characters "FN" are placed, indicating the end of the data transfer. On the Arduino side, a protocol is implemented that recognizes the input data. In the "void loop" block, a loop is organized to check the availability of data in the serial port buffer using the Serial.Available function. This function returns "True" as soon as the Arduino receives data.

4. Results

4.1. Correlation Analysis of Dataset SARS-CoV-2-RBV1

Figure 2 presents the results of the correlation analysis of the diagnosis–feature and feature–feature pairs in the form of a "heatmap" over the entire volume of the SARS-CoV-2-RBV1 database. The first column of Table 3 shows the features most highly associated with the survivors and non-survivors of COVID-19 with a point-biserial correlation (r_{pb}) coefficient exceeding 0.5. Here, the negative or positive result of the point-biserial correlation coefficient provides information about the direction of the relationship between the diagnosis of the disease and the quantitative characteristics. As seen in the first column of Table 3, the features most associated with disease diagnosis are MCHC, HDL-C, cholesterol and LDH. The second column of Table 3 shows the accuracy of the cut-off values calculated by the threshold approach [12] for each trait in classifying COVID-19 patients. The features presented in the second column are the predictors that classify patients with the highest accuracy. For comparison, the results of the threshold classification A_{th} from [12] are presented, and features with $A_{th} \geq 70\%$ are shown. The threshold classification method and the point-biserial correlation method give an intersecting set of features, but the threshold classification provides more diagnosis-related features. While the point-biserial correlation coefficient reveals the level of association between living and deceased COVID-19 patient traits, the diagnosis has only two values (1 and 0). However, when separating these two classes, the threshold method considers all the data of the relevant feature, and it has high sensitivity.

Table 3. Features most strongly correlated with the diagnosis according to the point-biserial correlation coefficient and the threshold correlation method.

Feature (Point-Biserial Correlation Coefficient (r_{pb}))	Feature (Threshold Accuracy of Classification A_{th} from [12])
MCHC (0.8)	MCHC (94.35%)
HDL-C (−0.77)	HDL-C (94.73%)
Cholesterol (−0.71)	Cholesterol (94.47%)
LDL (−0.68)	LDL (96.47%)
	Triglyceride (90.96%)
	Amylase (85.1%)
	UA (81.12%)
	TP (79.68%)
	CK-MB (78.91%)
	LDH (74.98%)
	Albumin (72.91%)

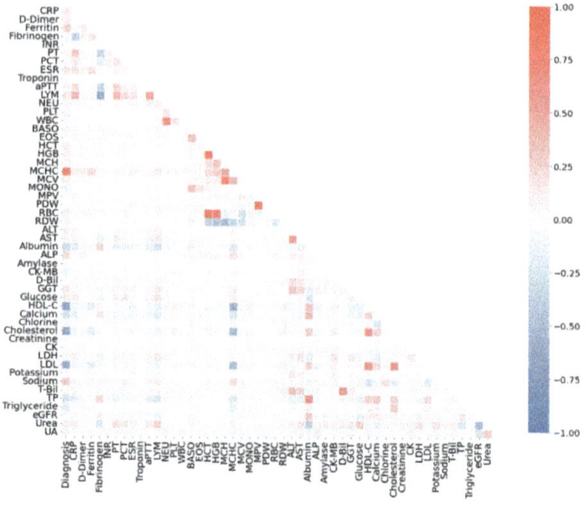

Figure 2. Correlation of the SARS-CoV-2-RBV1 dataset for diagnosis–feature (point-biserial correlation) and feature–feature pairs (Pearson coefficient).

An analysis of the correlation of features among themselves (Figure 2) reveals several features that are linearly dependent on each other. The most strongly correlated pairs with the Pearson coefficient exceeding 0.6 modulo are shown in Table 4. The same table presents Pearson's coefficients separately for a variety of COVID-19 positive and negative participants. Full heatmaps by class (COVID-19, non-COVID-19) are shown in Figures 3 and 4.

Table 4. The features most strongly correlated with each other by the Pearson coefficient for the entire database and separately for classes (positive or negative COVID-19 status).

Pair Feature–Feature	Pearson's Coefficient for COVID-19 Diagnosis	Pearson's Coefficient for Positive COVID-19	Pearson's Coefficient for Negative COVID-19
		Type High–High	
HCT–HGB	0.96	0.95 (High)	0.97(High)
MPV–PDW	0.93	0.94	0.92
HCT–RBC	0.87	0.88	0.87
MCH–MCV	0.84	0.84	0.84
HGB–RBC	0.83	0.83	0.83
NEU–WBC	0.74	0.71	0.81
Albumin–TP	0.64	0.67	0.5
MCH–MCHC	0.53	0.62	0.99
MCH–RDW	−0.55	−0.61	−0.51
		Type High–Low	
Fibrinogen–LYM	−0.77	−0.78 (High)	−0.01 (Low)
Cholesterol–LDL	0.65	0.59	0.012
Cholesterol–HDL-C	0.64	0.39	−0.024
Chlorine–Sodium	0.18	0.63	−0.025
		Type Low–High	
MCHC–MCV	0.41	0.09 1(Low)	0.84 (High)
ALT–AST	0.6	0.48	0.76
eGFR–Urea	−0.55	−0.49	−0.63
INR–PT	0.12	0.075	1
D-Bil–T-Bil	0.6	0.33	0.91
HDL-C–LDL	0.63	0.19	0.3

Three main types of pair correlations can be distinguished. The High–High type is the pairs of features for which the correlation has a high value does not depend on the presence or absence of COVID-19 disease. The High–Low type is the pairs of features that are highly correlated only in sick patients. The Low–High type is the pairs of features that are highly correlated only in healthy patients. In general, the features are more correlated in patients with COVID-19 (Figure 3). From a medical point of view, pair correlation will be reviewed in the Discussion Section.

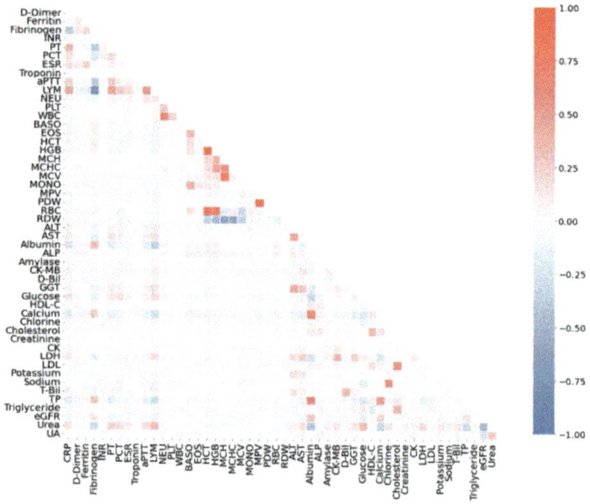

Figure 3. Pearson correlation analysis results for positive diagnoses for COVID-19 from the SARS-CoV-2-RBV1 dataset.

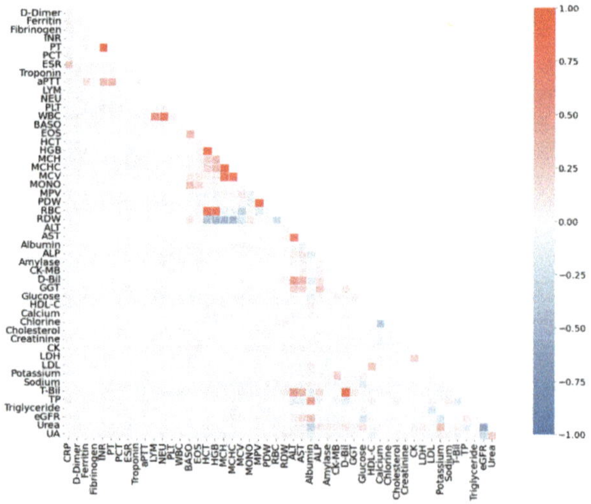

Figure 4. Pearson correlation analysis results for negative diagnoses for COVID-19 from the SARS-CoV-2-RBV1 dataset.

4.2. Classification Results for Dataset SARS-CoV-2-RBV1

Table 5 presents the results of the machine learning algorithms optimized to obtain the maximum classification values using 51 features. The results are sorted in descending order of algorithm efficiency. For each algorithm, the average training and inference time of the model and methods for preprocessing of the input data are given.

Table 5. Results of assessing the classification accuracy of machine learning models for the SARS-CoV-2-RBV1 dataset.

Classification Algorithm	Average Model Accuracy A_{51},%	Average Learning Time, s	Average Inference Time, µs	Normalization Method	Methods for Generating Additional Features
Histogram-based Gradient Boosting	100	6.39	11.6	-	-
Random Forest	99.943	13.15	21.9	QT	-
K-nearest neighbors	99.924	3.17	22.1	QT	ETP
Extra Trees classifier	99.905	18.73	24.5	RS	-
Multilayer Perceptron	99.886	3.99	2.2	RS	LSVMP
Multinomial Naive Bayes	99.792	2.48	11.7	QT	RTE
Linear Discriminant Analysis	99.773	9.15	7.5	QT	PN
Support Vector Machine with non-linear kernel	99.754	222.41	43.2	QT	NS
Decision Tree	99.660	1.46	1.2	RS	LSVMP
Passive-Aggressive	99.641	2.91	13.1	QT	RTE
Bernoulli Naive Bayes	99.622	2.59	11.3	QT	RTE
Support Vector Machine with linear kernel	99.584	5.21	1242	MM	PN
Gaussian Naive Bayes	98.565	1.68	3.5	QT	ICA
LogNNet [12]	99.509	100	3	-	-

The accuracy of the algorithms A_{51} ranged from 98.56% to 100%, indicating that all models were good at identifying the association of features with the diagnosis of COVID-19. The most efficient model is based on the histogram-based gradient boosting classifier with a 100% accuracy.

Figure 5 presents the learning curves for the HGB model using all the features from the dataset. The red curve (training accuracy) shows the training ability of the model, and the green curve (cross-validation accuracy) shows the generalization ability of the model depending on the number of training examples. Each point on the graph was obtained using five different splits into a test (20%) and training (80%) subsets.

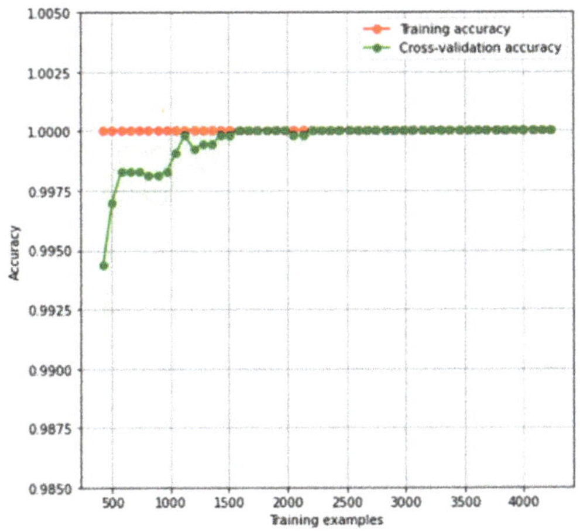

Figure 5. Learning curves for the histogram-based gradient boosting classifier model using 51 features from the SARS-CoV-2-RBV1 dataset.

The red curve represents the accuracy of the model on the training samples. The model has sufficient complexity to recognize all training samples with a 100% accuracy. The green curve represents the accuracy of the model on the test subset, the samples of which were not involved in model training. With an increase in training samples, the cross-validation accuracy of the model grows. The curves converge with each other and completely coincide when the number of training samples is more than 2500. The dots on the graph represent the average accuracy using five different splits, and the shaded areas represent the standard deviation.

Unlike other models, HGB does not require data preprocessing. The training time of the HGB model is about 6 s, which makes it possible to effectively use it to enumerate input features when searching for optimal combinations. The LogNNet model was used to implement the classification on the Arduino board, so its algorithm has a compact form suitable for IoT devices.

The HGB model was used to study the most significant combinations of the first, second and third features.

4.2.1. Investigation of the Effectiveness of the HGB Model Operating on One Feature

Table 6 presents the classification result of the SARS-CoV-2-RBV1 dataset for the HGB model using a single input feature. The features are sorted in descending order of A_1 classification accuracy. The most effective features are the first six features: LDL (№ 43), cholesterol (№ 39), HDL-C (№ 36), MCHC (№ 20), triglyceride (№ 48) and amylase (№ 31). The same features are dominant in assessing the correlation between the sign and the diagnosis from Table 3.

Table 6. Classification efficiency of SARS-CoV-2-RBV1 datasets using the single feature for the Histogram-based Gradient Boosting classifier.

№	Feature	A_1,%	№	Feature	A_1,%	№	Feature	A_1,%	№	Feature	A_1,%
43	LDL	96.84	4	Fibrinogen	76.03	50	Urea	68.10	21	MCV	56.43
39	Cholesterol	95.07	29	Albumin	75.3	7	PCT	63.25	22	MONO	56.26
36	HDL-C	94.99	44	Potassium	75.22	27	ALT	62.33	5	INR	56.19
20	MCHC	94.35	3	Ferritin	74.45	35	Glucose	62.17	6	PT	56.04
48	Triglyceride	93.76	38	Chlorine	73.18	49	eGFR	62.04	17	HCT	55.75
31	Amylase	90.01	46	T-Bil	72.77	14	WBC	61.91	26	RDW	55.62
51	UA	87.91	34	GGT	72.62	16	EOS	61.40	9	Troponin	54.07
42	LDH	85.76	41	CK	70.97	13	PLT	61.25	18	HGB	53.94
47	TP	80.41	2	D-Dimer	70.46	28	AST	60.55	25	RBC	53.43
37	Calcium	80.40	33	D-Bil	70.37	8	ESR	59.12	23	MPV	53.13
32	CK-MB	79.73	11	LYM	69.90	15	BASO	58.72	24	PDW	53.09
1	CRP	77.81	45	Sodium	69.35	12	NEU	57.51	19	MCH	52.13
30	ALP	77,71	40	Creatinine	69,24	10	aPTT	56.53			

4.2.2. Investigation of the Effectiveness of the HGB Model Operating on Two Features

Table 7 presents the classification result of the SARS-CoV-2-RBV1 dataset for the HGB model using two input features. The pairs of features are sorted in descending order of classification accuracy A_2.

Table 7. Classification efficiency of SARS-CoV-2-RBV1 dataset using 2 features for the Histogram-based Gradient Boosting classifier.

№	First Feature	Second Feature	Average Accuracy A_2,%
20-19	MCHC	MCH	99.81
43-32	LDL	CK-MB	99.62
36-32	HDL-C	CK-MB	99.49
48-32	Triglyceride	CK-MB	99.45
43-39	LDL	Cholesterol	99.43
43-20	LDL	MCHC	99.22
39-36	Cholesterol	HDL-C	99.18
39-48	Cholesterol	Triglyceride	99.11
43-42	LDL	LDH	99.05
43-31	LDL	Amylase	99.03
36-20	HDL-C	MCHC	98.98
43-51	LDL	UA	98.86
36-31	HDL-C	Amylase	98.81
39-20	Cholesterol	MCHC	98.73
20-48	MCHC	Triglyceride	98.65
39-38	Cholesterol	Chlorine	98.62
43-38	LDL	Chlorine	98.43
20-31	MCHC	Amylase	98.28
36-42	HDL-C	LDH	98.16
48-42	Triglyceride	LDH	98.14

The resulting pairs contain the most effective features: LDL (№ 43), cholesterol (№ 39), HDL-C (№ 36), MCHC (№ 20), triglyceride (№ 48) and amylase (№ 31), which have the best A_1 score (Table 7). The best result (A_2 = 99.81) was obtained for the MCHC–MCH feature pair. At the same time, the pair contains the MCH (№ 19) feature with low efficiency (A_1 = 52.13) and Pearson correlation ~0.041. Such a combination of features with high and low correlation is observed very often, and this combination results in a high classification efficiency. Among the features from Table 7, the following have a low linear correlation with the diagnosis: MCH (0.041), UA (0.066), amylase (0.03) and LDH (0.071). Pearson's coefficient from the distribution in Figure 3 is indicated in brackets.

There are pairs consisting entirely of effective features, for example, LDL–MCHC (№ 43-№ 20), HDL-C–MCHC (№ 36-№ 20), etc. Figure 6 shows the relationship between the feature pairs for the top 50 results. The main six features are in the center. Asterisks indicate the features that most often form a pair with the main features: UA (№ 51), LDH (№ 42), CK-MB (№ 32) and ALP (№ 30). The main feature LDL (№ 43) forms the largest number of effective pairs for classification.

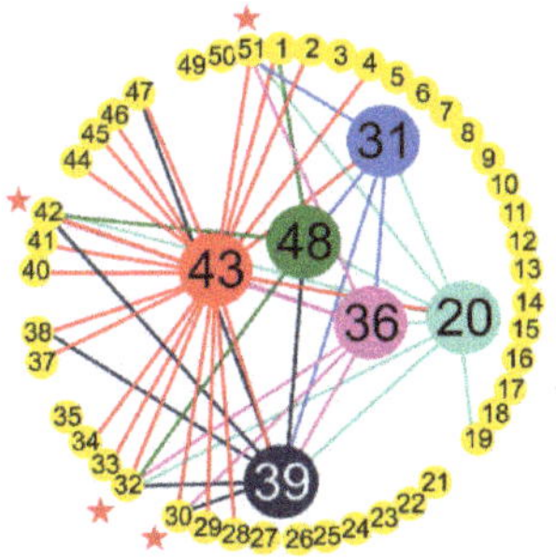

Figure 6. Pairs of features with high classification efficiency SARS-CoV-2-RBV1 dataset for the Histogram-based Gradient Boosting classifier.

To find the reasons for the effectiveness of the pairs of features from Table 7, two-dimensional distributions of the diagnosis (attractors) were constructed for the first six pairs (Figure 7). For the healthy patients (non-COVID-19), there are clear linear and cruciform attractors, while for people diagnosed with COVID-19, these attractors shift and become chaotic. This difference in the shape of the attractors allows for classifiers to effectively distinguish between the two classes. The best separation of attractor shapes is observed for the MCHC–MCH pair (Figure 7a) that explains its highest classification ability. For the pairs in Figure 7b–e, shifted cruciform attractors are observed, which also contributes to their effective separation by classifiers. In Figure 7f, two attractors are blurred, but due to their weak intersection, the classification efficiency is high.

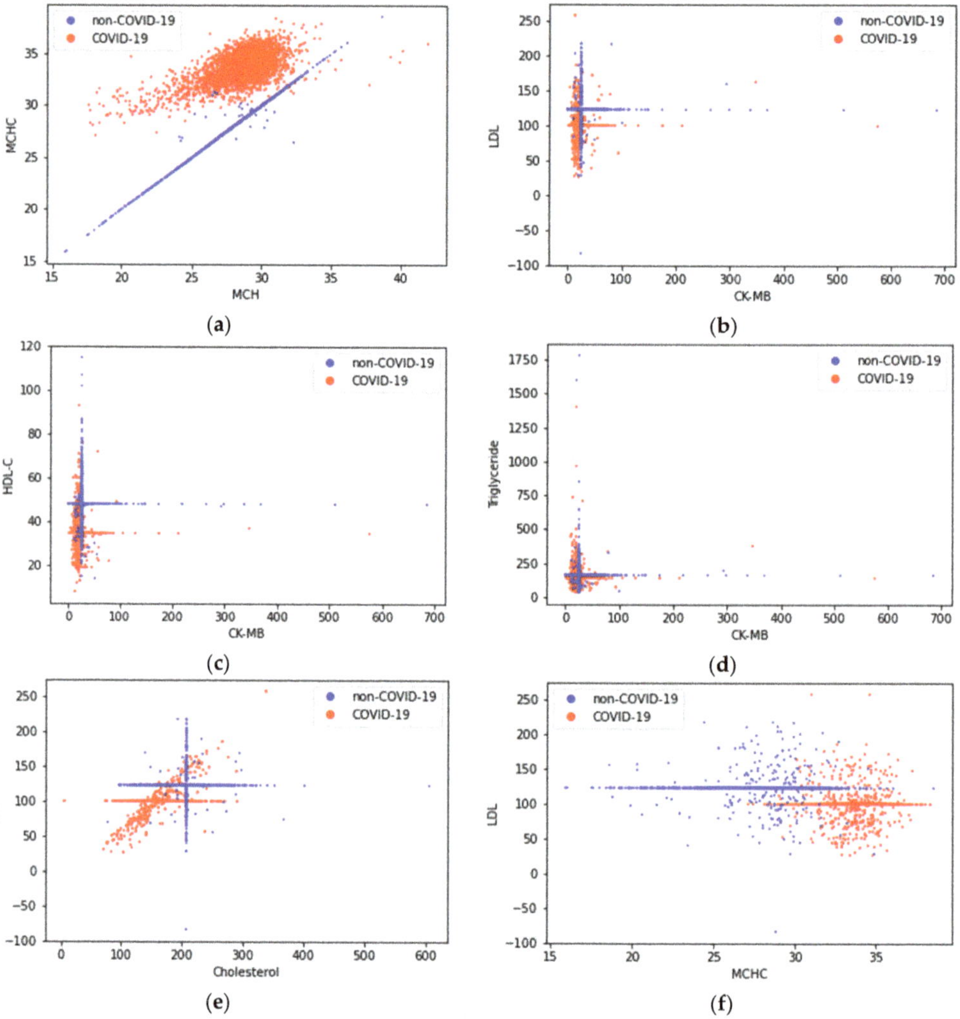

Figure 7. Two-dimensional distributions (attractors) of a COVID-19 and non-COVID-19 diagnosis in the coordinates of feature pairs MCHC–MCH (**a**), LDL–CK-MB (**b**), HDL-C–CK-MB (**c**), Triglyceride–CK-MB (**d**), LDL–Cholesterol (**e**), LDL–MCHC (**f**).

When using two features, the maximum accuracy is A_2 = 99.81% and this value is lower than when using the 51 features A_{51} = 100%. However, feature reduction is important to simplify the classification of patients in practical terms. More accurate models can be obtained using three features.

4.2.3. The Study of the Most Significant Combination of Three Features of the HGB Model

Table 8 presents the classification result of the SARS-CoV-2-RBV1 dataset for the HGB model using three input features.

Table 8. Classification efficiency of SARS-CoV-2-RBV1 dataset using 3 features for the Histogram-based Gradient Boosting classifier.

№	First Feature	Second Feature	Third Feature	Average Accuracy A_3,%
39-48-32	Cholesterol	Triglyceride	CK-MB	99.91
39-36-32	Cholesterol	HDL-C	CK-MB	99.91
43-20-19	LDL	MCHC	MCH	99.91
20-31-19	MCHC	Amylase	MCH	99.85
43-51-32	LDL	UA	CK-MB	99.85
39-20-19	Cholesterol	MCHC	MCH	99.83
48-42-32	Triglyceride	LDH	CK-MB	99.83
36-20-19	HDL-C	MCHC	MCH	99.79
36-42-32	HDL-C	LDH	CK-MB	99.79
43-38-51	LDL	Cholesterol	UA	99.79
20-48-19	MCHC	Triglyceride	MCH	99.77
39-48-31	Cholesterol	Triglyceride	Amylase	99.77
39-36-38	Cholesterol	HDL-C	Chlorine	99.75
36-31-51	HDL-C	Amylase	UA	99.75
39-36-42	Cholesterol	HDL-C	LDH	99.75
20-51-19	MCHC	UA	MCH	99.74
39-48-38	Cholesterol	Triglyceride	Chlorine	99.72
39-31-51	Cholesterol	Amylase	UA	99.70
39-48-42	Cholesterol	Triglyceride	LDH	99.66
48-31-42	Triglyceride	Amylase	LDH	99.51

An analysis of Table 8 reveals that no new features have been added in the first twenty most accurate models compared to Table 7. The MCH and MCHC features are found only in pairs. With the addition of the third feature, the maximum classification efficiency increased from A_2 = 99.81% to A_3 = 99.91%.

4.2.4. The Study of the Most Significant Combination of 11 Features of the HGB Model

Tables 7 and 8 include only 11 features: LDL (№ 43), cholesterol (№ 39), HDL-C (№ 36), MCHC (№ 20), triglyceride (№ 48), amylase (№ 31), UA (№ 51), LDH (№ 42), CK-MB (№ 32), ALP (№ 30) and MCH (№ 19). The classification accuracy of the HGB model using 11 features was A_{11} = 100%. Therefore, 11 features are sufficient to determine the presence of COVID-19 using machine learning methods based on the histogram-based gradient boosting classifier.

4.3. LogNNet Implementation on Arduino for Edge Computing

A compact 77-line LogNNet algorithm was created for diagnosing and predicting COVID-19 disease using routine blood values on an Arduino controller.

LogNNet testing on Arduino revealed an accuracy of A_{51} = 99.7%, which coincides with the accuracy on the model computer program [46]. The classification time for the input vector is about 0.1 s. An estimate of the RAM used by the Arduino controller is shown in Figure 8.

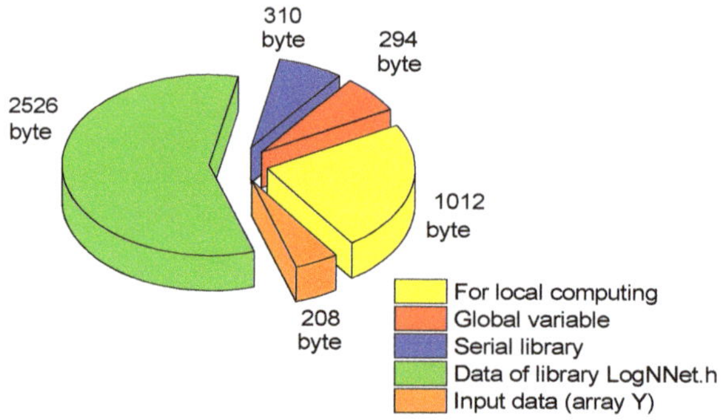

Figure 8. Estimation of the RAM used by the Arduino controller when working with the neural network LogNNet 51:50:20:2.

Global variables (arrays S_h, S_{h2} and variables) occupy 294 bytes of RAM, and incoming data is written to array Y, which occupies 208 bytes. The Arduino uses the Serial system library to operate the serial port. It is loaded at initiation in the "void setup" block and takes 310 bytes of RAM. The data stored in the LogNNet.h library are also loaded into the RAM during the program's initialization and take 2526 bytes, the maximum contribution made by the matrix W_1—2142 bytes. For local computations within functions and procedures, at least 1012 bytes must be reserved. The total RAM consumption is of 4350 bytes.

4.4. Machine Learning COVID-19 Sensor for IoT

The LogNNet network can be easily imported to various microcontrollers and used to predict a diagnosis based on blood biochemical parameters. However, our experimental results in Sections 3.2 and 3.3 are significantly inferior in accuracy to resource-intensive machine learning algorithms. Therefore, we proposed two architectures of the IoT system (Figure 9), which include an IoT device with LogNNet implementation (edge computing) and a cloud service containing a trained HGB model (AI computing). These configurations implement the prognosis of the disease in offline and online modes with ML sensors for diagnosis of the COVID-19 disease (Sensor 1.0 type).

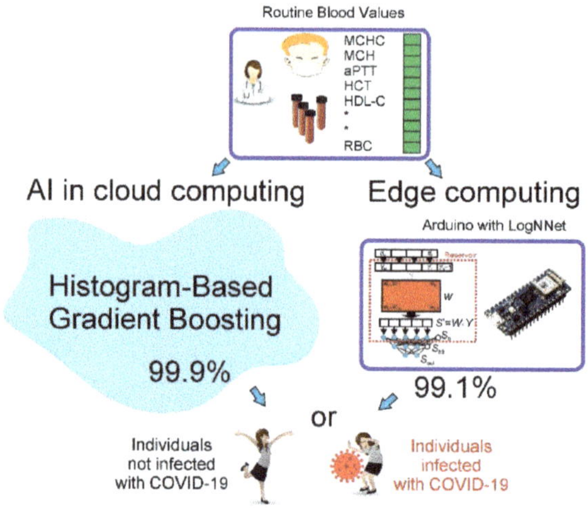

Figure 9. Two architectures of the IoT system, which includes an IoT device with LogNNet implementation (edge computing) and a cloud service containing a trained HGB model (AI computing).

In the IoT device, the results of a biochemical blood test are entered manually or transmitted directly from the laboratory equipment. If the cloud service is unavailable or if the blood tests are performed on site using a mobile laboratory in remote areas, the diagnosis is made by the LogNNet network. If the IoT device has access to the network, it sends a network request to the cloud service, wherein the diagnosis is determined using the HGB model. The cloud service sends a response with a diagnosis, which is displayed on the IoT device using an LED indication or on an LCD display.

5. Discussion

5.1. Analysis of Results from a Medical Perspective

COVID-19 has a higher mortality and infectivity than influenza [3,13]. The disease still causes death and continues to spread [1,6,15]. The use of vaccines did not stop the spread of the disease, and important mutations were detected in the structure of the virus during the epidemic [1]. Most of the infected patients had mild symptoms and a good prognosis. However, some patients developed severe symptoms, such as severe pneumonia, acute respiratory distress syndrome (ARDS) and multiple organ dysfunction syndromes (MODSs) [2,5,24]. A need for studies to determine the prognosis and immune conditions of the COVID-19 disease remains [3,74]. Therefore, the early evaluation of patients who need intensive care and have high mortality expectations as well as the effective identification of relevant biomarkers are important to reduce the mortality of the disease [5,6,25].

Various complications may be encountered during the treatment process of COVID-19 and, therefore, the course of the disease should be predicted earlier [64,77]. It is important to diagnose and predict the prognosis of the disease at an early stage so that the first response to severely infected COVID-19 patients can be conducted properly [2,5].

Although many studies on COVID-19 have been published, the relationships between the pathological aspects of the disease and routine blood values have not been fully determined [77]. Previous studies have reported that changes in many RBVs and hematological abnormalities are observed during the course of the disease [14,77].

In this study, according to the A_{th} threshold classification result based on [12], the most effective features in the diagnosis of the disease were found to be LDL with 96.47%, HDL-C with 94.73%, cholesterol with 94.47% and MCHC with 94.35% (Table 3). Indeed, in previous studies, large changes in these features were reported in severe and fatal COVID-19 patients, and these features may be important biomarkers for the prognosis of the disease [1,2,5,14].

Considering the linear dependency structures of the features among each other, the most effective combinations of dual features in the diagnosis of the disease were obtained and the Pearson correlation values were calculated (Table 4). The highly positive linear correlation structure of some trait pairs with positive and negative individuals was remarkable. The highest positive and negative linearly correlated trait pairs (High–High) were HCT–HGB, MPV–PDW and HCT–RBC (96%, 93% and 87%, respectively). These features vary greatly in severe COVID-19 patients and may be associated with the prognosis and mortality of the disease [1,2,14]. The high positive association of trait pairs expressed as the High–High type with both positive and negative COVID-19 individuals led us to believe that various comorbidities such as hypertension, obesity and diabetes may exist in our negative COVID-19 population. Considering hospital admissions of negative COVID-19 patients, these trait pairs are highly associated not only with COVID-19 but also with various inflammatory syndromes and infections [1,2,78]. Djakpo et al. [79] stated that the abnormalities of HGB, HCT and RBC or anemia observed in patients with comorbidities are due to the inability of the bone marrow to produce enough RBCs to carry oxygen and lung damage caused by COVID-19 which complicates gas exchange.

Considering the relationship of the patients with these features, the presence of possible comorbid conditions prevents erythrocyte production due to existing inflammation. Since the variation in these trait pairs is hypersensitive to the immune response in individuals, these trait pairs were highly correlated with sick and healthy individuals. The MCH–MCHC trait pair was found to be highly positively correlated, especially with healthy individuals, and this pair may be used as an important marker to distinguish healthy individuals in the diagnosis of the disease. Changes in these characteristics may indicate the suppression of lymphocytic and erythrocyte series or platelet and erythrocyte deformities [1]. In addition, in this study, a highly positive association of the MCH–MCV trait pair with COVID-19 was found. Mertoğlu et al. [2], Huyut et al. [14] and Karakike et al. [21] stated that this was due to the decrease in the size of erythrocytes and anisocytosis in patients. The high positive association of the HGB–RBC trait pair with sick individuals may be related to impaired erythropoiesis in the later stages of the disease. The High–High type feature set provides important clues in the isolation of both sick and healthy individuals.

In Table 4, a high (77%) negative relationship between the fibrinogen–LYM feature pair and COVID-19 patients is seen, and we believe that this level of relationship is due to the fibrinogen feature. Indeed, Winata and Kurniawan [28] noted that the degradation product of fibrinogen (FBU) was increased in all patients in the late stage of COVID-19 and that this was significantly associated with coagulation. In addition, the high correlation of the cholesterol–LDL, cholesterol–HDL-C and chlorine-sodium trait pairs (High–Low type in Table 4) with sick individuals showed that these trait pairs were important markers in identifying sick individuals. Fang et al. [80] and Mertoğlu et al. [1] stated that this feature set may be associated with multi-organ involvement in COVID-19 and the widespread distribution of angiotensin-converting enzyme receptors in the body.

The fact that the Low–High trait pair MCHC–MCV was found to be highly positively correlated with COVID-19 negative individuals in Table 4 suggested the importance of the size of erythrocyte and anisocytosis in healthy individuals [80]. In addition, the functional properties of the ALT–AST, eGFR–Urea and D-Bil–T-Bil pairs were found to be important markers in the isolation of COVID-19 negative individuals. Mertoğlu et al. [1], Huyut et al. [14] and Zhou et al. [27] stated that the decrease in ALT, AST, GGT, total bilirubin and eGFR indicated that the patients had serious damage to organs such as pancreas and kidney. In another study, Bertolini et al. [81] stated that AST, GGT, ALP and bilirubin may be frequently elevated in COVID-19 and that the main underlying causes of this condition may be hyper inflammation and thrombotic microangiopathy. In addition, the high positive correlation of the INR–PT trait pair with negative COVID-19 individuals suggested that it is important to monitor these individuals for the development of disseminated intravascular coagulopathy and acute respiratory distress [80,82].

In this study, 13 popular classifier machine learning models and the LogNNet neural network model were run on 51 routine blood values to detect patients infected with COVID-19. Histogram-based gradient boosting (HGB) was the model with the fastest and highest accuracy in determining the diagnosis of the disease (accuracy: 100%, time: 6.39 sec).

For the HGB model using a single input feature (A_1), the most effective features in the diagnosis of the disease were LDL 96.87% (№ 43), cholesterol 9507% (№ 39), HDL-C 94.99% (№ 36), MCHC 94.35% (№ 20), triglyceride (№ 48) and amylase (№ 31) (Table 6). For the HGB model using the dual entry feature (A_2), the most effective trait pair in the diagnosis of the disease was MCHC–MCH (A_2 = 99.81) (Table 7). The success of MCH as a single-entry feature in the diagnosis of the disease is low (A_1 = 52.13). Huyut and Velichko [12] found an accuracy rate of 99.1% in the diagnosis of the disease by running the MCHC–MCH features with LogNNet. The HGB model operated with MCHC–MCH was found to be more successful than the LogNNet model in the diagnosis of the disease.

Since low values of MCH and high values of MCHC were associated with COVID-19 [83], it was expected that the use of these two features together in the diagnosis of the disease would produce higher classification success. The most effective dual trait pairs (Table 7) were similar to the most effective single traits (Table 6) for the HGB model for the diagnosis of the disease. This provides important information about the functional properties of the binary trait pairs obtained with the HGB model in the diagnosis of the disease. Six basic features, that is LDL (№ 43), cholesterol (№ 39), HDL-C (№ 36), MCHC (№ 20), triglyceride (№ 48) and amylase (№ 31), among the combinations of binary features used in the diagnosis of the disease and four features, that is UA (№ 51), LDH (№ 42),

CK-MB (№ 32) and ALP (№ 30), that most frequently pair with these features are given in Figure 6. The main feature LDL (№ 43) generated the largest number of effective pairs for classification. The effectiveness of these feature pairs (Table 7) in detecting patients is visualized in two-dimensional space (Figure 7). Classification is most clearly visible in the MCHC–MCH pair (Figure 7a), which explains the higher classification ability.

In the binary feature combinations used by HGB in the diagnosis of the disease, the maximum accuracy was A_2 = 99.81% which is slightly lower than the use of 51 features (A_{51} = 100%). However, feature reduction provides more cost effective and rapid results in interpreting the classification of patients from a practical point of view and identifying the most effective features. The highest classification success obtained for the HGB model using three feature combinations was A_3 = 99.91 (Table 8).

Analysis of Table 8 showed that no new features were added to the top twenty models with the highest accuracy compared to Table 7. The binary combinations in Table 7 were sufficient for the diagnosis of the disease. In addition, the co-existence of MCH and MCHC features in all combinations reveals hidden association structures between these features and contains important clues in the diagnosis of the disease.

In this study, the most important 11 biomarkers were found with the HGB model used to determine the diagnosis of the disease, and with these features, all patients and healthy individuals were correctly identified with high performance (A11 = 100%). In addition, the importance of various combinations of these features in the diagnosis of the disease was recognized. The performance of these 11 features, namely LDL (№ 43), cholesterol (№ 39), HDL-C (№ 36), MCHC (№ 20), triglyceride (№ 48), amylase (№ 31), UA (№ 51), LDH (№ 42), CK-MB (№ 32), ALP (№ 30) and MCH (№ 19) and their various combinations in the diagnosis of the disease was higher than the individual performances, suggesting that there is a high level of confidential information between these feature combinations and COVID-19.

Kocar et al. [84] and Zinellu et al. [85] presented evidence of significant changes in the lipid profile of severe COVID-19 patients, particularly in total cholesterol, LDL and HDL-C concentrations. They also reported that increased cholesterol concentrations in the cell membrane increased the binding activity of SARS-CoV-2, facilitated membrane fusion and enabled the successful entry of the virus into the host. Therefore, Kocar et al. [84] and Wei et al. [86] indicated that total cholesterol, LDL and HDL-C characteristics may aid in early risk stratification and clinical decisions. However, conflicting results have been reported for changes in triglyceride levels of severe COVID-19 patients [85]. Stephens et al. [87] stated that in severe COVID-19 patients, the elevated serum amylase value is often not attributable to acute pancreatitis or a clinically significant pancreatic injury, but is more likely to be a nonspecific manifestation of shock/critical illness. Mao et al. [83] stated that changes in leukocytes, neutrophils, lymphocytes, platelets, hemoglobin levels, MCV and MCHC are generally associated with lung involvement, oxygen demand and disease activity. They also noted that high MCV and low MCHC are associated with advanced anemia and are independent predictors of disease worsening [83].

Wu et al. [88] stated that an increase or decrease in LDH is indicative of radiographic progression or improvement. They also demonstrated the potential usefulness of serum LDH as a marker for assessing clinical severity, monitoring treatment response and thus aiding risk stratification and early intervention in COVID-19 pneumonia. Hu et al. [89] stated that SARS-CoV-2 infection is associated with low serum uric acid (SUA) levels, and this feature may be an independent risk factor for the disease. They also noted that male patients with COVID-19 accompanied by low SUA levels are at higher risk of developing severe symptoms than those with high SUA levels at admission. Zinellu et al. [90] found that high CK-MB concentrations were significantly associated with severe morbidity and mortality in COVID-19 patients. They stated that this biomarker of myocardial damage may be useful for the classification of patients with severe COVID-19, and that high CK-MB values may reflect excessive inflammation status. They also stated that the evaluation of CK-MB in COVID-19 patients provides specific clinical information for early risk stratification, independent of myocardial necrosis and cardiac complications. Afra et al. [91] showed the incidence of abnormal liver tests in severe COVID-19 patients and reported the association of elevated AST, ALT and total bilirubin levels with liver injury in severe COVID-19 patients [13,91,92]. However, conflicting results have been reported regarding the ALP levels of mild and severe COVID-19 patients [91]. In addition, Afra et al. [91] showed that elevated liver enzymes can effectively predict hospital-critical COVID-19 cases.

The accuracy of ML algorithms is difficult to determine when used without any physician input [93,94]. A major limitation of ML is that it is difficult to explain how these algorithms arrive at their conclusions [95]. An ML algorithm can be likened to a black box that takes inputs and produces outputs without any explanation as to how it produces the outputs [94].

Additionally, if an algorithm misdiagnoses a malignant lesion, the algorithm cannot explain why it chose a particular diagnosis [94,95]. While the printouts can aid interpretation, it can be a potential danger and problem to the patient if the model fails to explain to a patient why he or she has diagnosed a lesion as benign or malignant, or how it has chosen a particular treatment [94].

Physician interpretation is necessary for choosing a diagnosis or treatment. In addition to the black box nature of these algorithms, machine learning is also prone to the "garbage in, garbage out" motto [94]. This maxim indicates that the quality of the dataset input determines the quality of the output. Therefore, if the data inputs are badly labeled, the outputs of the algorithm will reflect these inaccuracies [93–95].

In addition, all the devices should be evaluated in prospective clinical trials and made publicly available in the peer-reviewed literature.

5.2. *Analysis of Results from IoT Perspective*

The aim of this study is the feasibility analysis of a fast, reliable and cost-effective digital tool for the diagnosis of COVID-19 based on the RBV values measured at admission. The proposed solution is based on the concept of ML sensors for diagnosis of the COVID-19 disease (Sensor 1.0 type). The concept makes a step towards "smart sensorics of human" with promising opportunities for AI applications in healthcare.

In our study, we are not targeting IoT systems for telemedicine, wherein any procedure is performed by a physician using telecommunication means of transmitting medical data. Solutions of clinical telemedicine are subject to strict certification. Telemedicine is prescribed by a doctor and is administered via a medical device (never via a smartphone). Instead, we focus on promising IoT systems for telehealth/telecare and mobile health (m-Health) [45]. First, data from ML sensors support the prognosis of the disease in offline and online modes. Second, ML sensors can be used in AAL and other IoT environments to support a person in his/her everyday life. Importantly, COVID-19 is not the only disease to apply ML sensors in IoT systems.

AI methods become effective for the prognosis of various diseases. COVID-19 has opened the new era for AI methods to mitigate future pandemics. The rapidly growing number of publications confirms the potential of ML sensors for collecting datasets for further analysis with AI methods. Predictive analytics uses available retrospective data and various predictive models (including ML-constructed) to aid in answering the question "What could happen?". Prognosis from the sensed data is required not only for clinical medicine (to support clinical medical decisions). Managerial predictive analytics supports managers in healthcare at various levels to assess possible scenarios for the development of diseases, the budgets of medical organizations, the need for medicines, etc.

In AAL, ML sensors are useful in personal use as digital assistance (recommendations, including prognosis). In fact, the five natural human sensors (vision, hearing, touch, smell, taste) are extended by ML sensors. A person can develop health insight from their own RBVs in real time or collect the data for retrospective analysis. Humans themselves can act as complicated sensors [44]. A human traditionally finds a way to enhance her/his function, e.g., glasses (optical tool) to advance the vision or thermometer (physical tool) to regularly sense body temperature. Now the era of digital tools for personal health assistance is coming.

The implemented prototype of the diagnosis tool demonstrates that the LogNNet network can be imported to various microcontrollers. Many IoT devices can be made smarter, opening a way to develop advanced AmI healthcare with essential parts of IoT and edge intelligence [96]. A LogNNet-equipped ML sensor can be effectively employed in future IoT applications for healthcare and for other problem domains that require active digitalization and emerging AmI methods [46].

The LogNNet network can be used to predict a diagnosis based on blood biochemical parameters. This result is an important step in smart human sensors for IoT application, as the COVID-19 status and other blood-related health parameters are difficult to analyze on the IoT edges (in contrast to more widespread parameters, such as temperature or heartbeat) [97–99]. Our approach is applicable to the development of personalized bionic systems (smart suit for a person or AmI environment with people), wherein disease status recognition is a regular digital service for healthcare or well-being applications in everyday life [45].

Although the small IoT devices cannot provide such high accuracy as resource-intensive ML algorithms on powerful computer systems, AAL systems are intended for everyday life settings (e.g., at home, workspace, outdoor). Where strict medical decisions and critical medical support are not mandatory, the digital services may provide attention points and optional recommendations for personal use. We believe this type of smart human sensors will soon diffuse from the restricted medical lab setting toward the wide market of smart consumer electronics and digital services [100].

6. Limitations of the Study

The data primarily represent a single institution (EBYU-MG) and the Turkish population. Secondly, our dataset does not include comorbidities of patients and other diagnostic information of patient subgroups. In practice, the data in retrospective studies collected in a certain period cannot meet all data sample requirements. We suggest the findings in this study be supported by a retrospective cohort study setup.

7. Conclusions and Future Studies

Determining a COVID-19 infected status with diagnostic tests and imaging results is costly and time-consuming. If this process is prolonged, the patient's health may be at greater risk by being exposed to different complications. This study provides a fast, reliable and cost-effective alternative mobile tool for the diagnosis of COVID-19 based on the RBVs measured at the time of admission.

In this study, 13 popular classifier machine learning models and the LogNNet neural network model were run on 51 routine blood values to detect patients infected with COVID-19. The histogram-based gradient boosting (HGB) model was the most successful classification model in terms of accuracy and time in detecting the diagnosis of the disease (accuracy: 100%, time: 6.39 s). In addition, the absence of any normalization method and additional feature selection procedure for the HGB model contributes to the speed and efficiency of the model.

The eleven most important biomarkers in the diagnosis of the disease were found with the HGB classifier: LDL (№ 43), cholesterol (№ 39), HDL-C (№ 36), MCHC (№ 20), triglyceride (№ 48), amylase (№ 31), UA (№ 51), LDH (№ 42), CK-MB (№ 32), ALP (№ 30) and MCH (№ 19). Using only these 11 RBVs features, the HGB model accurately detected all COVID-19 patients (A_{11} = 100%).

The high accuracy of the single, double and triple combinations of these 11 features selected by the HGB model in the diagnosis of the disease showed the importance of these features in the diagnosis of the disease. In addition, the performance of double and triple combinations of these features in the detection of sick and healthy individuals was higher than the individual performances, suggesting that there is a high level of hidden information between these blood feature combinations and COVID-19.

The HGB model reveals that 11 features are sufficient for the diagnosis of the presence of COVID-19 using the HGB classifier. These features and their binary combinations are an important source of variation in the diagnosis of COVID-19. We propose to use these features and their binary combinations to be run with HGB as important biomarkers in the diagnosis of the disease.

The study results can be effectively used in IoT medical edge devices with low RAM resources, ML sensors, portable point-of-care blood testing devices [101], decision support systems, telecare and m-Health. This opportunity empowers the development of many innovative applications for predictive analytics in clinical MIS or everyday AAL systems.

The artificial intelligence models for the early prediction of the diagnosis and progression of COVID-19 and other diseases produce satisfactory results. Future artificial intelligence studies for the early diagnosis and prognosis of fatal, costly and severe diseases will ease the burden of healthcare professionals and increase patient comfort. In addition, the use the physiological, comorbidity and demographic features of the patients together with the RBVs data may provide interesting insights. Testing the results of this study on multi-racial, multi-center and larger patient groups may improve the generalizability of the findings. In this context, this study may pave the way for many exciting subsequent investigations.

Author Contributions: Conceptualization, M.T.H. and A.V.; methodology, A.V., M.T.H., M.B., Y.I. and D.K.; software, A.V., M.T.H., M.B. and Y.I.; validation, M.T.H. and A.V.; formal analysis, A.V., M.T.H., M.B, Y.I. and D.K.; investigation, A.V.; resources, M.T.H.; data curation, M.T.H.; writing—original draft preparation, A.V., M.T.H., M.B., Y.I. and D.K.; writing—review and editing, A.V., M.T.H., M.B., Y.I. and D.K.; visualization, A.V. and M.B.; supervision, D.K.; project administration, D.K.; funding acquisition, D.K. All authors have read and agreed to the published version of the manuscript.

Funding: The research is implemented with financial support by Russian Science Foundation, project no. 22-11-20040 (https://rscf.ru/en/project/22-11-20040/ (accessed on 14 September 2022)) jointly with Republic of Karelia and funding from Venture Investment Fund of Republic of Karelia (VIF RK).

Institutional Review Board Statement: The dataset used in this study was collected in order to be used in various studies in the estimation of the diagnosis, prognosis and mortality of COVID-19. The necessary permissions for the collected dataset were given by the Ministry of Health of the Republic of Turkey and the Ethics Committee of Erzincan Binali Yıldırım University. This study was conducted in accordance with the 1989 Declaration of Helsinki. Erzincan Binali Yıldırım University Human Research Health and Sports Sciences Ethics Committee Decision Number: 2021/02-07.

Informed Consent Statement: In this study, a dataset including only routine blood values, RT-PCR results (positive or negative) and treatment units of the patients was downloaded retrospectively from the information system of our hospital in a digital environment. A new sample was not taken from the patients. There is no information in the dataset that includes identifying characteristics of individuals. It was stated that routine blood values would only be used in academic studies, and written consent was obtained from the institutions for this. In addition, therefore, written informed consent was not administered for every patient.

Data Availability Statement: The data used in this study can be shared with the parties, provided that the article is cited.

Acknowledgments: We thank the method of Erzincan Mengücek Gazi Training and Research Hospital for their support in reaching the material used in this study. Special thanks to the editors of the journal and to the anonymous reviewers for their constructive criticism and improvement suggestions.

Conflicts of Interest: The authors declare no conflict of interest.

Appendix A

Algorithm A1. LogNNet neural network executable code on Arduino Nano IoT

```
#include "LogNNet.h"

float Y[S+1];
float Sh[P+1];
float Sh2[M+1];

int i = 0;
String data;

float Fun_activ(float x) {
  return 1 / (1 + exp(-1*x));
}

void Reservoir(float *Y) {
  long W = C;
  Sh[0] = 1;
  for (int j = 1; j <= P; j++) {
    Sh[j] = 0;
    for (int i = 0; i <= S; i++) {
      W = (D - K * W) % L;
      Sh[j] = Sh[j] + ((float)W/L) * Y[i];
    }
    Sh[j] = ((Sh[j] - (float)minS[j-1]/
        scale_factor) /
((float)(maxS[j-1]
        - minS[j-1])/scale_factor)) - 0.5
        -
(float)meanS[j-1]/(scale_factor*10);
  }
}

void Hidden_Layer() {
  Sh2[0] = 1;
  for (int j = 1; j <= M; j++) {
    Sh2[j] = 0;
    for (int i = 0; i <= P; i++)
      Sh2[j] = Sh2[j] + Sh[i] *
((float)W1[i][j]/scale_factor);
    Sh2[j] = Fun_activ(Sh2[j]);
  }
}

byte Output_Layer() {
  float Sout[N+1]; byte digit = 0;
  for (int j = 0; j <= N; j++) {
    Sout[j] = 0;
    for (int i = 0; i <= M; i++)
      Sout[j] = Sout[j] + Sh2[i] *
((float)W2[i][j]/scale_factor);
    Sout[j] = Fun_activ(Sout[j]);
  }
  for (int j = 0; j <= N; j++) {
    if (Sout[j] > Sout[digit])
      digit = j;
  }
  return digit;
}

void setup() {
  Serial.begin(115200);
}

void loop() {
  if (Serial.available() > 0) {
      data = Serial.readStringUntil('T');

      if (data != "FN") {
          Y[i] = data.toFloat();
          i++;
      }
      else {
          i = 0;
          Reservoir(Y);
          Hidden_Layer();
          byte Digit = Output_Layer();
          Serial.print(String(Digit));
      }
  }
}
```

References

1. Mertoglu, C.; Huyut, M.; Olmez, H.; Tosun, M.; Kantarci, M.; Coban, T. COVID-19 Is More Dangerous for Older People and Its Severity Is Increasing: A Case-Control Study. *Med. Gas Res.* **2022**, *12*, 51–54. [CrossRef]
2. Mertoglu, C.; Huyut, M.T.; Arslan, Y.; Ceylan, Y.; Coban, T.A. How Do Routine Laboratory Tests Change in Coronavirus Disease 2019? *Scand. J. Clin. Lab. Investig.* **2021**, *81*, 24–33. [CrossRef]
3. Zhou, C.; Chen, Y.; Ji, Y.; He, X.; Xue, D. Increased Serum Levels of Hepcidin and Ferritin Are Associated with Severity of COVID-19. *Med. Sci. Monit.* **2020**, *26*, e926178. [CrossRef]
4. Huyut, M.T.; Huyut, Z. Forecasting of Oxidant/Antioxidant Levels of COVID-19 Patients by Using Expert Models with Biomarkers Used in the Diagnosis/Prognosis of COVID-19. *Int. Immunopharmacol.* **2021**, *100*, 108127. [CrossRef]
5. Huyut, M.T.; İlkbahar, F. The Effectiveness of Blood Routine Parameters and Some Biomarkers as a Potential Diagnostic Tool in the Diagnosis and Prognosis of Covid-19 Disease. *Int. Immunopharmacol.* **2021**, *98*, 107838. [CrossRef]

6. Huyut, M.; Üstündağ, H. Prediction of Diagnosis and Prognosis of COVID-19 Disease by Blood Gas Parameters Using Decision Trees Machine Learning Model: A Retrospective Observational Study. *Med. Gas Res.* **2022**, *12*, 60–66. [CrossRef] [PubMed]
7. Cabitza, F.; Campagner, A.; Ferrari, D.; Di Resta, C.; Ceriotti, D.; Sabetta, E.; Colombini, A.; De Vecchi, E.; Banfi, G.; Locatelli, M.; et al. Development, Evaluation, and Validation of Machine Learning Models for COVID-19 Detection Based on Routine Blood Tests. *Clin. Chem. Lab. Med.* **2021**, *59*, 421–431. [CrossRef] [PubMed]
8. Vogels, C.B.F.; Brito, A.F.; Wyllie, A.L.; Fauver, J.R.; Ott, I.M.; Kalinich, C.C.; Petrone, M.E.; Casanovas-Massana, A.; Catherine Muenker, M.; Moore, A.J.; et al. Analytical Sensitivity and Efficiency Comparisons of SARS-CoV-2 RT–QPCR Primer–Probe Sets. *Nat. Microbiol.* **2020**, *5*, 1299–1305. [CrossRef]
9. Booth, A.L.; Abels, E.; McCaffrey, P. Development of a Prognostic Model for Mortality in COVID-19 Infection Using Machine Learning. *Mod. Pathol.* **2021**, *34*, 522–531. [CrossRef]
10. Ko, J.; Baldassano, S.N.; Loh, P.-L.; Kording, K.; Litt, B.; Issadore, D. Machine Learning To Detect Signatures of Disease in Liquid Biopsies-A User's Guide Graphical Abstract HHS Public Access. *Lab Chip* **2018**, *18*, 395–405. [CrossRef]
11. Huyut, M.T. Automatic Detection of Severely and Mildly Infected COVID-19 Patients with Supervised Machine Learning Models. *IRBM* **2022**, *1*, 35673548. [CrossRef]
12. Huyut, M.T.; Velichko, A. Diagnosis and Prognosis of COVID-19 Disease Using Routine Blood Values and LogNNet Neural Network. *Sensors* **2022**, *22*, 4820. [CrossRef] [PubMed]
13. Chen, N.; Zhou, M.; Dong, X.; Qu, J.; Gong, F.; Han, Y.; Qiu, Y.; Wang, J.; Liu, Y.; Wei, Y.; et al. Epidemiological and Clinical Characteristics of 99 Cases of 2019 Novel Coronavirus Pneumonia in Wuhan, China: A Descriptive Study. *Lancet* **2020**, *395*, 507–513. [CrossRef]
14. Tahir Huyut, M.; Huyut, Z.; İlkbahar, F.; Mertoğlu, C. What Is the Impact and Efficacy of Routine Immunological, Biochemical and Hematological Biomarkers as Predictors of COVID-19 Mortality? *Int. Immunopharmacol.* **2022**, *105*, 108542. [CrossRef] [PubMed]
15. Huyut, M.T.; Kocaturk, İ. The Effect of Some Symptoms and Features During the İnfection Period on the Level of Anxiety and Depression of Adults After Recovery From COVID-19. *Curr. Psychiatry Res. Rev.* **2022**, *18*, 151–163. [CrossRef]
16. Guan, W.; Ni, Z.; Hu, Y.; Liang, W.; Ou, C.; He, J.; Liu, L.; Shan, H.; Lei, C.; Hui, D.S.C.; et al. Clinical Characteristics of Coronavirus Disease 2019 in China. *N. Engl. J. Med.* **2020**, *382*, 1708–1720. [CrossRef]
17. Banerjee, A.; Ray, S.; Vorselaars, B.; Kitson, J.; Mamalakis, M.; Weeks, S.; Baker, M.; Mackenzie, L.S. Use of Machine Learning and Artificial Intelligence to Predict SARS-CoV-2 Infection from Full Blood Counts in a Population. *Int. Immunopharmacol.* **2020**, *86*, 106705. [CrossRef] [PubMed]
18. Huyut, M.T.; Soygüder, S. The Multi-Relationship Structure between Some Symptoms and Features Seen during the New Coronavirus 19 Infection and the Levels of Anxiety and Depression Post-Covid. *East. J. Med.* **2022**, *27*, 1–10. [CrossRef]
19. Perricone, C.; Bartoloni, E.; Bursi, R.; Cafaro, G.; Guidelli, G.M.; Shoenfeld, Y.; Gerli, R. COVID-19 as Part of the Hyperferritinemic Syndromes: The Role of Iron Depletion Therapy. *Immunol. Res.* **2020**, *68*, 213–224. [CrossRef] [PubMed]
20. Mehta, P.; McAuley, D.F.; Brown, M.; Sanchez, E.; Tattersall, R.S.; Manson, J.J. COVID-19: Consider Cytokine Storm Syndromes and Immunosuppression. *Lancet* **2020**, *395*, 1033–1034. [CrossRef]
21. Karakike, E.; Giamarellos-Bourboulis, E.J. Macrophage Activation-like Syndrome: A Distinct Entity Leading to Early Death in Sepsis. *Front. Immunol.* **2019**, *10*, 55. [CrossRef]
22. Tural Onur, S.; Altın, S.; Sokucu, S.N.; Fikri, B.İ.; Barça, T.; Bolat, E.; Toptaş, M. Could Ferritin Level Be an Indicator of COVID-19 Disease Mortality? *J. Med. Virol.* **2021**, *93*, 1672–1677. [CrossRef] [PubMed]
23. Rosário, C.; Zandman-Goddard, G.; Meyron-Holtz, E.G.; D'Cruz, D.P.; Shoenfeld, Y. The Hyperferritinemic Syndrome: Macrophage Activation Syndrome, Still's Disease, Septic Shock and Catastrophic Antiphospholipid Syndrome. *BMC Med.* **2013**, *11*, 185. [CrossRef]
24. Lippi, G.; Plebani, M.; Henry, B.M. Thrombocytopenia Is Associated with Severe Coronavirus Disease 2019 (COVID-19) Infections: A Meta-Analysis. *Clin. Chim. Acta* **2020**, *506*, 145–148. [CrossRef] [PubMed]
25. Cheng, L.; Li, H.; Li, L.; Liu, C.; Yan, S.; Chen, H.; Li, Y. Ferritin in the Coronavirus Disease 2019 (COVID-19): A Systematic Review and Meta-Analysis. *J. Clin. Lab. Anal.* **2020**, *34*, e23618. [CrossRef] [PubMed]
26. Feld, J.; Tremblay, D.; Thibaud, S.; Kessler, A.; Naymagon, L. Ferritin Levels in Patients with COVID-19: A Poor Predictor of Mortality and Hemophagocytic Lymphohistiocytosis. *Int. J. Lab. Hematol.* **2020**, *42*, 773–779. [CrossRef] [PubMed]
27. Zhou, F.; Yu, T.; Du, R.; Fan, G.; Liu, Y.; Liu, Z.; Xiang, J.; Wang, Y.; Song, B.; Gu, X.; et al. Clinical Course and Risk Factors for Mortality of Adult Inpatients with COVID-19 in Wuhan, China: A Retrospective Cohort Study. *Lancet* **2020**, *395*, 1054–1062. [CrossRef]
28. Winata, S.; Kurniawan, A. Coagulopathy in COVID-19: A Systematic Review. *Medicinus* **2021**, *8*, 72. [CrossRef]
29. Hariyanto, T.I.; Japar, K.V.; Kwenandar, F.; Damay, V.; Siregar, J.I.; Lugito, N.P.H.; Tjiang, M.M.; Kurniawan, A. Inflammatory and hematologic markers as predictors of severe outcomes in COVID-19 infection: A systematic review and meta-analysis. *Am. J. Emerg. Med.* **2021**, *41*, 110–119. [CrossRef]
30. Remeseiro, B.; Bolon-Canedo, V. A Review of Feature Selection Methods in Medical Applications. *Comput. Biol. Med.* **2019**, *112*, 103375. [CrossRef]
31. Guyon, I.; Gunn, S.; Nikravesh, M.; Zadeh, L.A. *Feature Extraction: Foundations and Applications*; Studies in Fuzziness and Soft Computing; Springer: Berlin/Heidelberg, Germany, 2008; ISBN 9783540354888.

32. Jiang, S.Q.; Huang, Q.F.; Xie, W.M.; Lv, C.; Quan, X.Q. The Association between Severe COVID-19 and Low Platelet Count: Evidence from 31 Observational Studies Involving 7613 Participants. *Br. J. Haematol.* **2020**, *190*, e29–e33. [CrossRef] [PubMed]
33. Zheng, Y.; Zhang, Y.; Chi, H.; Chen, S.; Peng, M.; Luo, L.; Chen, L.; Li, J.; Shen, B.; Wang, D. The Hemocyte Counts as a Potential Biomarker for Predicting Disease Progression in COVID-19: A Retrospective Study. *Clin. Chem. Lab. Med.* **2020**, *58*, 1106–1115. [CrossRef] [PubMed]
34. Hall, M.A. Correlation-Based Feature Selection for Machine Learning. Ph.D. Thesis, The University of Waikato, Hamilton, New Zealand, 1999.
35. Dash, M.; Liu, H. Consistency-Based Search in Feature Selection. *Artif. Intell.* **2003**, *151*, 155–176. [CrossRef]
36. Zhao, Z.; Liu, H. Searching for Interacting Features. In Proceedings of the 20th International Joint Conference on Artificial Intelligence, Hyderabad, India, 6–12 January 2007; pp. 1156–1161.
37. Hall, M.A.; Smith, L.A. Practical Feature Subset Selection for Machine Learning. In Proceedings of the the 21st Australasian Computer Science Conference ACSC'98, Perth, Australia, 4–6 February 1998; Volume 20, pp. 181–191.
38. Kononenko, I. *Estimating Attributes: Analysis and Extensions of RELIEF. Machine Learning: ECML-94*; Lecture Notes in Computer Science; Springer: Berlin/Heidelberg, Germany, 1994; Volume 784, pp. 171–182. [CrossRef]
39. Le Thi, H.A.; Nguyen, V.V.; Ouchani, S. *Gene Selection for Cancer Classification Using DCA. Advanced Data Mining and Applications*; Lecture Notes in Computer Science; Springer: Berlin/Heidelberg, Germany, 2008; Volume 5139, pp. 62–72. [CrossRef]
40. Tibshirani, R. Regression Shrinkage and Selection via the Lasso. *J. R. Stat. Society. Ser. B Methodol.* **1996**, *58*, 267–288. [CrossRef]
41. Zhu, J.S.; Ge, P.; Jiang, C.; Zhang, Y.; Li, X.; Zhao, Z.; Zhang, L.; Duong, T.Q. Deep-Learning Artificial Intelligence Analysis of Clinical Variables Predicts Mortality in COVID-19 Patients. *J. Am. Coll. Emerg. Physicians Open* **2020**, *1*, 1364–1373. [CrossRef] [PubMed]
42. Meigal, A.Y.; Korzun, D.G.; Moschevikin, A.P.; Reginya, S.; Gerasimova-Meigal, L.I. Ambient Assisted Living At-Home Laboratory for Motor Status Diagnostics in Parkinson's Disease Patients and Aged People. In *Research Anthology on Supporting Healthy Aging in a Digital Society*; IGI Global: Hershey, PA, USA, 2022; pp. 836–862. Available online: https://services.igi-global.com/resolvedoi/resolve.aspx?doi=10.4018/978-1-6684-5295-0.ch047 (accessed on 1 October 2022). [CrossRef]
43. Fernandes, J.M.; Silva, J.S.; Rodrigues, A.; Boavida, F. A Survey of Approaches to Unobtrusive Sensing of Humans. *ACM Comput. Surv.* **2022**, *55*, 1–28. [CrossRef]
44. Kostakos, V.; Rogstadius, J.; Ferreira, D.; Hosio, S.; Goncalves, J. *Participatory Sensing, Opinions and Collective Awareness*, 1st ed.; Loreto, V., Haklay, M., Hotho, A., Servedio, V.D.P., Stumme, G., Theunis, J., Tria, F., Eds.; Springer International Publishing: Cham, Switzerland, 2017; pp. 69–92. ISBN 978-3-319-25658-0.
45. Korzun, D.G. Internet of Things Meets Mobile Health Systems in Smart Spaces: An Overview. In *Internet of Things and Big Data Technologies for Next Generation Healthcare*; Bhatt, C., Dey, N., Ashour, A.S., Eds.; Springer International Publishing: Cham, Switzerland, 2017; pp. 111–129. ISBN 978-3-319-49736-5.
46. Korzun, D.; Balandina, E.; Kashevnik, A.; Balandin, S.; Viola, F. *Ambient Intelligence Services in IoT Environments: Emerging Research and Opportunities*; IGI Global: Hershey, PA, USA, 2019; ISBN 9781522589730.
47. Warden, P.; Stewart, M.; Plancher, B.; Banbury, C.; Prakash, S.; Chen, E.; Asgar, Z.; Katti, S.; Reddi, V.J. Machine Learning Sensors. *arXiv* **2022**. [CrossRef]
48. Chinchole, S.; Patel, S. Artificial Intelligence and Sensors Based Assistive System for the Visually Impaired People. In Proceedings of the 2017 International Conference on Intelligent Sustainable Systems (ICISS), Palladam, India, 7–8 December 2017; pp. 16–19.
49. Gulzar Ahmad, S.; Iqbal, T.; Javaid, A.; Ullah Munir, E.; Kirn, N.; Ullah Jan, S.; Ramzan, N. Sensing and Artificial Intelligent Maternal-Infant Health Care Systems: A Review. *Sensors* **2022**, *22*, 4362. [CrossRef]
50. Machine Learning Sensors: Truly Data-Centric AI | Towards Data Science. Available online: https://towardsdatascience.com/machine-learning-sensors-truly-data-centric-ai-8f6b99904633a (accessed on 23 August 2022).
51. Ma, Y.; Hou, L.; Yang, X.; Huang, Z.; Yang, X.; Zhao, N.; He, M.; Shi, Y.; Kang, Y.; Yue, J.; et al. The Association between Frailty and Severe Disease among COVID-19 Patients Aged over 60 Years in China: A Prospective Cohort Study. *BMC Med.* **2020**, *18*, 274. [CrossRef]
52. Fan, B.E. Hematologic Parameters in Patients with COVID-19 Infection: A Reply. *Am. J. Hematol.* **2020**, *95*, E215. [CrossRef]
53. Ferrari, D.; Motta, A.; Strollo, M.; Banfi, G.; Locatelli, M. Routine Blood Tests as a Potential Diagnostic Tool for COVID-19. *Clin. Chem. Lab. Med.* **2020**, *58*, 1095–1099. [CrossRef] [PubMed]
54. Wu, J.; Zhang, P.; Zhang, L.; Meng, W.; Li, J.; Tong, C.; Li, Y.; Cai, J.; Yang, Z.; Zhu, J.; et al. Rapid and Accurate Identification of COVID-19 Infection through Machine Learning Based on Clinical Available Blood Test Results. *medRxiv* **2020**. [CrossRef]
55. Shakeel, P.M.; Burhanuddin, M.A.; Desa, M.I. Lung Cancer Detection from CT Image Using Improved Profuse Clustering and Deep Learning Instantaneously Trained Neural Networks. *Meas. J. Int. Meas. Confed.* **2019**, *145*, 702–712. [CrossRef]
56. Cui, H.; Wang, X.; Feng, D. Automated Localization and Segmentation of Lung Tumor from PET-CT Thorax Volumes Based on Image Feature Analysis. In Proceedings of the 2012 Annual International Conference of the IEEE Engineering in Medicine and Biology Society, San Diego, CA, USA, 28 August–1 September 2012; pp. 5384–5387. [CrossRef]
57. Tomita, K.; Nagao, R.; Touge, H.; Ikeuchi, T.; Sano, H.; Yamasaki, A.; Tohda, Y. Deep Learning Facilitates the Diagnosis of Adult Asthma. *Allergol. Int.* **2019**, *68*, 456–461. [CrossRef]
58. Ryu, K.S.; Lee, S.W.; Batbaatar, E.; Lee, J.W.; Choi, K.S.; Cha, H.S. A Deep Learning Model for Estimation of Patients with Undiagnosed Diabetes. *Appl. Sci.* **2020**, *10*, 421. [CrossRef]

59. Kolachalama, V.B.; Singh, P.; Lin, C.Q.; Mun, D.; Belghasem, M.E.; Henderson, J.M.; Francis, J.M.; Salant, D.J.; Chitalia, V.C. Association of Pathological Fibrosis With Renal Survival Using Deep Neural Networks. *Kidney Int. Rep.* **2018**, *3*, 464–475. [CrossRef] [PubMed]
60. Wu, C.C.; Yeh, W.C.; Hsu, W.D.; Islam, M.M.; Nguyen, P.A.A.; Poly, T.N.; Wang, Y.C.; Yang, H.C.; Li, Y.C.J. Prediction of Fatty Liver Disease Using Machine Learning Algorithms. *Comput. Methods Programs Biomed.* **2019**, *170*, 23–29. [CrossRef] [PubMed]
61. Oguntimilehin, A.; Adetunmbi, A.O.; Abiola, O.B. A Machine Learning Approach to Clinical Diagnosis of Typhoid Fever. *Int. J. Comput. Inf. Technol.* **2013**, *4*, 671–676.
62. Kouchaki, S.; Yang, Y.Y.; Walker, T.M.; Walker, A.S.; Wilson, D.J.; Peto, T.E.A.; Crook, D.W.; Clifton, D.A.; Hoosdally, S.J.; Gibertoni Cruz, A.L.; et al. Application of Machine Learning Techniques to Tuberculosis Drug Resistance Analysis. *Bioinformatics* **2019**, *35*, 2276–2282. [CrossRef]
63. Taylor, R.A.; Moore, C.L.; Cheung, K.H.; Brandt, C. Predicting Urinary Tract Infections in the Emergency Department with Machine Learning. *PLoS ONE* **2018**, *13*, e0194085. [CrossRef]
64. Yang, H.S.; Hou, Y.; Vasovic, L.V.; Steel, P.A.D.; Chadburn, A.; Racine-Brzostek, S.E.; Velu, P.; Cushing, M.M.; Loda, M.; Kaushal, R.; et al. Routine Laboratory Blood Tests Predict SARS-CoV-2 Infection Using Machine Learning. *Clin. Chem.* **2020**, *66*, 1396–1404. [CrossRef] [PubMed]
65. Brinati, D.; Campagner, A.; Ferrari, D.; Locatelli, M.; Banfi, G.; Cabitza, F. Detection of COVID-19 Infection from Routine Blood Exams with Machine Learning: A Feasibility Study. *J. Med. Syst.* **2020**, *44*, 135. [CrossRef]
66. Zhang, S.; Huang, S.; Liu, J.; Dong, X.; Meng, M.; Chen, L.; Wen, Z.; Zhang, L.; Chen, Y.; Du, H.; et al. Identification and Validation of Prognostic Factors in Patients with COVID-19: A Retrospective Study Based on Artificial Intelligence Algorithms. *J. Intensive Med.* **2021**, *1*, 103–109. [CrossRef]
67. Alle, S.; Karthikeyan, A.; Kanakan, A.; Siddiqui, S.; Garg, A.; Mehta, P.; Mishra, N.; Chattopadhyay, P.; Devi, P.; Waghdhare, S.; et al. COVID-19 Risk Stratification and Mortality Prediction in Hospitalized Indian Patients: Harnessing Clinical Data for Public Health Benefits. *PLoS ONE* **2022**, *17*, e0264785. [CrossRef] [PubMed]
68. Gao, Y.; Chen, L.; Chi, J.; Zeng, S.; Feng, X.; Li, H.; Liu, D.; Feng, X.; Wang, S.; Wang, Y.; et al. Development and Validation of an Online Model to Predict Critical COVID-19 with Immune-Inflammatory Parameters. *J. Intensive Care* **2021**, *9*, 19. [CrossRef]
69. Vaishnav, P.K.; Sharma, S.; Sharma, P. Analytical Review Analysis for Screening COVID-19 Disease. *Int. J. Mod. Res.* **2021**, *1*, 22–29.
70. Kukar, M.; Gunčar, G.; Vovko, T.; Podnar, S.; Černelč, P.; Brvar, M.; Zalaznik, M.; Notar, M.; Moškon, S.; Notar, M. COVID-19 Diagnosis by Routine Blood Tests Using Machine Learning. *Sci. Rep.* **2021**, *11*, 10738. [CrossRef] [PubMed]
71. Mei, X.; Lee, H.C.; Diao, K.Y.; Huang, M.; Lin, B.; Liu, C.; Xie, Z.; Ma, Y.; Robson, P.M.; Chung, M.; et al. Artificial Intelligence–Enabled Rapid Diagnosis of Patients with COVID-19. *Nat. Med.* **2020**, *26*, 1224–1228. [CrossRef] [PubMed]
72. Gómez-Pastora, J.; Weigand, M.; Kim, J.; Wu, X.; Strayer, J.; Palmer, A.F.; Zborowski, M.; Yazer, M.; Chalmers, J.J. Hyperferritinemia in Critically Ill COVID-19 Patients—Is Ferritin the Product of Inflammation or a Pathogenic Mediator? *Clin. Chim. Acta* **2020**, *509*, 249–251. [CrossRef]
73. Boslaugh, S. *Statistics in a Nutshell*, 2nd ed.; O'Reilly Media, Incorporated: Newton, MA, USA, 2012; ISBN 9781449361129.
74. Weiss, G.; Ganz, T.; Goodnough, L.T. Anemia of Inflammation. *Blood* **2019**, *133*, 40–50. [CrossRef]
75. Harrington, P. *Machine Learning in Action*; Simon and Schuster: New York, NY, USA, 2012; ISBN 978-1617290183.
76. Feurer, M.; Eggensperger, K.; Falkner, S.; Lindauer, M.; Hutter, F. Auto-Sklearn 2.0: Hands-Free AutoML via Meta-Learning. *arXiv* **2020**, arXiv:2007.04074.
77. Kim, S.; Kim, D.-M.; Lee, B. Insufficient Sensitivity of RNA Dependent RNA Polymerase Gene of SARS-CoV-2 Viral Genome as Confirmatory Test Using Korean COVID-19 Cases. *Preprints* **2020**, 1–14. [CrossRef]
78. Teymouri, M.; Mollazadeh, S.; Mortazavi, H.; Naderi Ghale-noie, Z.; Keyvani, V.; Aghababaei, F.; Hamblin, M.R.; Abbaszadeh-Goudarzi, G.; Pourghadamyari, H.; Hashemian, S.M.R.; et al. Recent Advances and Challenges of RT-PCR Tests for the Diagnosis of COVID-19. *Pathol. Res. Pract.* **2021**, *221*, 153443. [CrossRef]
79. Djakpo, D.K.; Wang, Z.; Zhang, R.; Chen, X.; Chen, P.; Ketisha Antoine, M.M.L. Blood Routine Test in Mild and Common 2019 Coronavirus (COVID-19) Patients. *Biosci. Rep.* **2020**, *40*, BSR20200817. [CrossRef]
80. Fang, B.; Meng, Q.H. The Laboratory's Role in Combating COVID-19. *Crit. Rev. Clin. Lab. Sci.* **2020**, *57*, 400–414. [CrossRef]
81. Bertolini, A.; van de Peppel, I.P.; Bodewes, F.A.J.A.; Moshage, H.; Fantin, A.; Farinati, F.; Fiorotto, R.; Jonker, J.W.; Strazzabosco, M.; Verkade, H.J.; et al. Abnormal Liver Function Tests in Patients With COVID-19: Relevance and Potential Pathogenesis. *Hepatology* **2020**, *72*, 1864–1872. [CrossRef]
82. Terpos, E.; Ntanasis-Stathopoulos, I.; Elalamy, I.; Kastritis, E.; Sergentanis, T.N.; Politou, M.; Psaltopoulou, T.; Gerotziafas, G.; Dimopoulos, M.A. Hematological Findings and Complications of COVID-19. *Am. J. Hematol.* **2020**, *95*, 834–847. [CrossRef] [PubMed]
83. Mao, J.; Dai, R.; Du, R.C.; Zhu, Y.; Shui, L.P.; Luo, X.H. Hematologic Changes Predict Clinical Outcome in Recovered Patients with COVID-19. *Ann. Hematol.* **2021**, *100*, 675–689. [CrossRef]
84. Kočar, E.; Režen, T.; Rozman, D. Cholesterol, Lipoproteins, and COVID-19: Basic Concepts and Clinical Applications. *Biochim. Biophys. Acta Mol. Cell Biol. Lipids* **2021**, *1866*, 209–214. [CrossRef]

85. Zinellu, A.; Paliogiannis, P.; Fois, A.G.; Solidoro, P.; Carru, C.; Mangoni, A.A. Cholesterol and Triglyceride Concentrations, COVID-19 Severity, and Mortality: A Systematic Review and Meta-Analysis With Meta-Regression. *Front. Public Health* **2021**, *9*, 705916. [CrossRef]
86. Wei, X.; Zeng, W.; Su, J.; Wan, H.; Yu, X.; Cao, X.; Tan, W.; Wang, H. Hypolipidemia Is Associated with the Severity of COVID-19. *J. Clin. Lipidol.* **2020**, *14*, 297–304. [CrossRef] [PubMed]
87. Stephens, J.R.; Wong, J.L.C.; Broomhead, R.; Mpfle, R.S.; Waheed, U.; Patel, P.; Brett, S.J.; Soni, S. Raised Serum Amylase in Patients with COVID-19 May Not Be Associated with Pancreatitis. *Br. J. Surg.* **2021**, *108*, e152–e153. [CrossRef]
88. Wu, M.Y.; Yao, L.; Wang, Y.; Zhu, X.Y.; Wang, X.F.; Tang, P.J.; Chen, C. Clinical Evaluation of Potential Usefulness of Serum Lactate Dehydrogenase (LDH) in 2019 Novel Coronavirus (COVID-19) Pneumonia. *Respir. Res.* **2020**, *21*, 171. [CrossRef] [PubMed]
89. Hu, F.; Guo, Y.; Lin, J.; Zeng, Y.; Wang, J.; Li, M.; Cong, L. Association of Serum Uric Acid Levels with COVID-19 Severity. *BMC Endocr. Disord.* **2021**, *21*, 97. [CrossRef] [PubMed]
90. Zinellu, A.; Sotgia, S.; Fois, A.G.; Mangoni, A.A. Serum CK-MB, COVID-19 Severity and Mortality: An Updated Systematic Review and Meta-Analysis with Meta-Regression. *Adv. Med. Sci.* **2021**, *66*, 304–314. [CrossRef]
91. Afra, H.S.; Amiri-Dashatan, N.; Ghorbani, F.; Maleki, I. Positive Association between Severity of COVID-19 Infection and Liver Damage: A Systematic Review and Meta-Analysis. *Gastroenterol. Hepatol. Bed Bench* **2020**, *13*, 292–304. [CrossRef]
92. Huang, Y.; Yang, R.; Xu, Y.; Gong, P. Clinical Characteristics of 36 Non-Survivors with COVID-19 in Wuhan, China. *medRxiv* **2020**. [CrossRef]
93. González-Cruz, C.; Jofre, M.A.; Podlipnik, S.; Combalia, M.; Gareau, D.; Gamboa, M.; Vallone, M.G.; Faride Barragán-Estudillo, Z.; Tamez-Peña, A.L.; Montoya, J.; et al. Machine Learning in Melanoma Diagnosis. Limitations About to Be Overcome. *Actas Dermo-Sifiliográficas (Engl. Ed.)* **2020**, *111*, 313–316. [CrossRef] [PubMed]
94. Chan, S.; Reddy, V.; Myers, B.; Thibodeaux, Q.; Brownstone, N.; Liao, W. Machine Learning in Dermatology: Current Applications, Opportunities, and Limitations. *Dermatol. Ther.* **2020**, *10*, 365–386. [CrossRef] [PubMed]
95. Sáez, C.; Romero, N.; Conejero, J.A.; García-Gómez, J.M. Potential Limitations in COVID-19 Machine Learning Due to Data Source Variability: A Case Study in the NCov2019 Dataset. *J. Am. Med. Inform. Assoc.* **2021**, *28*, 360–364. [CrossRef]
96. Amin, S.U.; Hossain, M.S. Edge Intelligence and Internet of Things in Healthcare: A Survey. *IEEE Access* **2021**, *9*, 45–59. [CrossRef]
97. Sruthi, P.L.; Raju, K.B. Prediction of the COVID-19 Pandemic with Machine Learning Models. In Proceedings of the 2021 Fifth International Conference on I-SMAC (IoT in Social, Mobile, Analytics and Cloud) (I-SMAC), Palladam, India, 11–13 November 2021; pp. 474–481.
98. Anjum, N.; Alibakhshikenari, M.; Rashid, J.; Jabeen, F.; Asif, A.; Mohamed, E.M.; Falcone, F. IoT-Based COVID-19 Diagnosing and Monitoring Systems: A Survey. *IEEE Access* **2022**, *10*, 87168–87181. [CrossRef]
99. Mukati, N.; Namdev, N.; Dilip, R.; Hemalatha, N.; Dhiman, V.; Sahu, B. Healthcare Assistance to COVID-19 Patient Using Internet of Things (IoT) Enabled Technologies. *Mater. Today Proc.* **2021**. [CrossRef]
100. Meigal, A.Y.; Korzun, D.G.; Gerasimova-Meigal, L.I.; Borodin, A.V.; Zavyalova, Y.V. Ambient Intelligence At-Home Laboratory for Human Everyday Life. *Int. J. Embed. Real-Time Commun. Syst.* **2019**, *10*, 117–134. Available online: https://services.igi-global.com/resolvedoi/resolve.aspx?doi=10.4018/IJERTCS.2019040108 (accessed on 14 September 2022). [CrossRef]
101. Vetter, B.; Sampath, R.; Carmona, S. *Landscape of Point-of-Care Devices for Testing of Cardiometabolic Diseases*; FIND: Geneva, Switzerland, 2020.

sensors

MDPI

Article

Gait Characteristics Analyzed with Smartphone IMU Sensors in Subjects with Parkinsonism under the Conditions of "Dry" Immersion

Alexander Y. Meigal [1,*], Liudmila I. Gerasimova-Meigal [1], Sergey A. Reginya [2], Alexey V. Soloviev [2] and Alex P. Moschevikin [2]

[1] Medical Institute, Petrozavodsk State University, 33, Lenina pr., 185910 Petrozavodsk, Russia
[2] Physical-Technical Institute, Petrozavodsk State University, 33, Lenina pr., 185910 Petrozavodsk, Russia
* Correspondence: meigal@petrsu.ru; Tel.: +7-911-402-9908

Abstract: Parkinson's disease (PD) is increasingly being studied using science-intensive methods due to economic, medical, rehabilitation and social reasons. Wearable sensors and Internet of Things-enabled technologies look promising for monitoring motor activity and gait in PD patients. In this study, we sought to evaluate gait characteristics by analyzing the accelerometer signal received from a smartphone attached to the head during an extended TUG test, before and after single and repeated sessions of terrestrial microgravity modeled with the condition of "dry" immersion (DI) in five subjects with PD. The accelerometer signal from IMU during walking phases of the TUG test allowed for the recognition and characterization of up to 35 steps. In some patients with PD, unusually long steps have been identified, which could potentially have diagnostic value. It was found that after one DI session, stepping did not change, though in one subject it significantly improved (cadence, heel strike and step length). After a course of DI sessions, some characteristics of the TUG test improved significantly. In conclusion, the use of accelerometer signals received from a smartphone IMU looks promising for the creation of an IoT-enabled system to monitor gait in subjects with PD.

Keywords: inertial measurement unit; smartphone; accelerometry; TUG test; gait; Parkinson's disease; "dry" immersion

Citation: Meigal, A.Y.; Gerasimova-Meigal, L.I.; Reginya, S.A.; Soloviev, A.V.; Moschevikin, A.P. Gait Characteristics Analyzed with Smartphone IMU Sensors in Subjects with Parkinsonism under the Conditions of "Dry" Immersion. *Sensors* **2022**, 22, 7915. https://doi.org/10.3390/s22207915

Academic Editors: Raffaele Gravina and Leopoldo Angrisani

Received: 19 August 2022
Accepted: 14 October 2022
Published: 18 October 2022

1. Introduction

Parkinson's disease (PD) is very suitable for the application science-intensive instrumental research methods. PD is gradually becoming a kind of "model disease" for the testing of new technologies for PD diagnostics and escorting PD subjects [1]. For several reasons, PD is one of the most studied neural pathologies in humans. One of the reasons is that PD is a widespread neurodegenerative disease worldwide, and its prevalence is increasing [2]. Furthermore, PD exerts a high economic burden on society [3] and worsens the quality of life of patients with PD [4]. Next, PD is characterized by gradual progression over decades [5], and PD symptoms are reliably quantified using clinical scales, which allow for the mathematical modeling of PD evolvement [6]. In addition, PD seems to be an extremely informative research object, since it allows for the development of insights into such phenomena as muscle tone and tremor, motor commands, postural reactions, orientation in space and gait.

Earlier, we have shown that in subjects with PD that both single session of Earth-based microgravity—modeled with "dry" immersion conditions (DI) [7]—and a program of repeated DI sessions [8] attenuates muscle rigidity and tremors and improves some aspects of activity of daily living. Additionally, some motor-cognition tests [9] and characteristics of hemodynamics and heart rate variability were improved after a program of DI sessions [10]. On the other hand, the function of a patient's spatial orientation in a vertical stance and the function of postural transition proved non-responsive to the condition of DI [7]. Muscle rigidity is often associated with bradikinesia (slowness of movements) and akinesia (difficulties with starting motion), which is seen in the akinetic-rigid form of PD. This allows for the presumption that a decrease in muscle rigidity, provoked by DI conditions, may result in an improvement of gait characteristics, e.g., gait speed, cadence and length of steps.

The Timed Up-and-Go (TUG) test has proven to be reliable in many domains of neuromuscular and orthopedic pathology for assessing gait, basic mobility skill, strength, agility and balance [11]. It consists of five sequential phases: (1) standing up from a chair (Sit-to-Stand transition phase), (2) walking straight forward (Gait-Go phase, including stand-to-walk transition), (3) turning by 180° (U-turn phase), (4) walking back (Gait-Come phase), and (5) sitting down (Stand-to-Sit transition with a turn). In its classic 3 m form, the TUG test provides an immediate score, requires no training and only needs one tester [11]; however, the classic TUG test supplies little data on gait as it requires the patient to take only 4 to 6 steps in both directions. In addition, the first step, the step prior and right after the U-turn, and the last step are clearly specific by their biomechanical functionality (transition to locomotion, decelerating when approaching the U-turn point and the end-point of the test, correspondingly). To overcome this problem, longer (expanded) versions of the TUG test were invented. For example, Haas et al. [12] presented the so-called L-test, which includes longer walks and turning in both directions, and Galán-Mercant et al. [13] presented a 10 m version of the TUG test. Earlier, we proposed an even longer (extended) version of the TUG test (13 m long, which returns around 20 steps in one direction) to provide a more precise view of a self-paced walk at a comfortable speed in the middle of both the Gait-Go and Gait-Come phases [14].

Throughout the last decade, instrumented versions of the TUG test (iTUG) were increasingly invented. In most of these versions, varied numbers and positions of miscellaneous inertial measurement unit (IMU)-based wearable sensors (accelerometers) were used to discriminate between the phases of the TUG test [15,16]. The IMU is often fixed on a foot to obtain the exact position of a limb in real time. The quality of the sensor's trajectory restoration is often controlled by video capture, and its position accuracy is in the millimeter range [17,18]. One of the problems with such a system is the time synchronization of inertial sensor data and video flow [19]; some researchers use multi-IMU networks. For example, in the study by Qiu et al. [20], a system of 100 Hz IMUs connected via WiFi was applied for monitoring complex gait parameters, including knee angle dynamics. Bogaarts et al. [21] explored the impact of noise on gait features that had been extracted from smartphone sensor data. They created a model of a moving body, generated acceleration signals for plenty of the points on the body, then added noise to simulated signals and after that tried to extract the gait features. As a result, they showed that sensors in from-the-shelf smartphones are sufficient for registering acceleration signals, given that the sensor's noises introduce negligible impacts on the computation of step power and other similar parameters [21].

There is a multitude of technological approaches for studying PD. Among them are optical motion trackers, biopotential devices, audio and video recording, and, especially, wearable sensors, such as smart glasses, hats, insole sensors of ground-reaction force and smartphones [22]. Previously, we evaluated the effect of DI on PD subjects with conventional laboratory tools (EMG, reaction time, tapping test, posturography) [7–10].

According to the review by Deb et al. [22], wearable sensors are currently the most used (40% articles in the field), while smartphones are the least used; however, starting from the year 2020, there is a trend in the growing number of articles that have used smartphones for their research [22]. Among the application areas, the diagnosis and monitoring/prognosis of PD were the most studied, and among symptoms, the gait, tremor and speech of a subject were the most studied [22]. Smartphone applications have good to excellent ability for predicting and discriminating gait and postural instability between PD subjects and healthy controls, as well as the leg dexterity and gait cycle breakdown between PD subjects with different severities of the disease [23]. Thus, there is strong evidence regarding the potential use of smartphone applications to assess gait and balance among individuals with PD in the home or laboratory [22,23].

Smartphones are equipped with IMUs that consist of a 3-axis accelerometer, a 3-axis gyroscope and a digital magnetometer that is comparable in sensitivity to research-grade biomechanical instrumentation [24]. In the study by Manor et al. [24], smartphones were placed in the front pocket, which is relevant for non-laboratory settings. Typically, smartphones are secured to the trunk or lower extremities. In our earlier study, we suggested a method of reconstruction of the head trajectory in 3D-space using the IMU-based accelerometer and gyroscope of a smartphone, which was fixed on a subject's head [14]. We assumed that, in accordance with the concept of the "inverted pendulum model", the head produces the biggest displacement in the vertical axis [25]. Similarly, Hwang et al. [26] conducted research with a 60 Hz single IMU fixed on a head, which is similar to the method used in our study. They used a FIR low-pass filter to reduce the noise and applied threshold to capture the exact phases of a stride. Since a FIR filter introduces a certain latency in the processed series data, this fact should be considered in data analysis. The authors also presented comprehensible figures that demonstrated that a single sensor fixed on a head picks up acceleration signals from both legs, and further, they clarified how this obtained signal might be "decoded" and understood. Thus, a smartphone fixed on a subject's head can return meaningful information about gait. Still, the 100 Hz IMU of a smartphone does not allow for sufficiently precise tracking of the trajectory of the head.

The major hypothesis of the present study was that gait characteristics in patients with PD are responsive to the conditions of either one session of DI or a course of repeated DI sessions. To address this, we obtained up-sampled acceleration signals from smartphone-based 100 Hz IMU sensors attached to the subject's head during a 13 m TUG test before and after single session of DI and a program of seven DI sessions.

2. Materials and Methods

2.1. Subjects

Altogether, data from six PD subjects was collected in the study. Six subjects with PD participated in the study after providing their informed consent. Their anthropometric and clinical data and the medication they use is presented in Table 1. All of them are from the same cohort of subjects who participated in our earlier studies [7–10]. The data on gait characteristics presented in this article were obtained from these studies. All subjects signed their informed consent, and the protocol of the study was approved by the Local Ethical Committee (joint ethics committee of the Ministry of Healthcare of the Republic of Karelia and Petrozavodsk State University (Statement of approval No. 31, 18 December 2014)).

Table 1. The anthropometric and clinical data of the subjects with PD.

No. of Subject	Age (year) and Gender	Height (cm), Weight (kg)	Stage by Hoehn & Yahr	Clinical Form
1	47 M	182, 81	1	PD, AR
2	61 M	188, 83	1	PD, T
3	58 F	158, 65	2	PD, T
4	50 M	171, 94	2	PD, T
5	55 M	178, 86	2	PD, T
6	69 M	170, 95	2	PD, T

T—tremulous form, AR—akinetic-rigid form of PD. Subject 1 participated in 2 courses of DI sessions. Subject 6 did not participate in DI sessions.

2.2. Procedures

2.2.1. On-Earth Model of Microgravity

The on-Earth microgravity was modeled using the conditions of a "dry" immersion (DI). This method of DI has already been presented in detail in our earlier papers [7–10]. In brief, the condition of DI was created with the help of MEDSIM (Medical simulator of weightlessness, Center for Aerospace Medicine and Technology, IMBP, Moscow, Russia), which is housed in the Laboratory of Novel Methods in Physiology (Petrozavodsk State University). The MEDSIM facility uses a bathtub filled with 2 m^3 of fresh, thermally comfortable water stabilized at T = 32 °C. The water in the tub was periodically filtrated and aerated to prevent bacterial contamination. The water surface was covered with a large, square waterproof film (3×4 m^2), which was wrapped around the subject's body. The DI session was conducted at 9:30 AM, in the condition of "on-medication" in order to synchronize the effects of DI and the anti-PD therapy. The subjects usually took their medicines 2 h before the study, at 7:30 AM. Before DI, subjects were instructed to drink 200 mL of water and urinate due to the strong diuretic effect of DI [27]. Before immersion, subjects laid supine for approximately 10 min on a solid movable motor-driven platform on a cotton sheet in the MEDSIM facility in order to attach electrocardiogram electrodes, measure brachial blood pressure (BP), and familiarize (altogether around 5 min) and note ECG recordings in standard lead II (5 min). If after 10 min of lying supine the subject's BP was higher than 140/80 mm Hg, he/she was not allowed to enter DI and the study was postponed for another day. After that, the platform was driven to its bottom position, and subjects found themselves immersed in water without direct contact with the water; the head and upper chest were left above the water's surface. One DI session lasts for 45 min. BP and ECG were monitored at the 15th, 30th and 45th min. After the DI session, subjects laid motionless on the platform in its upper position for a further 5–7 min for re-adaptation to the pre-DI conditions and for ECG monitoring. Altogether, 22 measurements were successfully conducted: 10 measurements before/after a single session of DI (5 paired sets of data), and 12 measurements before and after a program of DI sessions (6 paired sets of data).

The program of DI consisted of seven 45 min DI sessions that were conducted twice a week for 25–30 days. The total DI dose during the course was $5\frac{1}{4}$ h.

2.2.2. Test Protocol: 13 m TUG Test

The TUG test was performed in its extended form (13 m instead of the conventional 3 m long test). Still, its phases were all the same: (1) standing up from a 46 cm high-chair (Sit-to-Stand phase), (2) walk straight (13 m, Gait-Go phase, including Stand-to-Walk transition), (3) turning by 180° (U-turn), (4) walking back (13 m, Gait-Come phase), and (5) sitting down (Stand-to-Sit transition with a turn). In addition, unlike the classic 3 m version, the 13 m version of the TUG test allowed for an analysis of the subject's steps (gait)—because subjects performed up to 20 steps in one direction, which is sufficient for analyzing gait [28]. The TUG test was performed 15 min prior and then 8–10 min after the DI session. A baseline gait analysis throughout the day was not conducted, neither was one conducted before or after the DI session. The TUG test was performed prior and 8–10 min after the DI session.

2.3. *Data Processing*

During the TUG test, the acceleration and rotation rate were measured with the sensor module in the smartphone Xiaomi Mi4 (Xiaomi Tech, Bejing, China 68.5 mm × 139.2 mm × 8.9 mm, 149 g). The obtained signals were further processed offline.

The subject was instructed to sit still and look forward before and after the test. In a motionless state, the shape of the accelerometer signal is formed by the current projections of the gravity vector, measurement noise and the existing zero-G offsets, as well as the head tremor. The beginning and end of the movement are characterized by a change in the x-, y- and z- components of the acceleration vector due to the inclination as well as the presence of linear accelerations while standing up and sitting down. For the gyroscope in a motionless state, the signal includes the sensor noise as well as the head tremor; however, it is characterized by the constancy of the mean value (measurement offset). The start and end points of the TUG test were selected manually by analyzing the change in the mean value due to the rotation of the head and body during inclination while standing up and sitting down.

The internal phases of the TUG test and step moments were determined automatically. For steps in a straight-line walk (15–17 more or less uniform steps in the middle of both the Gait-Go and Gait-Come phases), a set of gait features was calculated. Altogether, subjects performed 35–40 steps in both directions, of which 30–35 steps that were in the middle of the walk were analyzed.

2.4. Inertial Data Acquisition and Pre-Processing

The sampling rate of the inertial sensors—both the accelerometer and gyroscope—of the Xiaomi Mi4 smartphone that was used in the present study was 100 Hz (the period between data samples was $\Delta t = 10$ ms), which can be regarded as neither reliably accurate nor fast. The smartphone was fixed on the back of the head of a subject with an elastic band and, additionally, a tight-knitted hat; subjects felt comfortable with this kind of fixation and the smartphone never fell out of its position. Values for the acceleration and angular velocity were collected as a time-stamped data stream. Thus, the measurements were accompanied by timestamps from the smartphone's operating system timer. For further analysis, the accelerometer and gyroscope measurements with a time-stamp difference of less than 5 ms (half of the measurement period) were considered synchronous. In order to increase the time resolution and achieve a smoother distribution, the time series data were up-sampled to a 10-fold-higher frequency of 1 kHz ($\Delta t' = 1$ ms) (Figure 1). In addition, an increase in the time resolution allowed for the application of high-order digital filters to the obtained time series.

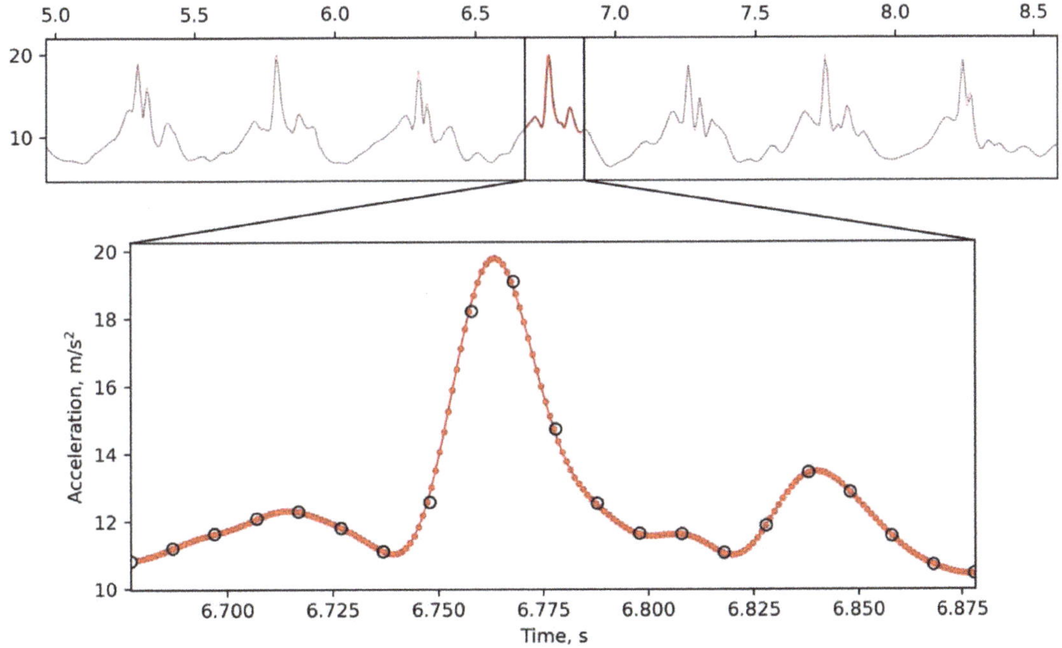

Figure 1. Up-sampling of a periodic signal obtained during walking. The black open circles on the bottom panel correspond to the real data sampled at a frequency of 100 Hz. The red points are new data points reconstructed with up-sampling. The red curve is a continuous signal passing through all the circles.

Since the analyzed signal tended to be periodic, the up-sampling, which used Fast Fourier Transform, could be applied. Furthermore, as long as the measurement signals are real-valued, the real (single-sided) FFT is suitable for conversion into the frequency domain. In the frequency domain, up-sampling means there is zero-padding at the end of the high frequency components of the signal. The up-sampling procedure included the following steps:

(1) forward Fourier transform of original signal X = F(x);
(2) zero-padding F(x) up to new length F(y);
(3) inverse Fourier transform of F(y) to obtain up-sampled signal y;
(4) scaling up-sampled signal y to preserve amplitudes.

A simple calibration of the zero offsets of the sensors was performed before the start of the test. To do this, we used the measurements obtained from a smartphone placed on a horizontal surface. It was noted that the sensor offsets were probably pre-calibrated by the Android OS. The bias instability and velocity/angle random walk for smartphone sensors was previously analyzed by us using the Allan variation [14]. The bias instabilities are (7.3, 8.2, 8) $\times$ 10^{-4} m/s^2 for the x-, y- and z-axis of the accelerometer, and (1.7, 5, 7) $\times$ 10^{-5} deg/s for the gyroscope. Since the test duration is less than 1 min, the bias drifts can be neglected.

The orientation of the smartphone was calculated using a well-known complementary filter proposed by Robert Mahony et al. [29] and is expressed in the form of a quaternion Q. Using Q, the acceleration and angular velocity measurement vectors were converted to a global coordinate system (global frame):

$$GV = Q \otimes SV \otimes Q^*, \quad (1)$$

where GV and SV are "pure" quaternions associated to the 3-dimensional measurement vector in the sensor frame and global frame, respectively; Q* is a conjugate of Q; and the $\otimes$ symbol represents the Hamilton product.

2.5. Turns (Rotation) Detection

Automatic detection of a turn was conducted by analyzing the projection of the angular velocity on the vertical axis. No additional filtering of measurements was performed. If the values of the amplitude and duration of the rotation rate exceeded certain threshold values, a rotation was considered to be detected (recorded). At the first stage, a comparison was made with the threshold value of the rotation rate (10 degrees per second). At the second stage, the rotation duration was estimated. Rotations lasting less than 1 s were discarded. If three or more turns were detected in the TUG test, the two longest turns were considered the 1st (at the U-turn phase) and 2nd (prior to sitting down on a chair) turn. According to the available experimental data, this algorithm was successful in 100% of cases for both turn events.

2.6. Step Detection

Step detection was automatically performed by analyzing the time series of the acceleration vector. Since the typical cadence of stepping is about two steps per second, the measurements were filtered with a forward–backward zero-phase low-pass filter (Butterworth, 10th order) with a cut-off frequency of 3 Hz, which allowed us to obtain the LPF time series data. After that, peak values of the filtered signal were detected. Moments where the acceleration magnitude reached 11 m/s^2 were taken as the approximate time-stamp of the initial contact of the foot with the ground (T′ point).

For each step, the revised time-stamp T_step of the heel strike and the corresponding maximum acceleration along the vertical axis were determined by searching for the maximum value in the $\pm$40 ms window near the T′ point. Not all steps taken during the TUG test were taken into account for gait analysis. The following local maxima that were obtained during the step detection procedure were discarded:

- the first peak corresponding to the moment of standing up and the second peak corresponding to the moment of the first step;
- steps during the first U-turn;
- steps from the moment of the second turn until the end of the whole test.

2.7. Gait Features

2.7.1. Duration of the TUG Test Phases (D-Parameters)

To estimate the duration of the entire TUG20 test and its phases, the following parameters were determined (Figure 2):

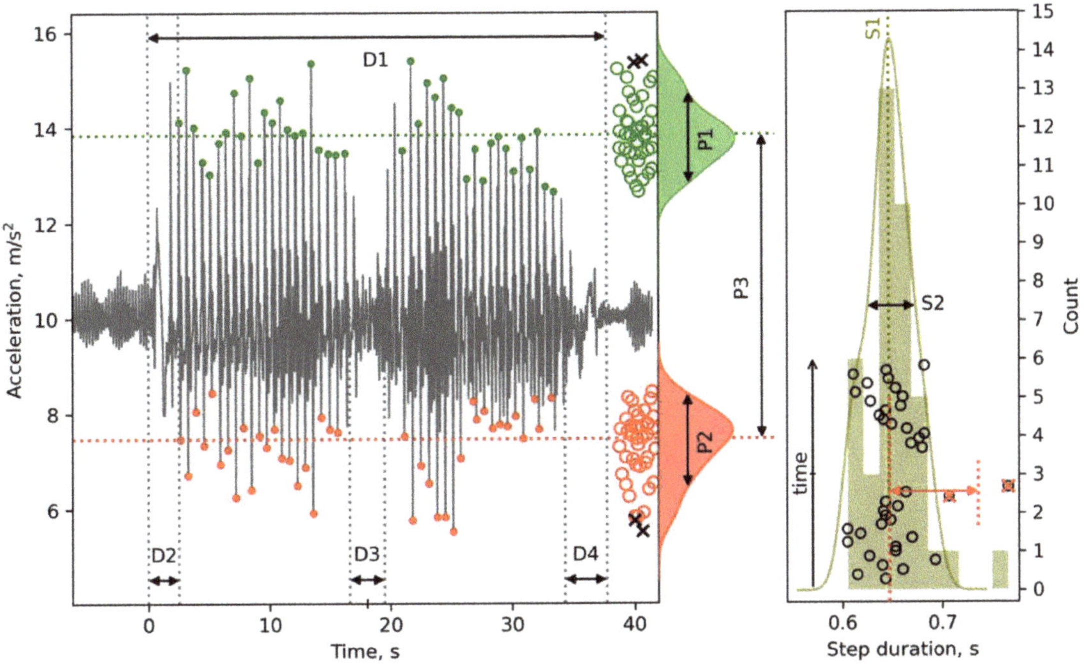

Figure 2. A representative plot of the 13 m TUG test with the phases (D1–D4) and parameters P1–P3 determined with an accelerometer (**left panel**) and the moments of step duration distribution (S1–S2, **right panel**) along progression of time.

D1 (The entire TUG test duration): the time from the very beginning of motion (the Sit-to-Stand movement) until the end of the test (sitting down on a chair).

D2 (Corresponds to the Sit-to-Stand phase plus the Stand-to-Walk period): the time from the start of the lifting to the moment of the heel strike on the second step.

D3 (U-turn phase, the 1st turn duration): the time to perform a 180° turn at the far turning point.

D4 (Walk-to-Sit phase, or the 2nd turn duration): the time from the beginning of the second turn until the end of the test.

2.7.2. Characteristics of the Temporal Stability of Stepping (S-Parameters)

For the analysis of gait stability, only straight-line, uniform steps were taken into account (see Section 2.6). The following parameters were computed:

S1 (Mean_step_duration, s): the duration of the step (dt) was determined as the difference between consecutive time-stamps of successive steps (T_{step} moments). Before calculating the average value, two points with the largest deviation from the median value of step duration were discarded (red crosses, see Figure 2).

S2 (Step_duration_std, s) (see Figure 2).

To calculate the cadence mean and standard deviation, the "instantaneous walking pace" was first estimated for each step (cadence = 60/dt); then two outliers should be discarded. Usually, these outliers were characteristic of the "transitional" moments during the TUG test (at the beginning and end of the Gait-Go and Gait-Come phases, and before the U-turn).

S3 (Cadence_mean, steps per min).

S4 (Cadence_std, steps per min).

S5 The ratio of the average deviation of the two largest outliers of the step duration to the standard deviation of the step duration without taking into account the two largest outliers (red double-sided arrow, see Figure 2). S5 reflects a tendency to take unusually long steps (LS).

S5 was calculated according to the following algorithm:

1. Select two outliers from "step duration" values;
2. Calculate D_{WO} as the mean value of the step durations without outliers;
3. For each outlier, calculate the absolute difference from D_{WO}, then calculate the mean of differences (D_{OUT});
4. Calculate D_{WO_STD} as the standard deviation of the step durations without outliers;
5. Calculate LS = D_{OUT}/D_{WO_STD}.

The estimates of the probability density functions of the step duration and the acceleration upper/lower peaks were obtained using kernel density estimation (KDE). KDE was computed using the Python scipy.stats.gaussian_kde function (written by Robert Kern, 2004, Enthought, Inc., Austin, TX, USA). As P1, P2 and S2 values are related to the width of the target variables' distributions, they are shown as the full width at half maximum. On the left panel, the red dots denote minimal acceleration when both feet were touching the floor, and the green dots denote heel strike. The open red and green circles represent these dots. Two outlier values are denoted with black crosses. On the right panel, the open black circles represent the individual step duration along the time course. The outlier values, denoted by red crosses (>0.7 s), represent unexpectedly longer steps right prior to U-turn. Furthermore, note that during the Gait-Come phase (upper group of open black circles), the length of the steps decreased roughly from 0.68 m to 0.6 m. For more information, see the text below; these data were obtained from Subject 6.

2.7.3. Characteristics of the Power Stability of Stepping (P-Parameters)

To analyze the power (amplitude) characteristics of each step, the following parameters were estimated:

P1 (Heel_strike_accel_std, m/s^2): the standard deviation of the vertical acceleration in Tstep moments. Two outliers were discarded. P1 characterizes the stability (uniformity) of the heel strike during stepping in the Gait-Go and Gait-Come phases (see Figure 2).

P2 (Swing_accel_std, m/s^2): standard deviation of the vertical acceleration minima that corresponds to the weight transfer phase. Two outliers were discarded. P2 characterizes the stability (uniformity) of the minima values when both feet made contact with the floor during the swing phase of stepping during the Gait-Go and Gait-Come phases (see Figure 2).

P3 (Peak-to-peak_vertical_acceleration_mean, m/s^2): the average difference between the minimum and maximum of the vertical accelerations in a series of straight steps.

All D- and P-parameters, and some of S-parameters, can be identified from Figure 2. The duration of the entire TUG test (D1) and its phases—D2, D3 and D4—shown on the left panel in Figure 2, were recognized automatically by analysis of the acceleration and rotation rate time series data. The upper peaks (green dots) correspond to heel strike moments and form a cloud of green open circles to the right. Their distribution is characterized by the P1 parameter. Similarly, P2 describes the width of distribution of the acceleration minima during the swing phase. The horizontal green and red dotted lines denote the medians for these sets. P3 is the difference between the medians. The right panel in Figure 2 describes the distribution of the performed steps over the step duration (histogram and kernel density estimation). S1 stands for the average step duration and S2 stands for the standard deviation. The black circles—from the lowest to the highest—correspond to the recognized steps from the first step to the last one in time. The two longest steps were excluded from the averaging statistics; however, they probably informed the light form of "freeze of gait".

2.8. Statistical Analysis

The analysis was executed with IBM SPSS Statistics 21.0 (SPSS, IBM Company, Chicago, IL, USA). The values of D1–4, S1–5 and P1–3 were compared in the pairs of conditions "before-after a single DI session" and "before-after a course of DI sessions" with the non-parametric paired Wilcoxon *t*-test.

3. Results

None of the D, P and S gait characteristics responded to the conditions of a single ("acute") DI session (Table 2); however, in each of the five examined subjects with PD, at least several—usually different—parameters were positively modified after a 45 min session of DI. Furthermore, at least in 2–4 measurements of 5, the gait parameters changed to better values. For example, in Subject 1, after a single session of DI, the D1 (duration of the entire TUG test) decreased by 5 s—from 30 to 25 s—and the subject's cadence increased from 88 to 100 steps/min. After another DI session with this subject, the values of the P1 parameter (heel strike) increased from 0.55 to 0.77 m/s^2, P2 increased (swing phase) from 0.50 to 0.82 m/s^2, and P3 increased from 8–9 to 10–11 m/s^2 (Figure 3), which provides insight into the increased variability of step length after DI and the stronger strike of the heel on the floor. In Subject 2, only the value of D4 decreased, which similarly occurred in Subject 3, wherein the value of S5 decreased (Figure 3). In addition, in all five cases of DI, the change in the distribution type of P2 from a unimodal distribution to a more bimodal one took place (see Figure 3). The individual data for all measurements are presented in Supplementary Material Table S1.

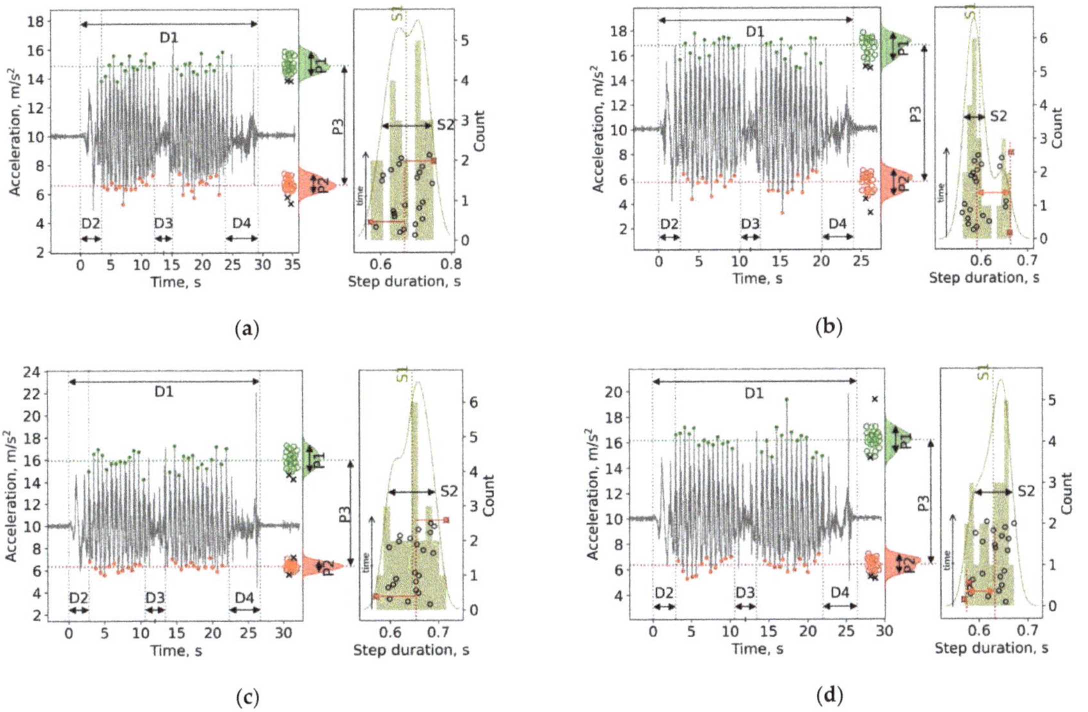

Figure 3. *Cont.*

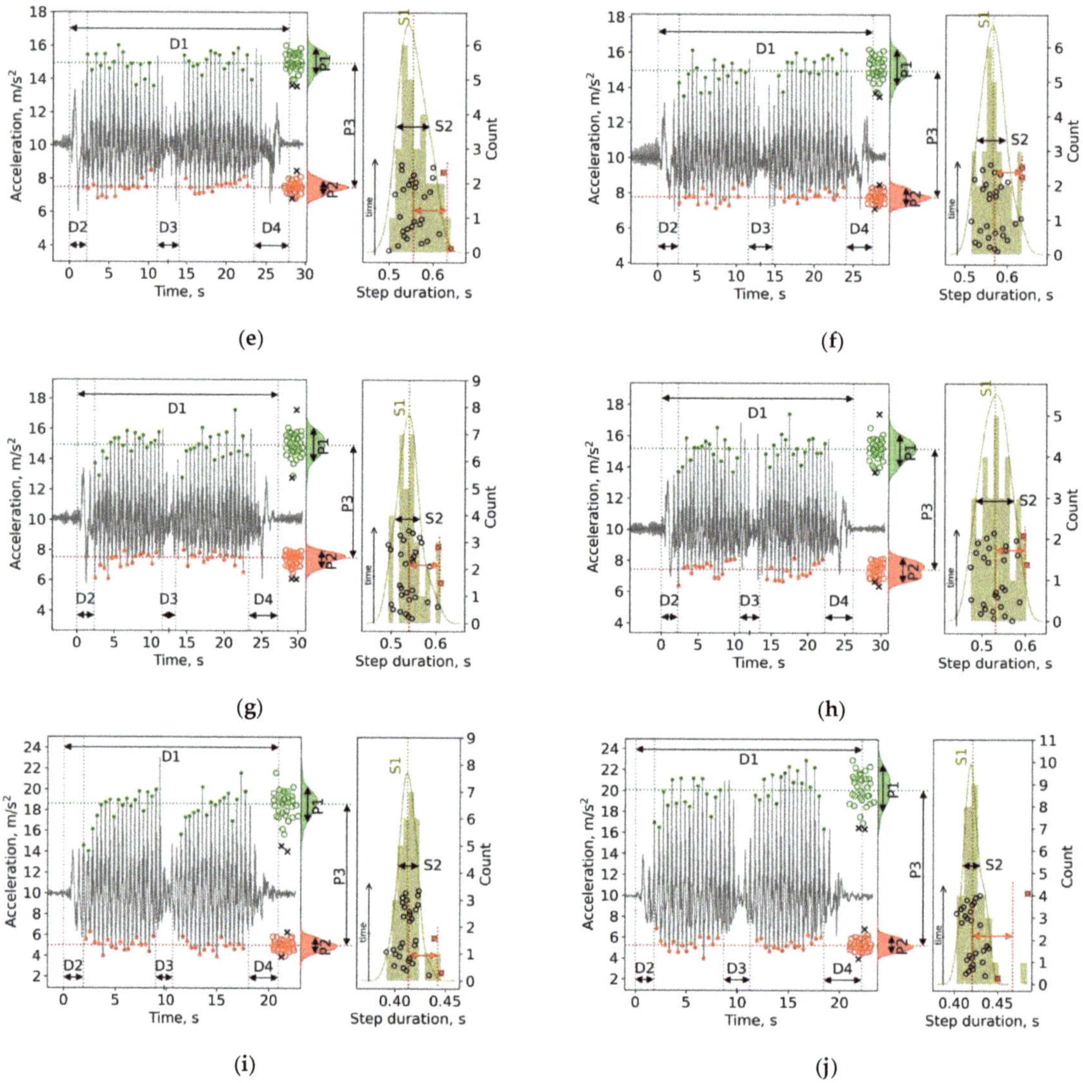

(e) (f) (g) (h) (i) (j)

Figure 3. Individual plots for five separate DI sessions in three subjects. For details, see Figure 2: (**a**) Subject 1 before and (**b**) after the 1st DI; (**c**) Subject 1 before and (**d**) after the 7th DI; (**e**) Subject 2 before and (**f**) after the 5th DI; (**g**) Subject 2 before and (**h**) after the 4th DI; (**i**) Subject 3 before and (**j**) after the 7th DI.

Unlike with a single DI session, a course of DI sessions exerted a significant influence on a few gait parameters, namely, D4 and S5 (see, Table 2), which means that subjects with PD performed sitting down on a chair with turning (D4 phase) faster, and there were unusually long steps after a course of DI sessions. The individual plots of stepping are presented in Figure 4.

Table 2. Gait characteristics before and after a single DI session and after a course of DI sessions.

Parameter	Before a Single DI Session	After a Single DI Session	*p*	Before a Course of DI Sessions	After a Course of DI Sessions	*p*
D1 (s)	26.4 ± 3.2	25.3 ± 2.1	0.35	26.5 ± 2.3	24.7 ± 2.6	0.173
D2 (s)	2.56 ± 0.61	2.50 ± 0.44	0.89	2.66 ± 0.56	2.44 ± 0.35	0.116
D3 (s)	2.36 ± 0.52	2.60 ± 0.23	0.50	2.44 ± 0.45	2.27 ± 0.39	0.249
D4 (s)	4.19 ± 0.92	4.69 ± 1.34	0.69	4.09 ± 0.89	3.51 ± 0.64	0.046
S1 (s)	0.56 ± 0.10	0.55 ± 0.08	0.35	0.54 ± 0.08	0.52 ± 0.07	0.688
S2 (s)	0.027 ± 0.013	0.025 ± 0.01	0.89	0.02 ± 0.014	0.018 ± 0.01	1.000
S3 (steps/min)	109.1 ± 22.6	111.2 ± 18.3	0.69	112.6 ± 18.0	116.4 ± 16.6	0.249
S4 (steps/min)	4.19 ± 0.92	4.69 ± 1.34	0.50	3.64 ± 1.39	3.76 ± 1.63	0.753
S5	2.65 ± 0.54	3.37± 0.27	0.23	2.66 ± 0.61	3.26 ± 0.39	0.028
P1 (m/s^2)	0.88 ± 0.40	0.95 ± 0.32	0.23	0.96 ± 0.40	0.92 ± 0.34	0.917
P2 (m/s^2)	0.46 ± 0.08	0.56 ± 0.18	0.23	0.46 ± 0.11	0.61 ± 0.19	0.075
P3 (m/s^2)	9.2 ± 2.26	9.9 ± 2.8	0.35	9.7 ± 2.35	10.75 ± 1.91	0.116

p—probability of difference in Wilcoxon test between "before" and "after" conditions. The meaning of D-, S- and P-parameters can be found in the text.

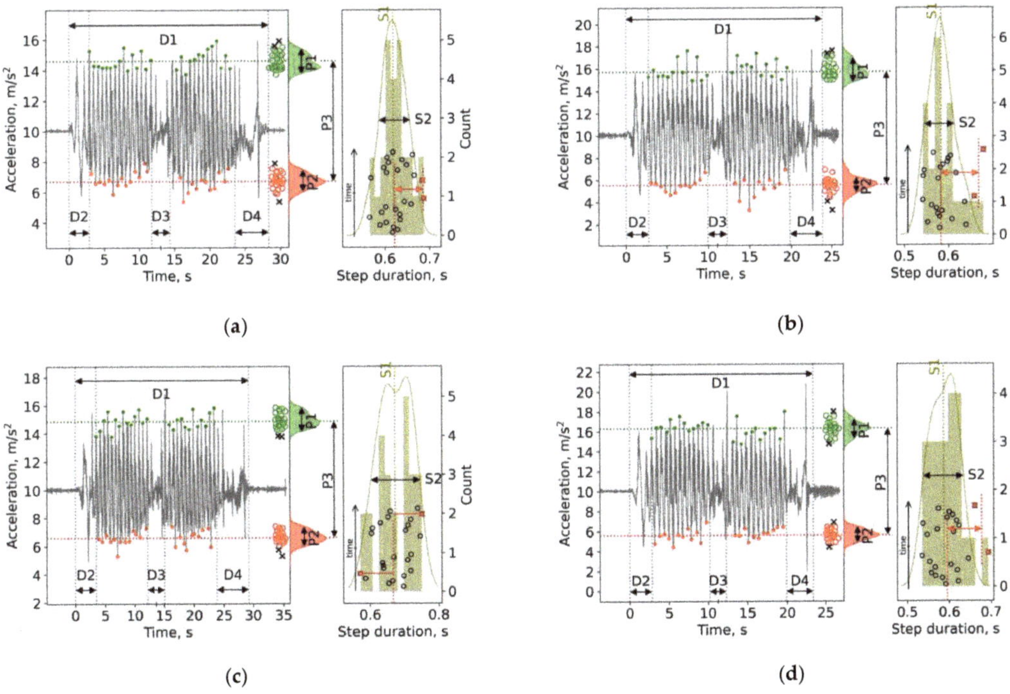

Figure 4. *Cont.*

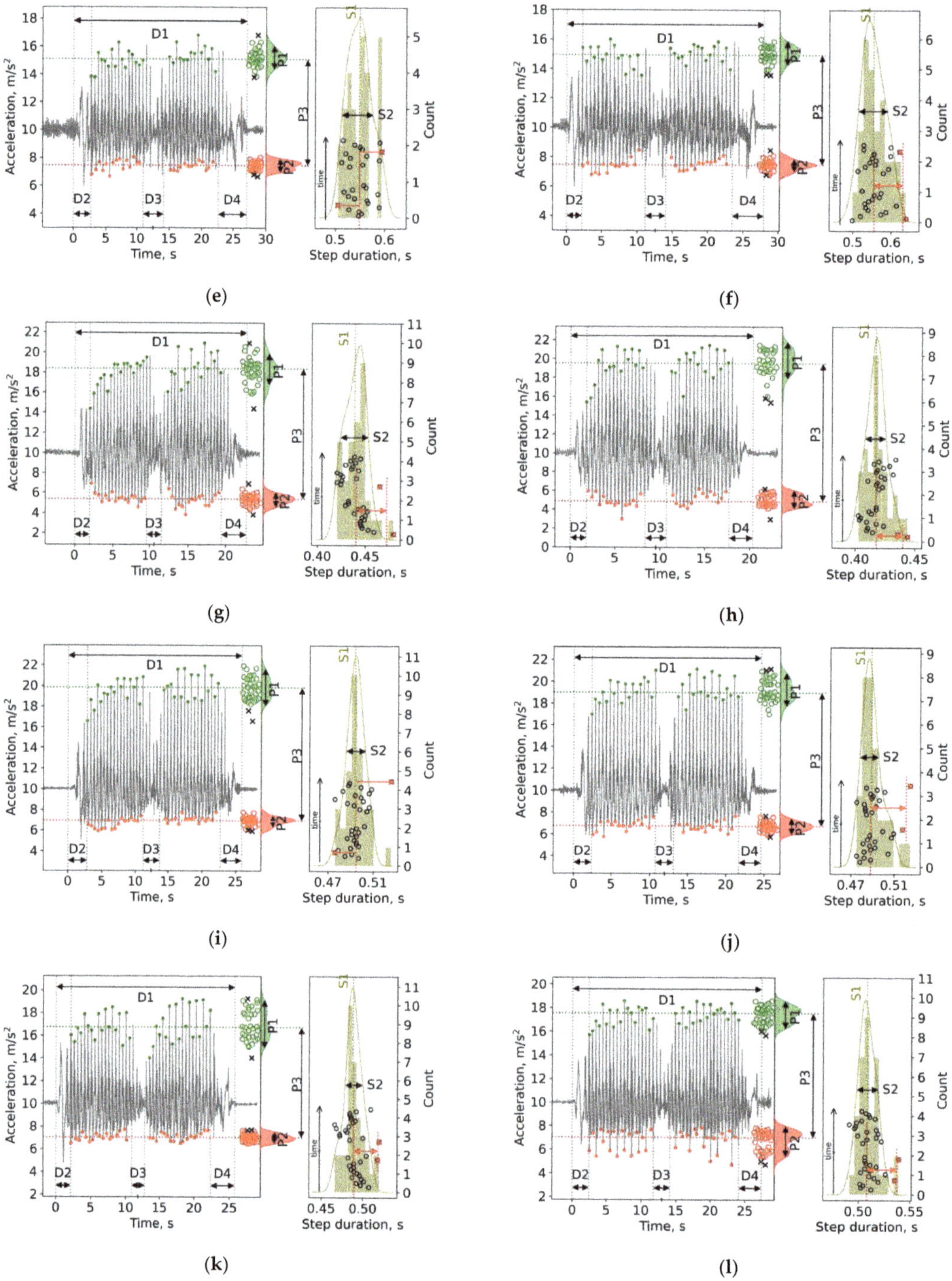

Figure 4. Individual plots for six courses of DI sessions in five subjects. For details, see Figure 2: (**a**) Subject 1 before and (**b**) after the 1st course of DI; (**c**) Subject 1 before and (**d**) after the 2nd course of DI; (**e**) Subject 2 before and (**f**) after the course of DI; (**g**) Subject 3 before and (**h**) after the course of DI; (**i**) Subject 4 before and (**j**) after the course of DI; (**k**) Subject 5 before and (**l**) after the course of DI.

4. Discussion

The purpose of this study was (1) to test the reliability of an assessment of stepping characteristics with an up-sampled IMU-based accelerometer signal and gyroscope of a smartphone when placed on the subject's head, and (2) with the help of the acceleration signal, to study the effect of a single DI session and a program of DI sessions on stepping in subjects with PD during a long version of the TUG test.

There are plenty of studies that have demonstrated sufficient reliability of iTUG test technologies based on a smartphone's IMU to recognize the phases of the TUG test [24,30–32]. It has been concluded that the iTUG test is relevant for self-administered TUG test [31,33] and has good agreement with 3D motion video capture analysis [34], and it is superior to stopwatch measurement [35]. As such, the recognition of sub-phases during the instrumented TUG test, either in its classic or extended versions, with smartphone accelerometers is not necessarily novel; however, most of these studies were conducted with the classic 3 m TUG test, with a smartphone attached to a belt and with a 100 Hz sampling rate.

Instead, in the present study, we focused on (1) the gait analysis during the Gait-Go and Gait-Come phases with the help of (2) the extended 13 m TUG test, and (3) with a smartphone fixed to the head. It has been found that the 13 m TUG test returns information about 16–21 steps in each direction (28–36 steps, altogether), of which 15–17 steps in the middle of the Gait-Go and Gait-Come phases of the TUG test were considered to be functionally uniform (straight walk). This number of steps is reliable, as data collected from 10–20 strides (20 steps) were reported to be sufficient for the reliable characterization of the gait speed and cadence of stepping [28]; however, the reliable evaluation of the variability of stepping requires much more data (hundreds of strides) [28]. In addition, we considered that the pre-processing of the time series with an up-sampling procedure (from 100 up to 1000 Hz) allowed us to increase the accuracy of the capture of stepping events (heel strike and swing phase). Moreover, we paid much attention to the step variability and evolution over time. For example, we introduced a special new parameter that measures the tendency to "freeze of gait"—i.e., unusually long steps, which can provide insights into the difficulties of performing a step.

From a technical point of view, the obtained parameters and graphical presentation of the TUG test can be regarded as reliable and demonstrative, as it allows for the tracing of individual features of the subject's gait and the recognition of graphical patterns of the subjects by eye. Furthermore, the position of the smartphone on the head can be regarded as a reliable site for the collection of information about a human's gait. This allows for a reduction in the number of IMUs to one that is placed on the head.

We found that a single ("acute") 45 min DI session exerted no effect on the studied parameters of gait across the entire group of subjects with PD, which is opposite to our original hypothesis. On the other hand, in each subject, an individual set of gait characteristics still changed. For example, in Subject 1 (see Figure 3), the entire duration of the TUG test (D1) decreased by 5 s (or, by 15%), and the time to perform the U-turn (D3 phase) decreased by 0.2–0.3 s, while the cadence (S1) increased by 3–12 steps/min. Furthermore, P1 (standard deviation of heel strike acceleration) and P2 (standard deviation of acceleration minima during the swing phase) increased by 0.2–0.3 m/s^2, and P3 (vertical acceleration range) increased by 2–3 m/s^2. As a whole, these changes suggest that after a single DI session, Subject 1 walked faster, performed faster turns and stepped more firmly on the floor. All these modifications can be regarded as positive. In Subjects 2 and 3, the effect of DI conditions was negligible, probably due to the relatively good initial values of their gait parameters, for example, in Subject 3, their cadence was 145 steps/min—in comparison to 90–112 steps/min in Subjects 1 and 2. In addition, Subject 1 did not take anti-PD medicine, which means that before the DI session he stood in the "off-medication" condition. As a result, the effect of DI was not inferred by anti-PD therapy.

The effect of a program of seven DI sessions was a bit more pronounced. At a minimum, the D4 and S5 parameters became significantly larger after a course of DI, and a change in P2 values resulted in an increase after a program of DI. The reaction to DI conditions was individually significant. Again, Subject 1 presented the most notable improvement in D1 (by 5–6 s, or by 20%), and almost in all other parameters. Subjects 2, 4 and 5 demonstrated moderate improvement of only some parameters, and Subject 3 demonstrated a notable improvement of gait.

The Internet of Things (IoT) is comprised of interconnected devices, machines, and servers with data storage that functioning through a network [36,37]. A smartphone can be considered an ideal measuring device for further instrumentation and incorporation into IoT-enabled systems since it already appears as a part of the Internet.

A smartphone is always "at hand" (in the pocket), it is not heavy or cost-effective, and it is already pre-set for data transfer to cloud-based storage [24]. Smartphones are already efficiently used to detect and monitor PD symptoms, e.g., with reaction time tests, tapping tests, and voice (speech), posture and gait tests [38], and there are smartphone applications that are available for self-testing [39]. In a sense, smartphones have undergone a kind of "instrumentalization" compared to regular consumer devices—for example, a treadmill [40]. Altogether, this makes smartphones a relevant candidate for the implementation of diagnostic and monitoring applications in PD. Smartphones are very suitable because, unlike wearable sensors, they do not need additional resources, as they are already a part of the Internet. In addition, smartphones are capable of performing online calculations.

Data collected on the gait of PD subjects with wearable accelerometers is suitable for Artificial Intelligence (AI) or IoT decisional support [36,41]. AI-based wearable gait monitoring is already used for optimization of Parkinson's disease management [41]. We figured that smartphone applications based on AI can be applied to monitor gait characteristics in PD subjects. Among the varied learning methods, deep learning may provide higher accuracy in PD assessment than machine learning [42].

The TUG20 test accelerometer signals have a repetitive structure and contain gait features. Furthermore, there are two ways that the methods of AI could be applied. First, it can be used to collect a database of signals and split this database into two parts: the training and test sets. To increase the adequacy of the model, this approach might be applied after investigation of more than 100 PD cases, which is difficult in real life. The second way is to investigate the gait features and to understand what features are significant, i.e., to exclude insignificant features and thus decrease the dimension of the model, and then apply these data to clustering. This approach requires less studied cases, and we would prefer to follow it in the future. The major limitation of this study was the insufficient number of study subjects and measurements, which did not allow for a more precise analysis of data to be conducted. Furthermore, control groups (young and older healthy subjects) were not formed. In future studies, we propose that more measurements should be conducted in control groups and subjects with PD, both under "dry" immersion conditions and non-DI conditions.

5. Conclusions

In conclusion, the data from smartphone-based IMU accelerometers allowed us to compute gait characteristics that are conventionally used in the field of locomotion physiology, such as step duration and cadence. Like other IMU-based analyzing systems, the presented method allowed for the recognition of the phases of the TUG test. The application of an extended version of the TUG test provided a sufficient number of steps to characterize gait, and it allowed for the visualization of the duration of individual steps during the process of locomotion. Furthermore, the presented method appears to be suitable for a fast visual evaluation of stepping patterns in PD subjects. Of note, some of the specific characteristics of Parkinsonism events were recognized with the IMU sensors—for example, unusually long steps, which were produced while walking.

For the entire group, the conditions of a single 45 min "dry" immersion affected none of the studied gait parameters derived with the help of smartphone-based IMU sensors; however, in one subject there was a clear increase in cadence, gait and turning speed. After a course of repeated DI sessions, some characteristics of the TUG test were improved; however, gait speed did not significantly change.

The presented method of gait analysis appears to be suitable for further instrumentation because a smartphone is perfectly suited for association in IoT-based networks.

Supplementary Materials: The following supporting information can be downloaded at: https://www.mdpi.com/article/10.3390/10.3390/s22207915/s1, Table S1: Individual values of gait characteristics at different study conditions.

Author Contributions: Conceptualization, A.Y.M. and L.I.G.-M.; methodology, A.Y.M. and A.P.M.; software, S.A.R., A.V.S. and A.P.M.; investigation, A.Y.M. and L.I.G.-M.; writing—original draft preparation, A.Y.M. and A.P.M.; writing, review and editing, A.Y.M., L.I.G.-M., A.P.M., S.A.R., A.V.S.; visualization, S.A.R.; supervision, A.Y.M. and A.P.M.; project administration, A.Y.M.; funding acquisition, A.Y.M. All authors have read and agreed to the published version of the manuscript.

Funding: The research was financially supported by the Ministry of Science and Higher Education of the Russian Federation (theme No. 0752-2020-0007, to AM).

Institutional Review Board Statement: The study was conducted in accordance with the Declaration of Helsinki, and approved by the Institutional Review Board (or Ethics Committee) of Ministry of health care of the Republic of Karelia and Petrozavodsk State University (Statement of approval No. 31, 18 December 2014).

Informed Consent Statement: Informed consent was obtained from all subjects involved in the study.

Data Availability Statement: The datasets generated for this study are available on request to the corresponding author.

Acknowledgments: The authors thank the subjects for their participation and engineer Kirill Prokchorov for assisting with conducting measurements.

Conflicts of Interest: The authors declare no conflict of interest.

References

1. Pasluosta, C.F.; Gassner, H.; Winkler, J.; Klucken, J.; Eskofier, B. Parkinson's disease as a working model for global healthcare restructuration: The internet of things and wearables technologies. In Proceedings of the 2015 International Conference on Wireless Mobile Communication and Healthcare, London, UK, 14–16 October 2015. [CrossRef]
2. Wirdefeldt, K.; Adami, H.O.; Cole, P.; Trichopoulos, D.; Mandel, J. Epidemiology and etiology of Parkinson's disease: A review of the evidence. *Eur. J. Epidemiol.* **2011**, *26* (Suppl. 1), 1. [CrossRef]
3. Martinez-Martin, P.; Macaulay, D.; Jalundhwala, Y.J.; Mu, F.; Ohashi, E.; Marshall, T.; Sail, K. The long-term direct and indirect economic burden among Parkinson's disease caregivers in the United States. *Mov. Disord.* **2019**, *34*, 236–245. [CrossRef] [PubMed]
4. Marras, C.; McDermott, M.P.; Rochon, P.A.; Tanner, C.M.; Naglie, G.; Lang, A.E.; Parkinson Study Group DATATOP Investigators. Predictors of deterioration in health-related quality of life in Parkinson's disease: Results from the DATATOP trial. *Mov. Disord.* **2008**, *23*, 653–659. [CrossRef] [PubMed]
5. Sveinbjornsdottir, S. The clinical symptoms of Parkinson's disease. *J. Neurochem.* **2016**, *139* (Suppl. 1), 318–324. [CrossRef]
6. Venuto, C.S.; Potter, N.B.; Dorsey, E.R.; Kieburtz, K. A review of disease progression models of Parkinson's disease and applications in clinical trials. *Mov. Disord.* **2016**, *31*, 947–956. [CrossRef] [PubMed]
7. Meigal, A.Y.; Tretjakova, O.G.; Gerasimova-Meigal, L.I.; Sayenko, I.V. Vertical spatial orientation in patients with parkinsonism under the state of single "dry" immersion and a course of immersions. *Hum. Physiol.* **2021**, *47*, 183–192. [CrossRef]
8. Meigal, A.; Gerasimova-Meigal, L.; Saenko, I.; Subbotina, N. Dry immersion as a novel physical therapeutic intervention for rehabilitation of Parkinson's disease patients: A feasibility study. *Phys. Med. Rehab. Kuror.* **2018**, *28*, 275–281. [CrossRef]
9. Meigal, A.Y.; Tretjakova, O.G.; Gerasimova-Meigal, L.I.; Sayenko, I.V. Program of seven 45-min dry immersion sessions improves choice reaction time in Parkinson's disease. *Front. Physiol.* **2021**, *11*, 621198. [CrossRef]
10. Gerasimova-Meigal, L.; Meigal, A.; Sireneva, N.; Saenko, I. Autonomic function in parkinson's disease subjects across repeated short-term dry immersion: Evidence from linear and non-linear HRV parameters. *Front. Physiol.* **2021**, *12*, 712365. [CrossRef]
11. Bennell, K.; Dobson, F.; Hinman, R. Measures of physical performance assessments: Self-Paced Walk Test (SPWT), Stair Climb Test (SCT), Six-Minute Walk Test (6MWT), Chair Stand Test (CST), Timed Up & Go (TUG), Sock Test, Lift and Carry Test (LCT), and Car Task. *Arthritis Care Res.* **2011**, *63* (Suppl. 11), S350–S370. [CrossRef]
12. Haas, B.; Clarke, E.; Elver, L.; Gowman, E.; Mortimer, E.; Byrd, E. The reliability and validity of the L-test in people with Parkinson's disease. *Physiotherapy* **2019**, *105*, 84–89. [CrossRef] [PubMed]

13. Galán-Mercant, A.; Barón-López, F.J.; Labajos-Manzanares, M.T.; Cuesta-Vargas, A.I. Reliability and criterion-related validity with a smartphone used in timed-up-and-go test. *Biomed. Eng. Online* **2014**, *13*, 156. [CrossRef] [PubMed]
14. Reginya, S.; Meigal, A.Y.; Gerasimova-Meigal, L.; Prokhorov, K.; Moschevikin, A. Using smartphone inertial measurement unit for analysis of human gait. *Int. J. Emb. Real-Time Commun. Syst.* **2019**, *10*, 101–117. [CrossRef]
15. Salarian, A.; Horak, F.B.; Zampieri, C.; Carlson-Kuhta, P.; Nutt, J.G.; Aminian, K. iTUG, a sensitive and reliable measure of mobility. *IEEE Trans. Neural Syst. Rehabil. Eng.* **2010**, *18*, 303–310. [CrossRef] [PubMed]
16. Caronni, A.; Sterpi, I.; Antoniotti, P.; Aristidou, E.; Nicolaci, F.; Picardi, M.; Pintavalle, G.; Redaelli, V.; Achille, G.; Sciumè, L.; et al. Criterion validity of the instrumented Timed Up and Go test: A partial least square regression study. *Gait Posture* **2018**, *61*, 287–293. [CrossRef] [PubMed]
17. Hori, K.; Mao, Y.; Ono, Y.; Ora, H.; Hirobe, Y.; Sawada, H.; Inaba, A.; Orimo, S.; Miyake, Y. Inertial Measurement Unit-based estimation of foot trajectory for clinical gait analysis. *Front. Physiol.* **2020**, *10*, 1530. [CrossRef]
18. Do, T.N.; Suh, Y.S. Gait analysis using floor markers and inertial sensors. *Sensors* **2012**, *12*, 1594–1611. [CrossRef]
19. Huynh-The, T.; Nguyen, T.V.; Pham, Q.V.; da Costa, D.B.; Kim, D.S. MIMO-OFDM modulation classification using three-dimensional convolutional network. *IEEE Trans. Veh. Technol.* **2022**, *71*, 6738–6743. [CrossRef]
20. Qiu, S.; Liu, L.; Zhao, H.; Wang, Z.; Jiang, Y. MEMS inertial sensors based gait analysis for rehabilitation assessment via multi-sensor fusion. *Micromachines* **2018**, *9*, 442. [CrossRef]
21. Bogaarts., G.; Zanon, M.; Dondelinger, F.; Derungs, A.; Lipsmeier, F.; Gossens, C.; Lindemann, M. Simulating the impact of noise on gait features extracted from smartphone sensor-data for the remote assessment of movement disorders. In Proceedings of the 2021 43rd Annual International Conference of the IEEE Engineering in Medicine & Biology Society (EMBC), Mexico, 1–5 November 2021; pp. 6905–6910. [CrossRef]
22. Deb, R.; An, S.; Bhat, G.; Shill, H.; Ogras, U.Y. A systematic survey of research trends in technology usage for Parkinson's disease. *Sensors* **2022**, *22*, 5491. [CrossRef]
23. Abou, L.; Peters, J.; Wong, E.; Akers, R.; Dossou, M.S.; Sosnoff, J.J.; Rice, L.A. Gait and balance assessments using smartphone applications in Parkinson's disease: A systematic review. *J. Med. Syst.* **2021**, *45*, 87. [CrossRef] [PubMed]
24. Manor, B.; Yu, W.; Zhu, H.; Harrison, R.; Lo, O.Y.; Lipsitz, L.; Travison, T.; Pascual-Leone, A.; Zhou, J. Smartphone app-based assessment of gait during normal and dual-task walking: Demonstration of validity and reliability. *JMIR Mhealth Uhealth* **2018**, *6*, e36. [CrossRef] [PubMed]
25. Mao, Y.; Ogata, T.; Ora, H.; Tanaka, N.; Miyake, Y. Estimation of stride-by-stride spatial gait parameters using inertial measurement unit attached to the shank with inverted pendulum model. *Sci. Rep.* **2021**, *11*, 1391. [CrossRef] [PubMed]
26. Huang, C.; Fukushi, K.; Wang, Z.; Nihey, F.; Kajitani, H.; Nakahara, K. Method for estimating temporal gait parameters concerning bilateral lower limbs of healthy subjects using a single in-shoe motion sensor through a gait event detection approach. *Sensors* **2022**, *22*, 351. [CrossRef] [PubMed]
27. Tomilovskaya, E.; Shigueva, T.; Sayenko, D.; Rukavishnikov, I.; Kozlovskaya, I. Dry immersion as a ground-based model of microgravity physiological effects. *Front. Physiol.* **2019**, *10*, 284. [CrossRef]
28. Hollman, J.H.; Childs, K.B.; McNeil, M.L.; Mueller, A.C.; Quilter, C.M.; Youdas, J.W. Number of strides required for reliable measurements of pace, rhythm and variability parameters of gait during normal and dual task walking in older individuals. *Gait Posture* **2010**, *32*, 23–28. [CrossRef]
29. Mahony, R.; Hamel, T.; Pflimlin, J.M. Nonlinear complementary filters on the special orthogonal group. *IEEE Trans. Autom. Control* **2008**, *53*, 1203–1218. [CrossRef]
30. Ponciano, V.; Pires, I.M.; Ribeiro, F.R.; Spinsante, S. Sensors are capable to help in the measurement of the results of the Timed-Up and Go test? A systematic review. *J. Med. Syst.* **2020**, *44*, 199. [CrossRef]
31. Hellmers, S.; Izadpanah, B.; Dasenbrock, L.; Diekmann, R.; Bauer, J.M.; Hein, A.; Fudickar, S. Towards an automated unsupervised mobility assessment for older people based on inertial TUG Measurements. *Sensors* **2018**, *18*, 3310. [CrossRef]
32. Su, D.; Liu, Z.; Jiang, X.; Zhang, F.; Yu, W.; Ma, H.; Wang, C.; Wang, Z.; Wang, X.; Hu, W.; et al. Simple smartphone-based assessment of gait characteristics in Parkinson disease: Validation study. *JMIR Mhealth Uhealth.* **2021**, *9*, e25451. [CrossRef]
33. van Lummel, R.C.; Walgaard, S.; Hobert, M.A.; Maetzler, W.; van Dieën, J.H.; Galindo-Garre, F.; Terwee, C.B. Intra-rater, inter-rater and test-retest reliability of an instrumented Timed Up and Go (iTUG) test in patients with Parkinson's disease. *PLoS ONE.* **2016**, *11*, e0151881. [CrossRef] [PubMed]
34. Beyea, J.; McGibbon, C.A.; Sexton, A.; Noble, J.; O'Connell, C. Convergent validity of a wearable sensor system for measuring sub-task performance during the Timed Up-and-Go test. *Sensors* **2017**, *17*, 934. [CrossRef] [PubMed]
35. Kleiner, A.F.R.; Pacifici, I.; Vagnini, A.; Camerota, F.; Celletti, C.; Stocchi, F.; De Pandis, M.F.; Galli, M. Timed Up and Go evaluation with wearable devices: Validation in Parkinson's disease. *J. Bodyw. Mov. Ther.* **2018**, *22*, 390–395. [CrossRef] [PubMed]
36. Bernardes, R.A.; Ventura, F.; Neves, H.; Fernandes, M.I.; Sousa, P. Wearable walking assistant for freezing of gait with environmental IoT monitoring: A contribution to the discussion. *Front. Public Health* **2022**, *10*, 861621. [CrossRef]
37. Sunny, A.I.; Zhao, A.; Li, L.; Sakiliba, S.K. Low-cost IoT-based sensor system: A case study on harsh environmental monitoring. *Sensors* **2021**, *21*, 214. [CrossRef]
38. Arora, S.; Venkataraman, V.; Zhan, A.; Donohue, S.; Biglan, K.M.; Dorsey, E.R.; Little, M.A. Detecting and monitoring the symptoms of Parkinson's disease using smartphones: A pilot study. *Parkinsonism Relat. Disord.* **2015**, *21*, 650–653. [CrossRef]

39. Orozco-Arroyave, J.R.; Vásquez-Correa, J.C.; Klumpp, P.; Pérez-Toro, P.A.; Escobar-Grisales, D.; Roth, N.; Ríos-Urrego, C.D.; Strauss, M.; Carvajal-Castaño, H.A.; Bayerl, S.; et al. *Apkinson*: The smartphone application for telemonitoring Parkinson's patients through speech, gait and hands movement. *Neurodegener. Dis. Manag.* **2020**, *10*, 137–157. [CrossRef]
40. Lesch, K.J.; Lavikainen, J.; Hyrylä, V.; Vartiainen, P.; Venojärvi, M.; Karjalainen, P.A.; Tikkanen, H.; Stenroth, L. A perturbed postural balance test using an instrumented treadmill—Precision and accuracy of belt movement and test-retest reliability of balance measures. *Front. Sports Act. Living* **2021**, *3*, 688993. [CrossRef]
41. Ileșan, R.R.; Cordoș, C.G.; Mihăilă, L.I.; Fleșar, R.; Popescu, A.S.; Perju-Dumbravă, L.; Faragó, P. Proof of concept in artificial-intelligence-based wearable gait monitoring for Parkinson's disease management optimization. *Biosensors* **2022**, *12*, 189. [CrossRef]
42. Rovini, E.; Maremmani, C.; Cavallo, F. How wearable sensors can support parkinson's disease diagnosis and treatment: A systematic review. *Front. Neurosci.* **2017**, *11*, 555. [CrossRef]

sensors

MDPI

Article

Predicting Chemical Carcinogens Using a Hybrid Neural Network Deep Learning Method

Sarita Limbu and Sivanesan Dakshanamurthy *

Lombardi Comprehensive Cancer Center, Georgetown University Medical Center, Washington, DC 20057, USA
* Correspondence: sd233@georgetown.edu

Abstract: Determining environmental chemical carcinogenicity is urgently needed as humans are increasingly exposed to these chemicals. In this study, we developed a hybrid neural network (HNN) method called HNN-Cancer to predict potential carcinogens of real-life chemicals. The HNN-Cancer included a new SMILES feature representation method by modifying our previous 3D array representation of 1D SMILES simulated by the convolutional neural network (CNN). We developed binary classification, multiclass classification, and regression models based on diverse non-congeneric chemicals. Along with the HNN-Cancer model, we developed models based on the random forest (RF), bootstrap aggregating (Bagging), and adaptive boosting (AdaBoost) methods for binary and multiclass classification. We developed regression models using HNN-Cancer, RF, support vector regressor (SVR), gradient boosting (GB), kernel ridge (KR), decision tree with AdaBoost (DT), KNeighbors (KN), and a consensus method. The performance of the models for all classifications was assessed using various statistical metrics. The accuracy of the HNN-Cancer, RF, and Bagging models were 74%, and their AUC was ~0.81 for binary classification models developed with 7994 chemicals. The sensitivity was 79.5% and the specificity was 67.3% for the HNN-Cancer, which outperforms the other methods. In the case of multiclass classification models with 1618 chemicals, we obtained the optimal accuracy of 70% with an AUC 0.7 for HNN-Cancer, RF, Bagging, and AdaBoost, respectively. In the case of regression models, the correlation coefficient (R) was around 0.62 for HNN-Cancer and RF higher than the SVM, GB, KR, DTBoost, and NN machine learning methods. Overall, the HNN-Cancer performed better for the majority of the known carcinogen experimental datasets. Further, the predictive performance of HNN-Cancer on diverse chemicals is comparable to the literature-reported models that included similar and less diverse molecules. Our HNN-Cancer could be used in identifying potentially carcinogenic chemicals for a wide variety of chemical classes.

Keywords: chemical carcinogens; machine learning; deep learning neural network; hybrid neural network; convolution neural network; fast forward neural network

Citation: Limbu, S.; Dakshanamurthy, S. Predicting Chemical Carcinogens Using a Hybrid Neural Network Deep Learning Method. *Sensors* **2022**, *22*, 8185. https://doi.org/10.3390/s22218185

Academic Editors: Dmitry Korzun, Andrei Velichko and Alexander Meigal

Received: 13 September 2022
Accepted: 23 October 2022
Published: 26 October 2022

1. Introduction

Substances capable of causing cancer are known as carcinogens. Carcinogenicity is a primary concern among all the toxicological endpoints due to the severity of its outcome. Carcinogens may be genotoxic, which induces DNA damage and cancer, or non-genotoxic, which uses other modes of action, such as tumor promotion, to exhibit their carcinogenic potential in humans [1]. Some of the genotoxic carcinogens are mutagens too. Many environmental chemicals have been identified as carcinogenic to humans [2,3]. The onset of cancer in humans depends on various factors, including the dose and duration of exposure to carcinogens. Identifying carcinogenic compounds is also an integral step during the drug development process. The two-year rodent carcinogenicity assay has been established as the standard to determine chemical carcinogenicity [4]. However, such animal testing is time-consuming, costly, and unethical. The experimentalists need to replace, reduce, and refine (3Rs) the use of animals as this 3Rs policy encourages alternative methods to minimize the unprincipled use of animals [5].

Computational methods for various toxicological endpoints prediction have now become a popular alternative to traditional animal testing. Numerous computational models using machine learning (ML) methods are developed to predict carcinogenicity based on the properties of chemicals. Computational models can be classification models (qualitative) that predict chemical is carcinogenic/noncarcinogenic (binary classification models) or that predict the degree of carcinogenicity (multiclass classification), and regression models (quantitative) that predict the dose of chemical required for carcinogenesis. Computational models based on structurally related congeneric chemicals are reported to have high predictive performance. Luan et al. reported an accuracy of 95.2% while predicting the carcinogenicity of N-nitroso compounds based on the support vector machine (SVM) method [6]. Ovidiu et al. presented a SVM-based model to predict the carcinogenicity of polycyclic aromatic hydrocarbons (PAH) with 87% accuracy [7]. Computational models based on non-congeneric chemicals are of interest due to their predictive ability for diverse chemicals. Fjodorova et al. predicted the carcinogenicity of non-congeneric chemicals with 68% accuracy using a counter propagation artificial neural network (CP ANN) [8]. Tanabe et al. reported an accuracy of 70% for non-congeneric chemicals based on SVM and improved the accuracy to 80% by developing models on the chemical subgroups based on their structure [9]. Zhang et al. presented binary classification models based on ensemble of the extreme gradient boosting (XGBoost) method that predicted the carcinogenicity of chemicals with 70% accuracy [10]. Li et al. used six different ML methods to generate the binary classification model with 83.91% accuracy and ternary (multiclass) classification models with 80.46% accuracy for the external validation set for the best model [11]. Toma et al. developed binary classification models with an accuracy of 76% and 74% and regression models with r^2 of 0.57 and 0.65 on oral and inhalation slope factors to predict carcinogenicity for the external validation set [12]. Fjodorova et al. reported a correlation coefficient of 0.46 for the test set for their regression models using counter propagation artificial neural network (CP ANN) [8]. Wang et al. constructed a deep learning model that requires fewer data and achieved 85% accuracy on the external validation set for carcinogenicity prediction [13].

Taken together, numerous carcinogenicity predictive models on congeneric and non-congeneric chemicals for binary classification and a few multiclass and regression models were reported [6–17]. However, there is a need for more non-congeneric computational models with a broad applicability domain for carcinogenicity prediction. In this study, to predict potential carcinogens, we developed a hybrid neural network method called, HNN-Cancer. Based on diverse non-congeneric chemicals, we have developed binary classification, multiclass classification, and regression models, using HNN-Cancer and other machine learning methods. We have used the binary classification to predict a chemical is carcinogenic or non-carcinogenic, the multiclass classification model to predict the severity of the chemical carcinogenicity, and the regression model to predict the median toxic dose.

2. Materials & Methods

2.1. Datasets

We have collected carcinogens from several different data sources detailed below.

1. Chemical Exposure Guidelines for Deployed Military Personnel Version 1.3 (MEG). We curated carcinogenic chemicals from the Technical Guide 230 (TG230): "Chemical Exposure Guidelines for Deployed Military Personnel" [18]. TG 230 provides military exposure guidelines (MEGs) for chemicals in the air, water, and soil, along with an assigned carcinogenicity group for each chemical. Chemicals are categorized into one of 5 groups: Group A (human carcinogen), Group B (probable human carcinogen), Group C (possible human carcinogen), Group D (not classifiable), and Group E (no evidence of carcinogenicity).
2. Environmental Health Risk Assessment and Chemical Exposure Guidelines for Deployed Military Personnel 2013 Revision (TG230). We curated carcinogenic chemicals

listed in the Technical Guide 230 (TG230): "Environmental Health Risk Assessment and Chemical Exposure Guidelines for Deployed Military Personnel" [19], which provides military exposure guidelines (MEGs).

3. National Toxicology Program (NTP). Carcinogenic chemicals were curated from the NTP [20]. NTP lists two groups of carcinogenic chemicals: (a) reasonably anticipated to be a human carcinogen and (b) known to be human carcinogens.
4. International Agency for Research on Cancer (IARC) Carcinogenic chemicals were curated from IARC [21]. IARC categorizes chemicals into one of the 5 groups: Group 1 (carcinogenic to humans), Group 2A (probably carcinogenic to humans), Group 2B (possibly carcinogenic to humans), Group 3 (not classifiable as to its carcinogenicity to humans), and Group 4 (probably not carcinogenic to humans).
5. The Japan Society for Occupational Health (JSOH) Carcinogenic chemicals were curated with the recommendation of Occupational Exposure Limits published by the JSOH [22], which are classified into one of the 3 groups: Group 1 (carcinogenic to humans), Group 2A (probably carcinogenic to humans), and Group 2B (possibly carcinogenic to humans).
6. The National Institute for Occupational Safety and Health (NIOSH) Carcinogenic chemicals curated from the NIOSH [23].
7. Carcinogenic Potency Database (CPDB)
    a. CPDB_CPE (CPDB CarcinoPred-EL) data: CPDB data for rat carcinogenicity were collected from the CarcinoPred-EL developed by Zhang et al. [10]. The list contains 494 carcinogenic and 509 non-carcinogenic chemicals.
    b. CPDB data: CPDB [24] data were collected and processed to obtain the median toxicity dose (TD50) for rat carcinogenicity. TD50 is the dose-rate in mg/kg body wt/day administered throughout life that induces cancer in half of the test animals. A total of 561 carcinogenic chemicals was obtained with TD50 values for rat carcinogenicity. A total of 605 noncarcinogenic chemicals was obtained for rat carcinogenicity. For 543 carcinogenic chemicals out of 561, the TD50 values in mmol/kg body wt/day were also obtained from the DSSTox database (https://www.epa.gov/chemical-research/distributed-structure-searchable-toxicity-dsstox-database; accessed on 30 September 2017).
8. Chemical Carcinogenesis Research Information System (CCRIS). Carcinogenesis data were collected from the CCRIS at ftp://ftp.nlm.nih.gov/nlmdata/.ccrislease/; accessed on 30 September 2017. The carcinogenicity and mutagenicity data were extracted. A total of 6833 chemicals was obtained after eliminating duplicates/conflicting data when compared to data sources 1 to 6, out of which 4054 were carcinogenic/mutagenic and 2779 were non-carcinogenic/mutagenic.
9. Drugbank 2018 The drug data were collected from the drug bank (www.drugbank.ca; accessed on 31 March 2018). The approved drugs predicted as carcinogenic by Zhang et al. [10] were removed, the remining 1756 approved drugs were considered non-carcinogenic.

2.1.1. Dataset I: Binary Classification Data

The two classes considered in the binary classification models were class 0 (non-carcinogen) and class 1 (carcinogen). Datasets used to train the models are listed below:

i. For binary classification of chemicals to predict the carcinogenic or non-carcinogenic category, 448 carcinogenic chemicals were obtained from data sources 1 to 6 above. Data 1 (MEG): The chemicals classified into Groups A, B, and C were considered as carcinogens. Data 2 (TG30): The chemicals listed as carcinogens were considered as carcinogens. Data 3 (NTP): The chemicals classified as either "reasonably anticipated to be a human carcinogen" or "known to be human carcinogens" were considered as carcinogens. Data 4 (IARC): The chemicals classified into Groups 1, 2A, and 2B were considered as carcinogens. Data 5 (JSOH): The chemicals classified into Groups

1, 2A, and 2B were considered as carcinogens. Data 6 (NIOSH): The carcinogenic chemicals listed were considered as carcinogens.

ii. CPDB_CPE chemicals from data source 7a contributed 320 carcinogenic and 458 non-carcinogenic additional data after comparing to the data from data sources 1 to 6 and removing duplicates and conflicting chemicals.

iii. The CCRIS mutagenicity/carcinogenicity data from data source 8 contributed 3868 mutagenic/carcinogenic data and 2500 non-mutagenic/carcinogenic data.

iv. A total of 400 non-carcinogenic approved drugs from data source nine was also used in this classification model.

For the binary classification model dataset, we used 7994 chemicals with 4636 carcinogenic and 3358 non-carcinogenic chemicals.

2.1.2. Dataset II: Multiclass Classification Data

The classes considered in the multiclass classification models were class 0 (non-carcinogen), 1 (possibly carcinogen and not classifiable chemicals), and 2 (carcinogen and probably carcinogen). Datasets used to train the models are listed below:

i. For multiclass classification, 882 carcinogenic and 2 non-carcinogenic chemicals were collected from data sources 1, 3, 4, and 5. There was a total of 2 in class 0, 604 in class 1, and 278 in class 2 in this dataset. Data 1 (MEG): The chemicals classified into Groups A and B were considered class 2. The chemicals classified into Groups C and D were considered class 1 carcinogens. Chemicals classified into group E are considered class 0 compounds. Data 3 (NTP): The chemicals classified as either "reasonably anticipated to be a human carcinogen" or "known to be human carcinogens" were considered class 2. Data 4 (IARC): The chemicals classified into Groups 1 and 2A were considered class 2 carcinogens, and those classified into Groups 2, B, and 3 were considered class 1 carcinogens. Data 5 (JSOH): The chemicals classified into Groups 1 and 2A were considered class 2 carcinogens, and those classified into Groups 2B were considered class 1 carcinogens. Considering Group D of MEG data as class 1 carcinogen along with Group C and considering Group 3 of IARC data as class 1 carcinogen along with Group 2B increased the multiclass data significantly in this dataset. In the case of binary classification, we discarded these groups.

ii. CPDB chemicals from data source 7b contributed 277 carcinogenic and 457 non-carcinogenic additional data after removing duplicates and conflicting chemicals compared to the data from data sources 1, 3, 4, and 5. The 277 carcinogenic chemicals were categorized into class 2, and 457 noncarcinogenic chemicals were categorized into class 0.

The dataset II for the multiclass classification models, we used a total of 459 chemicals data in class 0, 604 chemicals data in class 1, and 555 chemicals data in class 2.

2.1.3. Dataset III: Regression Data

Regression models were developed to predict the quantitative carcinogenicity or the median toxic dose (TD50) of the chemicals in the form of pTD50 (logarithm of the inverse of TD50). Dataset III for the regression models consisted of 561 TD50 data in mg/kg body wt/day converted to pTD50 from data source 7b. Independently, the regression models were also developed on 543 TD50 data in mmol/kg body wt/day converted to pTD50.

2.2. Descriptors

Mordred descriptor calculator [25] that calculates 1613 2D molecular descriptors from SMILES and is used for descriptor calculation. This descriptor calculator supports Python 3 that we used to run the Mordred locally. The final set of 653 descriptors was obtained with no missing calculated values for the entire datasets for which descriptors were calculated. The 653 descriptors were used as a final set of input features for the training and test data set for the machine learning models.

2.3. SMILES Preprocessing

The simplified molecular-input line-entry system (SMILES) uses ASCII strings for the 1D chemical structure representation of a compound and can be used to convert to its 2-D or 3-D representation. It is one of the key chemical attributes and is used in our deep learning model. Raw texts cannot be directly used as input for the deep learning models but should be encoded as numbers. Tokenizer class in python is used to encode the SMILES string. The SMILES preprocessing method that we used while predicting toxicity [17] created the index for the set of unique characters of SMILES from the training set only. If the training set consists of only two compounds "C=CC=C" and "O=CC, a dictionary would be created for only three distinct characters in the SMILES of the training set that would map C to 1, = to 2, and O to 3. Then, the vector output for the SMILES characters was one-hot encoded where the categorical value of each character in the SMILES is converted to binary vector with only the index set to 1. Thus, C, =, and O are represented by the vectors [1 0 0], [0 1 0], and [0 0 1], respectively. If a new character, such as 'N', which does not exist in the training set, appears in the SMILES of the test set, the character would be skipped. For the string C=CC#N, the SMILES vectorization method would output the following matrix of dimension LxM, where L = 325 is the allowed maximum length of the SMILES string and M is the number of the unique characters in the SMILES of the training set:

$$\begin{bmatrix} C \\ = \\ C \\ C \\ \# \\ N \end{bmatrix} = \begin{bmatrix} 1 & 0 & 0 \\ 0 & 1 & 0 \\ 1 & 0 & 0 \\ 1 & 0 & 0 \\ 0 & 0 & 0 \\ \vdots & \vdots & \vdots \\ 0 & 0 & 0 \end{bmatrix}$$

Here, in the modified vectorization method, we have created a unique index for 94 characters in the ASCII table. Hence, there is no possibility of missing out on creating an index of any character in the SMILES string represented in any format. A total of 94 characters in the ASCII table !, ", #, ... , =, >, ?, @, A, B, C, ... , |, }, ~ represented by decimal numbers 33, 34, 35, ... , 61, 62, 63, 64, 65, 66, 67, ... 124, 125, 126, respectively, made the vocabulary of the possible characters in the SMILES. Each of these 94 ASCII characters were obtained by looping through the numbers 33 through 126 and converting the number to the corresponding character using python function chr(). Then, the characters were mapped to indices 1, 2, 3, ... , 29, 30, 31, 32, 33, 34, 35, ... , 92, 93, 94 using the fit_on_texts() function of the Tokenizer module to create a dictionary.

Each character in the SMILES is converted to its corresponding index in the dictionary, and a vector is created for the SMILES of each compound. As an example, acrylonitrile-d3 with SMILES string C=CC#N is encoded as [35, 29, 35, 35, 3, 46]. As the SMILES length varies depending on the compound's length and properties, the length of the encoding results also varies. The resulting vector for the SMILES of every input compound is thus padded with 0s or truncated so that they are of uniform length, L. The SMILES for the input compounds are converted to a 2-D matrix of size K x L, where K is the number of input SMILES, and L = 325 is the allowed maximum length of the SMILES string used in the model. Thus, for the string C=CC#N, the current SMILES vectorization method would output the following vector of length 325:

[35, 29, 35, 35, 3, 46, 0, 0, ... , 0]

Our previous method [17] mapped the SMILES for the K number of chemicals to a one-hot encoded matrix of size KxLxM, where M is the number of the possible characters in the SMILES.

3. Machine Learning Models

3.1. Hybrid Neural Network Model

Hybrid neural network (HNN) model [17] that we developed for chemical toxicity prediction was used here by modifying the SMILES vectorization method. Then, the method by which the vectorized SMILES input is processed by the convolutional neural network (CNN) of the model. The model is developed in python using the Keras API with Tensorflow in the backend. The model consists of a CNN for deep learning based on structure attribute (SMILES) and a multilayer perceptron (MLP)-type feed-forward neural network (FFNN) for learning based on descriptors of the chemicals. To vectorize SMILES, each character in the SMILES string is converted to its positional index in the dictionary, as explained in the SMILES preprocessing section. The 2D array of vectorized SMILES strings was the input for the CNN. The embedding layer of Keras is used to convert the index of each character in the SMILES string into a dense vector. The embedding layer takes three arguments as input: input_dim is the vocabulary size of the characters in the SMILES string, output_dim is the size of the embedded output for each character, and input_length is the length of the SMILES string. In the model, we have embedded the index of each character in the SMILES to a vector of size 100 by setting the output_dim to 100. The embedding layer converts the input 2D array of size KxL, where K is the number of SMILES and L is the maximum length of SMILES, to a 3D array of size KxLx100.

The 1D convolution layer activation function ReLU represented mathematically as max(0, x), is used in the model that replaces all the negative values with zeros. The derivative of ReLU is always 1 for positive input, which counteracts the vanishing gradient problem during the backpropagation. The output of the pooling layer of the CNN, together with the FFNN, is connected to the final fully connected layer to perform the classification task.

3.2. Other Machine Learning Algorithms

To test the performance of HNN-Cancer for the case of binary classification and multiclass classification, the other machine learning algorithms random forest (RF), bootstrap aggregating (Bagging) using bagged decision tree, and adaptive boosting (AdaBoost), were used.

Random forest (RF): A bootstrap aggregating (bagging) model that uses ensemble decision trees to make final decisions. This algorithm uses only a subset of features to find the best feature to separate classes at each node of the tree. The regression model fits every feature, and the data are split at several points. The feature with the least error is selected as the node.

Bagged decision tree (Bagging): Bagging uses a bootstrap method to reduce variance and overfitting. It uses the ensemble method for the final decision. Bagging method uses all features to find the best feature for the splitting node of the tree.

Adaptive boosting (AdaBoost): AdaBoost is an ensemble machine learning method that uses weak classifiers to make stronger classifiers.

Support vector regressor (SVR): SVR depends on the subset of training data. SVR performs non-linear regression using kernel trick and transforms inputs into m-dimensional feature space.

Gradient boosting (GB): GB produces an ensemble of weak prediction models or regression trees in a stage-wise fashion. Each stage optimizes a loss function by choosing the function that points in the negative gradient direction.

Kernel ridge (KR): Ridge regression uses L2 regularization to limit the size of the coefficients of the model and eliminates the problem in the least square regression. The ridge method adds a penalty to the coefficients equal to the square of the magnitude of coefficients. Regularization parameter λ controls the penalty term. Kernel ridge uses kernel tricks to make the model non-linear.

Decision tree with AdaBoost (DT): The prediction of the decision tree was boosted with AdaBoost. The decision tree method predicts by learning decision rules from the training data. AdaBoost is a boosting algorithm introduced by Freund and Schapire [26]. AdaBoost makes final predictions from weighted voting of the individual predictions from weak learners. It implements AdaBoost.R2 algorithm [27].

KNeighbors (KN): Nearest neighbors find k number of training data closest to the test data for which prediction is made. Each closest neighbor contributes equally while making a prediction (default parameter).

3.3. Model Evaluation

All the statistical metric results presented for the model evaluation are the average of 10 repeats (in the case of binary classification models and regression models) and 30 repeats (in the case of multiclass classification models). Approximately 20% of data were separated randomly in each iteration as test sets and the remaining data as training sets, such as five-fold cross-validation, except that the test sets were randomly selected in each iteration. In the case of binary and multiclass classification, the performance of each model was evaluated based on accuracy and area under the receiver operating characteristic curve (AUC). The classification models were also assessed for sensitivity and specificity. The evaluation scores are calculated as:

$$Accuracy = \frac{TP + TN}{TP + TN + FN + FP} \times 100$$

$$Sensitivity\ (TPR) = \frac{TP}{TP + FN} \times 100$$

$$Specificity\ (TNR) = \frac{TN}{TN + FP} \times 100$$

For the five-fold cross-validation, we used 80:20 training to test set ratios, which are good numbers for the significant data size used in this study. Further, the data are shuffled in each iteration before separating the training and the test set to make sure the process does not end up with a dataset containing bias in both the training and the test set. Additionally, the average performance metrics were calculated from the outcome of 10 simulations in the case of binary classification models and regression models. Whereas for the multiclass classification models, the average performance metrics were calculated from the outcome of 30 simulations. The training on 80% of the data give more room for better performance (compared to 10-fold cross-validation with 90% data in the training set) while predicting for an external dataset using a model trained on 100% of the data.

In the multiclass classification, micro averaging is used to obtain the average of the metrics of all the classes. Micro averaging involves calculating the average by converting the data in multiple classes to binary classes and giving equal weight to each observation. In multiclass classification with the imbalanced dataset, micro averaging of any metric is preferred when compared to macro averaging, which involves calculating the metrics separately for each class and then averaging them by giving equal weight to each class. In the case of multiclass classification with *n* number of classes,

$$Acc_{micro} = \frac{(TP_1 + TP_2 + \cdots + TP_n) + (TN_1 + TN_2 + \cdots + TN_n)}{(TP_1 + \cdots + TP_n) + (TN_1 + \cdots + TN_n) + (FN_1 + \cdots + FN_n) + (FP_1 + \cdots + FP_n)}$$

$$Sensitivity_{micro} = \frac{TP_1 + TP_2 + \cdots + TP_n}{(TP_1 + TP_2 + \cdots + TP_n) + (FN_1 + FN_2 + \cdots + FN_n)} \times 100$$

$$Specificity_{micro} = \frac{TN_1 + TN_2 + \cdots + TN_n}{(TN_1 + TN_2 + \cdots + TN_n) + (FP_1 + FP_2 + \cdots + FP_n)} \times 100$$

where *TP* = true positive, *TN* = true negative, *FP* = false positive, *FN* = false negative, *TPR* = true positive rate, *TNR* = true negative rate.

The performance of each regression model was evaluated based on the coefficient of determination (R^2). The coefficient of determination gives the percentage of variation in the dependent variable that is predictable from the independent variable, or that is explained by the independent variable.

$$R^2 = \frac{ESS}{TSS} = \frac{\sum_{i=1}^{n} (\hat{y}_i - \overline{y})^2}{\sum_{i=1}^{n} (y_i - \overline{y})^2} \quad (1)$$

where ESS is explained as the sum of squares, and TSS is the total sum of squares; $\hat{y}_i$ is the predicted value of the ith dependent variable; y_i is the ith observed dependent variable; and $\overline{y}$ is the mean of the observed data.

4. Results and Discussion

It is a desperate need to efficiently evaluate potential carcinogenic compounds that humans are exposed to in preventing cancer incidence, progression, and high mortality. Several computational and machine learning models have been developed for the prediction of carcinogenic compounds [6–16,28–40]. However, most or all of the models are developed as binary or regression models, not as categorical multiclassification models or comprehensive classification models. Further, these models are limited to congeneric computational models with a limited applicability domain and small dataset; they lack chemical diversity and were applied to targeted organ systems for carcinogenicity prediction. To fill this gap, we developed HNN-Cancer, a deep learning-based hybrid neural network model and predicted the carcinogenicity in large scale with a variety of datasets. The HNN-Cancer combines two neural network models, the CNN and the FFNN. The HNN-Cancer model combines CNN for deep learning based on the structure attribute (SMILES) with a multilayer perceptron (MLP)-type feed-forward neural network (FFNN) for learning based on descriptors of the chemicals. We developed different classification models, such as binary classification, multiclass classification, and regression models based on diverse non-congeneric chemicals.

The HNN carcinogenicity prediction models are developed based on the hybrid neural network (HNN) architecture we reported previously for toxicity prediction [17]. To compare the HNN prediction performance, we also developed other machine learning models, such as random forest (RF), bootstrap aggregating (Bagging), and adaptive boosting (AdaBoost) for binary classification and multiclass classification. Several regression models were developed based on random forest (RF), support vector regressor (SVR), gradient boosting (GB), kernel ridge (KR), decision tree with AdaBoost (DT), and KNeighbors (KN) using the sklearn package in python to make the final consensus prediction of the median toxic dose (TD50). A consensus prediction was calculated based on the average of all seven predicted values. We used the modified version of the 3D array representation of 1D SMILES in the convolutional neural network (CNN) in the HNN models from our previous model [17]. The SMILES processing method included a vocabulary of 94 characters in the ASCII table so as not to miss any possible characters of SMILES in any format. Additionally, instead of using one-hot encoding to vectorize the characters in the 1-D SMILES, the embedding layer of the CNN was used.

4.1. Carcinogen Prediction Using Binary Classification

The binary classification models were developed for Dataset I comprising 7994 chemicals (4636 carcinogenic and 3358 noncarcinogenic) from 9 different sources. Out of 1613 descriptors calculated by the Mordred descriptor calculator, 653 descriptors with no missing values were used to develop the models. We used the SMILES string in addition to the 653 descriptors in the HNN model. The accuracy, AUC, sensitivity, and specificity of the HNN-Cancer, RF, and Bagging models were comparable, whereas AdaBoost statistical metrics were significantly lower (Figure 1). The accuracy of the three models was 74%, and their AUC was ~0.81. The sensitivity and specificity of the HNN model was 79.47% and 67.3%.

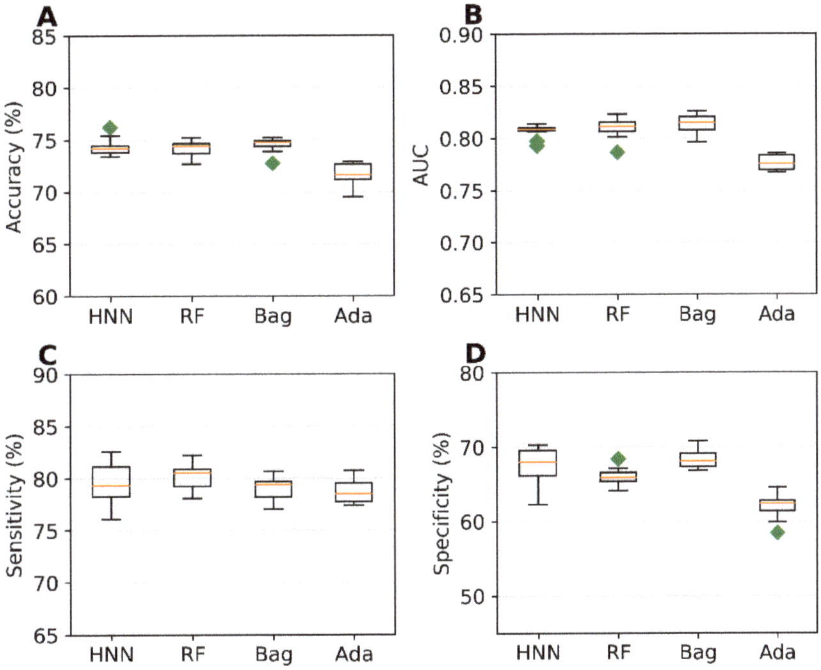

Figure 1. (**A**) accuracy, (**B**) AUC, (**C**) sensitivity, and (**D**) specificity for the dataset I as given by the binary classification models developed based on the HNN, RF, Bagging, and AdaBoost methods.

Zhang et al. [10] built several machine learning models on the CPDB's 1003 carcinogenic data on rats. The highest accuracy they reported was 70.1%, and an AUC of 0.765 for the five-fold cross-validation. Wang et al. [13] developed a deep learning tool CapsCarcino on the 1003 rat data from CPDB used by Zhang et al. For five-fold cross-validation, they reported accuracy of 74.5%, a sensitivity of 75%, and specificity of 74.2%. Li et al. developed 30 models on only 829 rat data from CPDB, with the highest accuracy of 89.29% on their test set. Tanabe et al. [9] developed an SVM model with an accuracy of 68.8% and an AUC of 0.683 for non-congeneric chemicals from six sources using dual cross-validation. They improved the accuracy by developing models on congeneric subgroups. Notably, these studies clearly demonstrate that models developed on more diverse chemicals result in reduced accuracy. In contrast, the predictive performance of our HNN-Cancer models based on a highly diverse set of chemicals is still good compared to the previously reported models with a high AUC. Hence, we expect the HNN-Cancer will rapidly make optimal carcinogen predictions for a wider variety of chemicals.

4.2. *Carcinogen Prediction Using Multiclass Classification*

The multiclass classification models were developed for Dataset II, containing 1618 chemicals with 459 chemicals in class 0, 604 in class 1, and 555 in class 2. In contrast, class 0 comprises non-carcinogens, class 1 comprises possible carcinogens and not classifiable chemicals, and class 2 comprises carcinogens and probable carcinogens. The overall accuracy is 50.58%, 54.73%, 55.52%, and 46.50%, the micro accuracy is 67.05%, 69.82%, 70.34%, and 64.33% whereas the average micro AUC is 0.68, 0.724, 0.725, and 0.653 for HNN-Cancer, RF, Bagging, and AdaBoost, respectively (Figure 2). As observed by Limbu et al. [17], the HNN-Cancer model is not performing better for the multiclass in comparison to RF and Bagging method. This is because the deep learning method performs best with a large dataset, and the dataset used in these two studies is not sufficiently large.

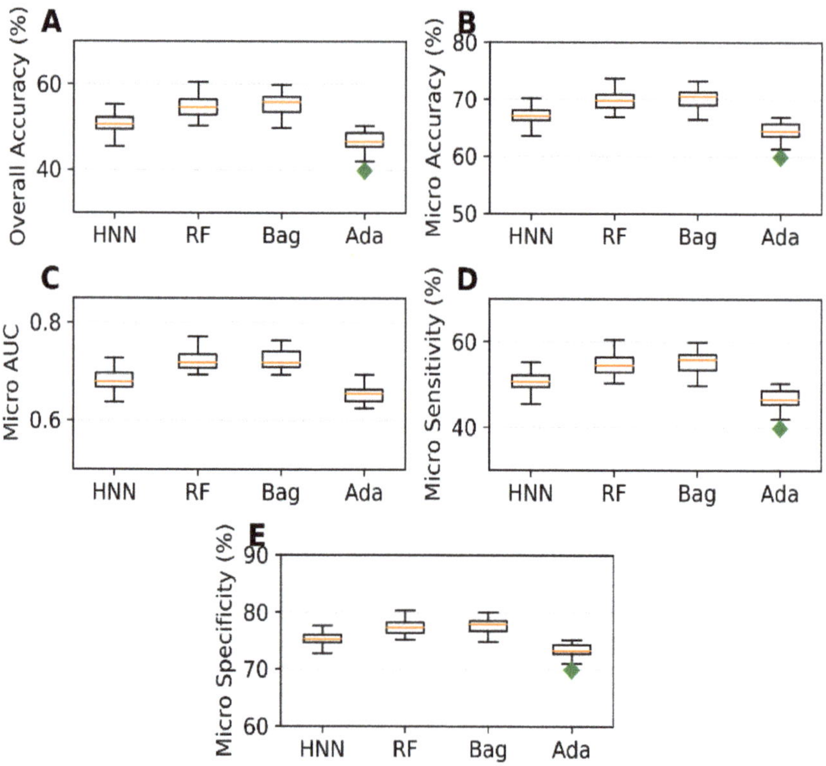

Figure 2. (**A**) Overall accuracy, (**B**) micro accuracy, (**C**) micro AUC, (**D**) micro sensitivity, and (**E**) micro specificity for the dataset II as given by the multiclass classification models developed based on HNN, RF, Bagging, and AdaBoost methods.

Li et al. developed 30 multiclass (ternary) classification models that categorized compounds into carcinogenic I (strongly carcinogenic), carcinogenic II (weakly carcinogenic), and non-carcinogens [11]. Their kNN model based on MACCS fingerprint with the best predictive performance achieved micro accuracy of 81.89%. The ternary classification of their data was based on the TD50 values where TD50 $\leq$ 10 mg/kg/day were carcinogenic I and TD50 > 10 mg/kg/day were carcinogenic II. Whereas the classification of data in our models is based on their category, they are class 2 if they are carcinogenic or probably carcinogenic, class 1 if they are possibly carcinogenic or not classifiable chemicals, class 0 if they are non-carcinogenic. All the data from CPDB with TD50 were classified as class 2, and non-carcinogens were classified as class 0; yet, none of them classified as class 1. However, we provided a complete classification range coverage when predicting the chemical carcinogenicity.

4.3. Carcinogenicity Prediction Using Regression

Regression models were developed for Dataset III comprising 561 TD50 chemicals. The models predicted carcinogenicity in the form of pTD50 (logarithm of the inverse of TD50), and the average of all seven predicted values was calculated as the final consensus prediction of the pTD50 value. The R^2 is 0.35, 0.36, 0.04, 0.33, 0.36, 0.39, and 0.21 for the HNN-Cancer, RF, SVM, GB, KR, DTBoost, and NN methods, respectively (Figure 3). The overall R^2 was slightly increased to 0.40 by the consensus prediction. The correlation coefficient (R) is 0.628, 0.611, 0.322, 0.588, 0.614, 0.636, 0.527, and 0.649 for the HNN, RF, SVM, GB, KR, DTBoost, NN, and consensus methods, respectively (Figure 4). The models were also developed for 543 TD50 data in mmol/kg body wt/day. The correlation coefficient (R) is 0.604, 0.601, 0.287, 0.577, 0.545, 0.617, 0.497, and 0.629 for the HNN-Cancer, RF, SVM, GB, KR, DTBoost, NN, and consensus methods, respectively (Figure 5).

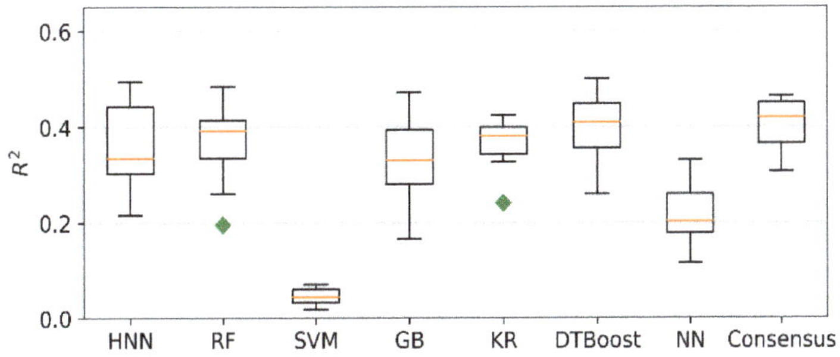

Figure 3. R^2 of regression models developed based on HNN-Cancer, RF, SVM, GB, KR, DTBoost, NN, and consensus methods.

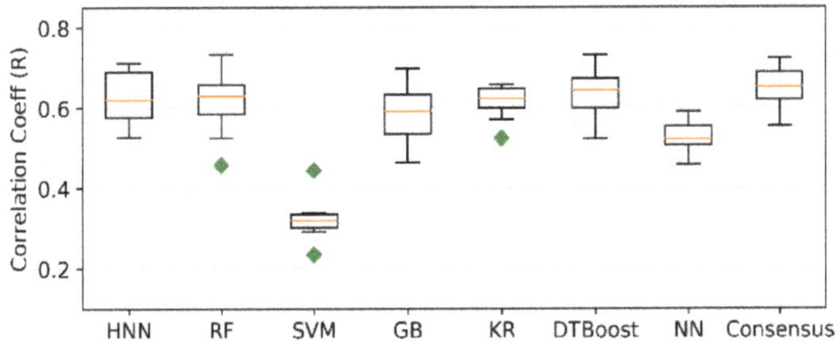

Figure 4. Correlation coefficient (R) of regression models developed based on HNN-Cancer, RF, SVM, GB, KR, DTBoost, NN, and consensus methods.

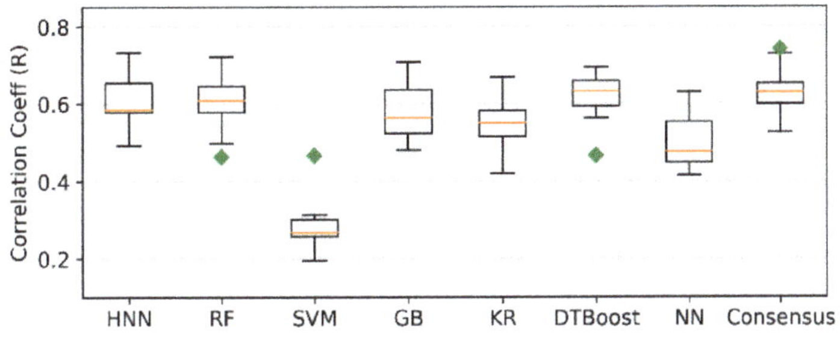

Figure 5. Correlation coefficient (R) of regression models developed based on HNN-Cancer, RF, SVM, GB, KR, DTBoost, NN, and consensus methods that predicts the carcinogenicity in mmol/kg body wt/day.

Fjodorova et al. [8] developed the quantitative models for carcinogenicity prediction on 805 rat data from CPDB using counter propagation artificial neural network (CP ANN) [8]. The correlation coefficient of the models was 0.46 for the test set. Toma et al. developed regression models to predict the carcinogenicity for external validation set with r^2 of 0.57 and 0.65 for models using oral and inhalation slope factor [12]. In the Toma et al. [12] study, only 315 out of 1110 oral and 263 out of 990 inhalation compounds were included in their final dataset after selecting compounds based on various criteria. The external validation set was randomly chosen from the finally obtained dataset with highly similar compounds. This may be the reason for a slightly better coefficient of determination reported by Toma et al. [12] compared to our models. Singh et al. [41] developed regression models based on generalized regression neural network (GRNN) to predict the carcinogenicity in mmol/kg body wt/day for 457 CPDB compounds and reported a correlation coefficient of 0.896 [41]. The high value of the correlation coefficient in comparison to our models could be attributed to the nine molecular descriptors selected for the regression models, and the GRNN method was used. Taken together, our model included the multi-classification models with full classification range coverage with diverse class of chemicals and provided optimal carcinogen predictive performance over the other methods.

5. Conclusions

Determining environmental chemical carcinogenicity is an urgent need. Though several machine learning models have been reported, there is a need for more non-congeneric computational models with a vast applicability domain for carcinogenicity prediction. In this study, we determined the carcinogenicity of thousands of wide-variety classes of real-life exposure chemicals. We have developed carcinogen prediction models based on our hybrid neural network (HNN) architecture method HNN-Cancer to determine chemical carcinogens. In the HNN-Cancer, we included new SMILES feature representation method. Using the HNN-Cancer and other machine learning methods, we predicted the carcinogen in terms of binary classification, multiclass classification, and regression models for the very diverse non-congeneric chemicals. Notably, the binary and multiclass classification models developed for the larger set of diverse chemicals were from diverse sources, most of which are human exposure-relevant chemicals.

The models based on the HNN-Cancer, RF, and Bagging methods predicted the carcinogens with an accuracy of 74% and an AUC of 0.81, which shows that the carcinogen predictions made by these models can be considered as optimal. Multiclass classification models to categorize the carcinogenicity of chemicals into one of the three classes: non-carcinogens, possible carcinogens/not classifiable chemicals, or carcinogens/probable carcinogens, were developed. The HNN-Cancer exhibited an accuracy of 50.58%, a micro accuracy of 67.05%, and a micro AUC of 0.68. Further, we developed regression models to predict the median toxic dose of chemicals in the form of pTD50. The consensus prediction achieved the overall R^2 of 0.40 by calculating the average of all the methods. Though our model included very diverse chemical categories and a larger number of chemicals from different data sources, still our models could be able to predict the binary, categorical (multiclass), and quantitative (regression) carcinogenicity comparable to the other literature reported models that included smaller and similar chemicals. Therefore, our HNN-Cancer can be used to identify the potential carcinogens for any chemical.

Several studies described the design of IoT-enabled environmental pollution and toxicology using the artificial intelligence technique to improve human health [42–47]. For example, Aisha et al. [42] proposed a neural network model that includes IoT-based sensor to sense eight pollutants and report the status of air quality in real-time by using a cloud server and informing the presence of hazardous pollutants levels in the air. Shukla et al. [46] and Memon et al. [47] employed artificial intelligence neural network IoT-enabled big data pipeline to the identification of breast cancer. Similarly, the HNN-Cancer could be integrated into the IoT-enabled sensors to inform the presence of carcinogens.

6. Limitations

The developed hybrid neural network method HNN-Cancer is first in class with developing various classification models, such as binary classification, multiclass classification, and regression models based on diverse non-congeneric chemicals. These models would enable the scientific community to classify chemicals carcinogenicity at specific doses or dose ranges. However, there are some potential limitations that exist in the prediction of carcinogens. Firstly, lack of a large dose-dependent chronic in vitro and in vivo carcinogen dataset to train the model. Secondly, the HNN-Cancer method needs several routines of optimization with further refinement. We will improve HNN-Cancer method carcinogen predictions further by including more experimentally determined carcinogenic dose data (in vitro and in vivo) that we obtained recently from the National Toxicology Program (NTP), bioinformatics and toxicology group.

Author Contributions: Conceptualization, S.D.; Data curation, S.L.; Formal analysis, S.L.; Funding acquisition, S.D.; Investigation, S.L. and S.D.; Methodology, S.L. and S.D.; Project administration, S.D.; Resources, S.D.; Software, S.L. and S.D.; Supervision, S.D.; Validation, S.L.; Writing—original draft, S.L. and S.D.; Writing—review & editing, S.D. All authors have read and agreed to the published version of the manuscript.

Funding: This research was funded in part by the United States Department of Defense (DOD) grant CA140882.

Institutional Review Board Statement: Not applicable.

Informed Consent Statement: Not applicable.

Data Availability Statement: Not applicable.

Acknowledgments: We acknowledges the support in part by the United States Department of Defense (DOD) grant CA140882, the GUMC Lombardi Comprehensive Cancer Center, and the GUMC Computational Chemistry Shared Resources (CCSR).

Conflicts of Interest: The authors declare no conflict of interest.

References

1. Hernández, L.G.; van Steeg, H.; Luijten, M.; van Benthem, J. Mechanisms of non-genotoxic carcinogens and importance of a weight of evidence approach. *Mutat. Res.* **2009**, *682*, 94–109. [CrossRef] [PubMed]
2. Wogan, G.N.; Hecht, S.S.; Felton, J.S.; Conney, A.H.; Loeb, L.A. Environmental and chemical carcinogenesis. *Semin. Cancer Biol.* **2004**, *14*, 473–486. [CrossRef] [PubMed]
3. Ledda, C.; Rapisarda, V. Occupational and Environmental Carcinogenesis. *Cancers* **2020**, *12*, 2547. [CrossRef] [PubMed]
4. Marone, P.A.; Hall, W.C.; Hayes, A.W. Reassessing the two-year rodent carcinogenicity bioassay: A review of the applicability to human risk and current perspectives. *Regul. Toxicol. Pharmacol.* **2014**, *68*, 108–118. [CrossRef] [PubMed]
5. Russell, W.; Burch, R. *The Principles of Humane Experimental Technique*; Methuen: London, UK, 1959; ISBN 0-900767-78-2.
6. Luan, F.; Zhang, R.; Zhao, C.; Yao, X.; Liu, M.; Hu, Z.; Fan, B. Classification of the Carcinogenicity of N-Nitroso Compounds Based on Support Vector Machines and Linear Discriminant Analysis. *Chem. Res. Toxicol.* **2005**, *18*, 198–203. [CrossRef]
7. Ivanciuc, O. Support Vector Machine Classification of the Carcinogenic Activity of Polycyclic Aromatic Hydrocarbons. *Internet Electron. J. Mol. Des.* **2002**, *1*, 203–218.
8. Fjodorova, N.; Vračko, M.; Tušar, M.; Jezierska, A.; Novič, M.; Kühne, R.; Schüürmann, G. Quantitative and qualitative models for carcinogenicity prediction for non-congeneric chemicals using CP ANN method for regulatory uses. *Mol. Divers.* **2010**, *14*, 581–594. [CrossRef]
9. Tanabe, K.; Kurita, T.; Nishida, K.; Lučić, B.; Amić, D.; Suzuki, T. Improvement of carcinogenicity prediction performances based on sensitivity analysis in variable selection of SVM models. *SAR QSAR Environ. Res.* **2013**, *24*, 565–580. [CrossRef]
10. Zhang, L.; Ai, H.; Chen, W.; Yin, Z.; Hu, H.; Zhu, J.; Zhao, J.; Zhao, Q.; Liu, H. CarcinoPred-EL: Novel models for predicting the carcinogenicity of chemicals using molecular fingerprints and ensemble learning methods. *Sci. Rep.* **2017**, *7*, 2118. [CrossRef]
11. Li, X.; Du, Z.; Wang, J.; Wu, Z.; Li, W.; Liu, G.; Shen, X.; Tang, Y. In Silico Estimation of Chemical Carcinogenicity with Binary and Ternary Classification Methods. *Mol. Inform.* **2015**, *34*, 228–235. [CrossRef]
12. Toma, C.; Manganaro, A.; Raitano, G.; Marzo, M.; Gadaleta, D.; Baderna, D.; Roncaglioni, A.; Kramer, N.; Benfenati, E. QSAR Models for Human Carcinogenicity: An Assessment Based on Oral and Inhalation Slope Factors. *Mol. Basel Switz.* **2020**, *26*, 127. [CrossRef] [PubMed]
13. Wang, Y.-W.; Huang, L.; Jiang, S.-W.; Li, K.; Zou, J.; Yang, S.-Y. CapsCarcino: A novel sparse data deep learning tool for predicting carcinogens. *Food Chem. Toxicol.* **2020**, *135*, 110921. [CrossRef] [PubMed]
14. Guan, D.; Fan, K.; Spence, I.; Matthews, S. Combining machine learning models of in vitro and in vivo bioassays improves rat carcinogenicity prediction. *Regul. Toxicol. Pharmacol.* **2018**, *94*, 8–15. [CrossRef] [PubMed]
15. Issa, N.T.; Wathieu, H.; Glasgow, E.; Peran, I.; Parasido, E.; Li, T.; Simbulan-Rosenthal, C.M.; Rosenthal, D.; Medvedev, A.V.; Makarov, S.S.; et al. A novel chemo-phenotypic method identifies mixtures of salpn, vitamin D3, and pesticides involved in the development of colorectal and pancreatic cancer. *Ecotoxicol. Environ. Saf.* **2022**, *233*, 113330. [CrossRef]
16. Li, N.; Qi, J.; Wang, P.; Zhang, X.; Zhang, T.; Li, H. Quantitative Structure-Activity Relationship (QSAR) Study of Carcinogenicity of Polycyclic Aromatic Hydrocarbons (PAHs) in Atmospheric Particulate Matter by Random forest (RF). *Anal. Methods* **2019**, *11*, 1816–1821. [CrossRef]

17. Limbu, S.; Zakka, C.; Dakshanamurthy, S. Predicting Environmental Chemical Toxicity Using a New Hybrid Deep Machine Learning Method. *ChemRxiv* **2021**. [CrossRef]
18. Hauschild, V.D. Chemical exposure guidelines for deployed military personnel. *Drug Chem. Toxicol.* **2000**, *23*, 139–153. [CrossRef]
19. USAPHC TG230 Environmental HRA and Chemical Military Exposure Guidelines (MEGs). Environmental Health Risk Assessment and Chemical Exposure Guidelines for Deployed Military Personnel. 2013 Revision. U.S. Army Public Health Command (USAPHC). Available online: https://phc.amedd.army.mil/PHC%20Resource%20Library/TG230-DeploymentEHRA-and-MEGs-2013-Revision.pdf (accessed on 12 September 2022).
20. National Toxicology Program: 14th Report on Carcinogens. Available online: https://ntp.niehs.nih.gov/go/roc14 (accessed on 5 March 2020).
21. List of Classifications–IARC Monographs on the Identification of Carcinogenic Hazards to Humans. Available online: https://monographs.iarc.who.int/list-of-classifications (accessed on 2 March 2020).
22. Recommendation of Occupational Exposure Limits (2018–2019). *J. Occup. Health* **2018**, *60*, 419–542. [CrossRef]
23. Carcinogen List-Occupational Cancer | NIOSH | CDC. Available online: https://www.cdc.gov/niosh/topics/cancer/npotocca.html (accessed on 28 February 2020).
24. Carcinogenic Potency Database. Available online: http://wayback.archive-it.org/org-350/20190628191644/https://toxnet.nlm.nih.gov/cpdb/chemicalsummary.html (accessed on 5 June 2018).
25. Moriwaki, H.; Tian, Y.-S.; Kawashita, N.; Takagi, T. Mordred: A molecular descriptor calculator. *J. Cheminform.* **2018**, *10*, 4. [CrossRef]
26. Freund, Y.; Schapire, R.E. A Decision-Theoretic Generalization of On-Line Learning and an Application to Boosting. *J. Comput. Syst. Sci.* **1997**, *55*, 119–139. [CrossRef]
27. Drucker, H. Improving Regressors Using Boosting Techniques. In Proceedings of the 14th International Conference on Machine Learning (ICML), Nashville, TN, USA, 8–12 July 1997; pp. 107–115.
28. Li, T.; Tong, W.; Roberts, R.; Liu, Z.; Thakkar, S. DeepCarc: Deep Learning-Powered Carcinogenicity Prediction Using Model-Level Representation. *Front. Artif. Intell.* **2021**, *4*, 757780. [CrossRef] [PubMed]
29. Li, T.; Tong, W.; Roberts, R.; Liu, Z.; Thakkar, S. DeepDILI: Deep Learning-Powered Drug-Induced Liver Injury Prediction Using Model-Level Representation. *Chem. Res. Toxicol.* **2021**, *34*, 550–565. [CrossRef] [PubMed]
30. Valerio, L.G., Jr.; Arvidson, K.B.; Chanderbhan, R.F.; Contrera, J.F. Prediction of rodent carcinogenic potential of naturally occurring chemicals in the human diet using high-throughput QSAR predictive modeling. *Toxicol. Appl. Pharmacol.* **2007**, *222*, 1–16. [CrossRef]
31. Jiao, Z.; Hu, P.; Xu, H.; Wang, Q. Machine Learning and Deep Learning in Chemical Health and Safety: A Systematic Review of Techniques and Applications. *ACS Chem. Health Saf.* **2020**, *27*, 316–334. [CrossRef]
32. Tan, N.X.; Rao, H.B.; Li, Z.R.; Li, X.Y. Prediction of chemical carcinogenicity by machine learning approaches. *SAR QSAR Environ. Res.* **2009**, *20*, 27–75. [CrossRef] [PubMed]
33. Tanabe, K.; Lučić, B.; Amić, D.; Kurita, T.; Kaihara, M.; Onodera, N.; Suzuki, T. Prediction of carcinogenicity for diverse chemicals based on substructure grouping and SVM modeling. *Mol. Divers* **2010**, *14*, 789–802. [CrossRef] [PubMed]
34. Toropova, A.P.; Toropov, A.A. CORAL: QSAR Models for Carcinogenicity of Organic Compounds for Male and Female Rats. *Comput. Biol. Chem.* **2018**, *72*, 26–32. [CrossRef]
35. Yauk, C.L.; Harrill, A.H.; Ellinger-Ziegelbauer, H.; van der Laan, J.W.; Moggs, J.; Froetschl, R.; Sistare, F.; Pettit, S. A Cross-Sector Call to Improve Carcinogenicity Risk Assessment through Use of Genomic Methodologies. *Regul. Toxicol. Pharmacol.* **2020**, *110*, 104526. [CrossRef]
36. Zhang, H.; Cao, Z.-X.; Li, M.; Li, Y.-Z.; Peng, C. Novel Naïve Bayes Classification Models for Predicting the Carcinogenicity of Chemicals. *Food Chem. Toxicol.* **2016**, *97*, 141–149. [CrossRef]
37. Wathieu, H.; Ojo, A.; Dakshanamurthy, S. Prediction of Chemical Multi-target Profiles and Adverse Outcomes with Systems Toxicology. *Curr. Med. Chem.* **2017**, *24*, 1705–1720. [CrossRef] [PubMed]
38. Issa, N.T.; Wathieu, H.; Ojo, A.; Byers, S.W.; Dakshanamurthy, S. Drug Metabolism in Preclinical Drug Development: A Survey of the Discovery Process, Toxicology, and Computational Tools. *Curr. Drug Metab.* **2017**, *18*, 556–565. [CrossRef] [PubMed]
39. Issa, N.T.; Stathias, V.; Schürer, S.; Dakshanamurthy, S. Machine and deep learning approaches for cancer drug repurposing. *Semin. Cancer Biol.* **2021**, *68*, 132–142. [CrossRef]
40. Glück, J.; Buhrke, T.; Frenzel, F.; Braeuning, A.; Lampen, A. In Silico genotoxicity and Carcinogenicity Prediction for Food-Relevant Secondary Plant Metabolites. *Food Chem. Toxicol.* **2018**, *116*, 298–306. [CrossRef]
41. Singh, K.P.; Gupta, S.; Rai, P. Predicting Carcinogenicity of Diverse Chemicals Using Probabilistic Neural Network Modeling Approaches. *Toxicol. Appl. Pharmacol.* **2013**, *272*, 465–475. [CrossRef] [PubMed]
42. Asha, P.; Natrayan, L.B.; Geetha, B.T.; Beulah, J.R.; Sumathy, R.; Varalakshmi, G.; Neelakandan, S. IoT enabled environmental toxicology for air pollution monitoring using AI techniques. *Environ. Res.* **2021**, *205*, 112574. [CrossRef] [PubMed]
43. Saravanan, D.; Kumar, D.K.S.; Sathya, R.; Palani, U. An iot based air quality monitoring and air pollutant level prediction system using machine learning approach–dlmnn. *Int. J. Future Gen. Commun. Netw.* **2020**, *13*, 925–945.
44. Satpathy, S.; Mohan, P.; Das, S.; Debbarma, S. A new healthcare diagnosis system using an IoT-based fuzzy classifier with FPGA. *J. Supercomput.* **2020**, *76*, 5849–5861. [CrossRef]

45. Senthilkumar, R.; Venkatakrishnan, P.; Balaji, N. Intelligent based novel embedded system based IoT enabled air pollution monitoring system. *Microprocess. Microsyst.* **2020**, *77*, 103172. [CrossRef]
46. Shukla, S.K.; Kumar, B.M.; Sinha, D.; Nemade, V.; Mussiraliyeva, S.; Sugumar, R.; Jain, R. Apprehending the Effect of Internet of Things (IoT) Enables Big Data Processing through Multinetwork in Supporting High-Quality Food Products to Reduce Breast Cancer. *J. Food Qual.* **2022**, *2022*, 2275517. [CrossRef]
47. Memon, M.H.; Li, J.P.; Haq, A.U.; Memon, M.H.; Zhou, W. Breast Cancer Detection in the IOT Health Environment Using Modified Recursive Feature Selection. *Wirel. Commun. Mob. Comput.* **2019**, *2019*, 5176705. [CrossRef]

sensors

MDPI

Article

Development of an Artificial Neural Network Algorithm Embedded in an On-Site Sensor for Water Level Forecasting

Cheng-Han Liu [1], Tsun-Hua Yang [1,*] and Obaja Triputera Wijaya [1,2]

[1] Department of Civil Engineering, National Yang Ming Chiao Tung University, Hsinchu 30010, Taiwan
[2] Department of Civil Engineering, Parahyangan Catholic University, Bandung 40141, Indonesia
* Correspondence: tshyang@nycu.edu.tw; Tel.: +886-3-571-3827

Abstract: Extreme weather events cause stream overflow and lead to urban inundation. In this study, a decentralized flood monitoring system is proposed to provide water level predictions in streams three hours ahead. The customized sensor in the system measures the water levels and implements edge computing to produce future water levels. It is very different from traditional centralized monitoring systems and considered an innovation in the field. In edge computing, traditional physics-based algorithms are not computationally efficient if microprocessors are used in sensors. A correlation analysis was performed to identify key factors that influence the variations in the water level forecasts. For example, the second-order difference in the water level is considered to represent the acceleration or deacceleration of a water level rise. According to different input factors, three artificial neural network (ANN) models were developed. Four streams or canals were selected to test and evaluate the performance of the models. One case was used for model training and testing, and the others were used for model validation. The results demonstrated that the ANN model with the second-order water level difference as an input factor outperformed the other ANN models in terms of RMSE. The customized microprocessor-based sensor with an embedded ANN algorithm can be adopted to improve edge computing capabilities and support emergency response and decision making.

Keywords: edge computing; ANN; microprocessor; water level prediction; decentralized

Citation: Liu, C.-H.; Yang, T.-H.; Wijaya, O.T. Development of an Artificial Neural Network Algorithm Embedded in an On-Site Sensor for Water Level Forecasting. *Sensors* **2022**, *22*, 8532. https://doi.org/10.3390/s22218532

Academic Editors: Andrei Velichko, Dmitry Korzun and Alexander Meigal

Received: 9 October 2022
Accepted: 3 November 2022
Published: 5 November 2022

1. Introduction

The Emergency Event Database (EM-DAT) includes records for 432 disastrous events related to natural hazards worldwide in 2021. Floods dominated these events, with 223 occurrences, with an average of 163 annual flood occurrences recorded in the 2001–2020 period [1]. The losses of life and property caused by floods are tremendous [2]. Structural and nonstructural measures have been devised to prevent or mitigate loss of life and property [3]. The development of early warning systems, which are nonstructural measures, was cited as a critical defense against floods [4]. These systems involve on-site facilities such as bubble gauges, float gauges and pressure sensors, which are installed to observe water level changes; then, these observations are used as indicators to assess the flood potential [5]. Accurate and cost-efficient water level monitoring sensors are required and must be deployed with very high intensity for detailed flood records [6–9]. Nevertheless, these sensors are only used for water level monitoring, and this kind of application provides limited lead time for decision makers to take response measures to mitigate the impact of disasters [7–11].

Edge computing is a distributed computing paradigm in which computations are largely or completely performed at distributed device nodes known as smart devices or edge devices, as opposed to computations in a centralized cloud environment [12]. By implementing edge computing on sensors, issues prevalent in centralized cloud systems, such as latency and network connection dependency, can be avoided [13]. Since system failure or other misinformation issues occur during the transmission process, which is common during disasters, simulation cannot be performed, resulting in delays in the emergency response and increasing the possibility of damage. Many studies in the fields such as medical care, manufacturing, and fault detection have developed sensors not only for monitoring but also implemented edge computing for applications that are close in proximity to the sources in case of need, e.g., [13–15]. In comparison with other applications, only a few studies have investigated edge computing in landslide- and flood-related applications [16–18]. People hesitate to apply edge computing in flood warning systems for the following possible reasons. First, most of the systems are still built based on traditional frameworks. If a prediction is performed in real time for operational purposes, the observed data from local monitoring devices are transmitted to the remote server through the internet. The server performs simulations and provides results to responders for decision making. This is called a centralized simulation approach. The monitoring devices are only capable of observing water levels without forecast functions. Therefore, there is no opportunity to implement edge computing until new sensors are developed and deployed. Second, to increase the lead time of the response, physically based models are used in the traditional framework for predictions. These systems consider different hydrological and inundation modeling components based on the specific target region, size of basins, available data and resources, and system development approach [19]. These physically based models considering detailed hydraulic processes (e.g., solving Saint-Venant equations) are complex and computationally intensive, causing limited applications in practical applications due to the availability of input data for parameterization and the detailed requirements of simulations [20–22]. None of these models are designed to be installed in sensors with limited computing power. In this regard, data-driven machine models that focus on the relationship between input factors (e.g., historical flow discharge and precipitation) and outputs (e.g., water level) are recommended as an alternative [23,24].

Related studies about the integration of customized sensors and data-driven models were examined. Customized ultrasonic sensors have been developed [5,10]. Warnings are issued when the monitored water levels are above a specific threshold. No extra calculation was performed on the sensors in these studies. Other studies used microcontroller-based sensors to collect environmental information and perform calculations in cloud-based neural networks to predict flood disaster conditions [25–27]. These studies confirmed the functionality of ANN models for water level predictions. However, the models were executed in the cloud-based server. Finally, Samikwa et al. [28] utilized edge computing for flood prediction and carried it on a low-power device within the IoT wireless sensor network. Long short-term memory (LSTM), a type of ANN, was applied in the study to predict one-hour ahead-of-time forecasts of water level. Similar to Bande and Shete [25], water level and rainfall were utilized as inputs in the study to train the ANN models to produce forecasts. However, the details of the input selection were not discussed in the study. Al Qundus et al. [29] deployed sensors to collect data such as water levels, temperature and wind speed. A support vector machine (SVM) algorithm was implemented at nodes (sensors). Only four features (temperature, humidity, wind speed, and water level) were selected to develop the SVM models. However, the details of feature selection were not discussed in the study.

This study proposed a novel decentralized flood warning system with edge computing. It consists of edge computing-enabled wireless water level monitoring sensors and a suitable forecasting algorithm that was embedded in these sensors. The newly developed sensor shifts applications, data, and computing power (services) away from centralized points to the logical extremes of a network. In other words, the sensor involves applications or general functionalities that are close in proximity to the sources of other processes, thus involving interactions between distributed systems technology and the physical world; this implies that the sensor can perform simulations and predictions directly at flood-prone locations with localized information. Therefore, situational and customized awareness is maintained during flooding, even if an internet connection is unavailable. As a result, the efficiency of the emergency response is increased. In addition, new flood prediction models are desperately needed to be performed on the computing power-limited sensors. ANN models were developed to determine the water level on the sensor. A detailed analysis regarding the correlation between input factors and output water levels was carefully conducted to maximize the efficiency of edge computing. Furthermore, special attention was given to extreme events such as typhoons during the development of the proposed system.

2. Study Areas

This study focused on three rivers and one artificial canal to develop the ANN model and evaluate the performance of the proposed system. The geographical locations of these study areas are shown in Figure 1.

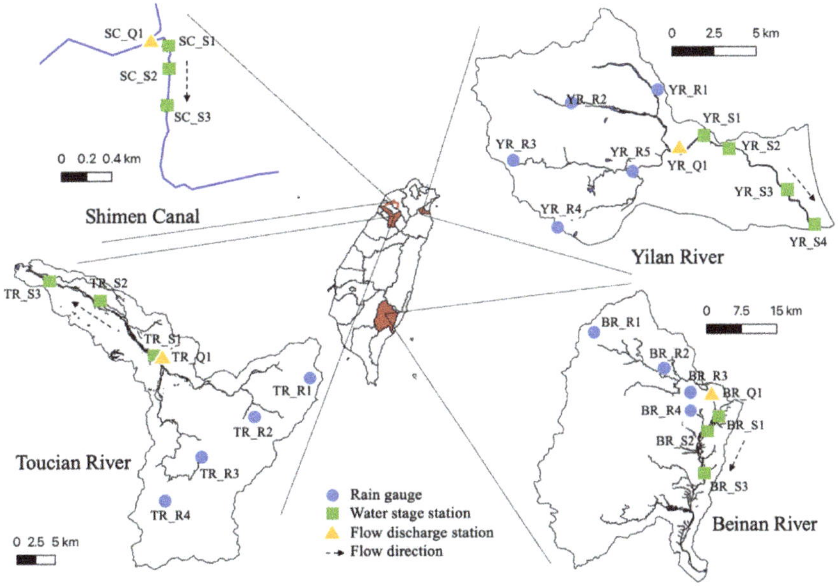

Figure 1. The four study areas are the Shimen canal in Taoyuan County (**upper left**), the Yilan River in Yilan County (**upper right**), the Beinan River in Taitung County (**bottom right**), and the Toucian River in Hsinchu County (**bottom left**), Taiwan.

The Yilan River Basin is located on northeastern Taiwan Island. Its main stream is approximately 24.4 km (km) long and covers an area of approximately 149.06 square km. The Yilan River Basin was first selected to train and test the ANN model for water level forecasting. This is because the precipitation, river stage, and flow velocity data have been carefully measured by the Water Resources Agency (WRA) and National Center for High-performance Computing (NCHC) since 2012 [30] for the Yilan River basin. In addition, there is no human interference, such as a reservoir upstream of the Yilan River, and there are no human operation-related factors considered among the ANN input factors in this study. Figure 1 (in a clockwise direction) shows the remaining two river basins, the Beinan River and Toucian River Basins, in eastern and western Taiwan and one artificial canal, Shimen Canal, in western Taiwan. The Beinan River is approximately 84 km long and flows through Taitung County to the Pacific Ocean. The Toucian River flows through Hsinchu County for 63 km to the west. Different from the Yilan River and Beinan River situations, there are also no human-made hydraulic structures upstream along the Toucian River, but there is an off-stream reservoir upstream of the river. These two rivers were selected because there was no human interference, such as reservoirs or gates, found in the rivers. For reference, the proposed system (integration of Raspberry Pi (RPi) sensors and an ANN model) was only implemented on-site in the Shimen Canal because of the limitations of devices and the need for permission to install equipment. Tests performed in the Beinan River and Toucian River were conducted offline.

3. System Development

In this study, a water level forecasting model is embedded in an RPi-based monitoring device that can provide real-time water level observations and support local calculations. The system structure and data processing flowchart are illustrated in Figure 2. The monitoring devices use ultrasonic waves to measure the water levels, and the observed data and other related information are preprocessed in the RPi platform. Thereafter, the water level predictions at specific locations are performed using the proposed ANN-based water level forecasting models. The details of each component in the structure are described in the following subsections.

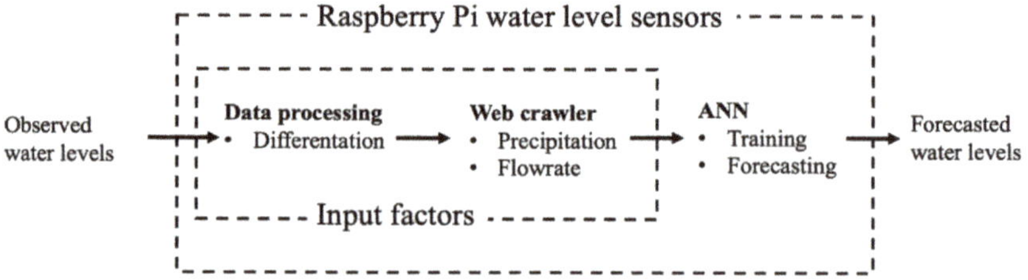

Figure 2. System data processing flowchart.

3.1. Raspberry Pi Water Level Sensor

Automatic water level sensors with wireless functions are usually costly. Therefore, low-cost, open-source, and low-energy-consumption sensors are always of interest for environmental monitoring [31]. The proposed sensor is shown in Figure 3.

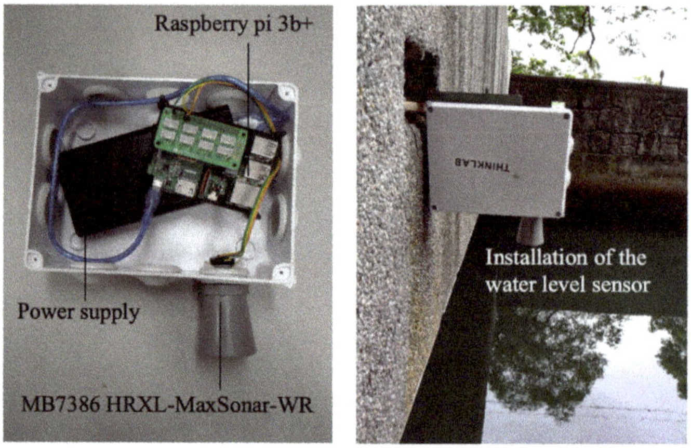

Figure 3. Details of the RPi-based ultrasonic water level sensor (**left**) and the installation of the sensor (**right**).

The RPi is a reliable, low-cost microcomputer (MCU) that was developed in 2006 by the University of Cambridge's Computer Department and has been produced by the Raspberry Pi Foundation since 2012. The RPi 3 Model B+ module, which was released in February 2018 with a 1.4 GHz 64-bit quad core processor, was used as a platform embedded with an ultrasonic sensor to measure water stages at a local site. The UNIX/Debian=based Raspian operating system supports the implementation of a Python programming language-based ANN module to forecast water levels with lead times. Many studies have successfully applied ultrasonic waves to measure water levels under severe environmental conditions [32,33]. The ultrasonic sensor used here is the high-performance ultrasonic distance sensor MB7386 HRXL-MaxSonar-WR from MaxBotix, Brainerd, MN, USA. The ultrasonic sensor emits sound waves at a frequency of 42 kHz with a 6 Hz sampling rate and detects the sound waves that bounce back. The distance can be estimated by the elapsed time between the generated and returning sound waves. Theoretically, the sensor is effective up to a maximum range of 10 m, with functions of temperature compensation and noise cancelation. However, the efficient measuring distance varies based on the size of the target and power supply to the sensor (usually within 5 m).

3.2. Artificial Neural Network Water Level Forecasting Algorithm

ANNs are inspired by the human central nervous system. ANNs usually consist of layers such as an input layer, one or more hidden layers, and an output layer. A three-layer ANN data processing flowchart is shown in Figure 4. The input layer comprises a number of nodes ($i = 1, 2, 3 \ldots n$). A node, also called an artificial neuron, connects to other nodes in the hidden layer and has an associated weight (w) and threshold (*bias*). When the incoming signals ($X_1, X_2, X_3 \ldots X_n$) are passed to the nodes ($j = 1, 2, 3 \ldots N$) in the next layer, they are multiplied by the weight of the connection. These weights describe the importance of any incoming signal, with larger weights contributing more significantly to the output compared to other signals. The effective signal (E_j) to node j shown in Equation (1) is the weighted sum of all incoming signals. In the first phase of training, the weights (i.e., w_{ji}) are set to random values.

$$E_j = \sum_{i=1}^{n} X_i w_{ji} + bias \quad (1)$$

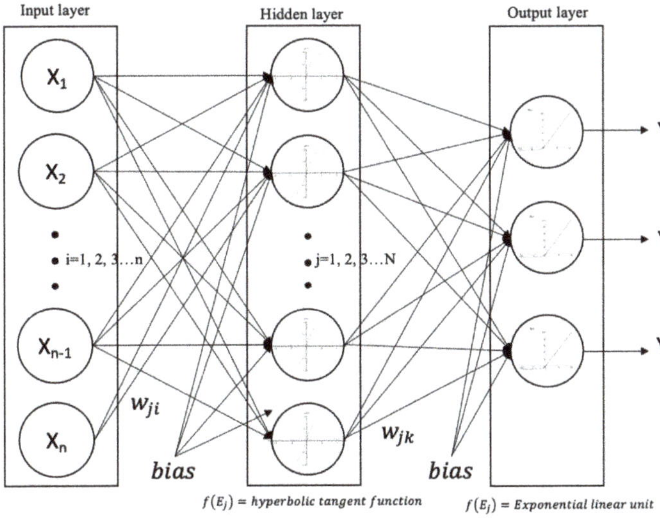

Figure 4. A three-layer ANN model and its data processing flowchart.

An activation function is used to transform the effective signal (E_j) into an output value to be fed to the next layer or as an output. In this study, hyperbolic tangent (tanh) and exponential linear unit (ELU) functions are used as the activation functions to transfer input signals to hidden and output layers, respectively. The tanh function has an S-shape similar to that of the sigmoid activation function, with a difference in the output range of -1 to 1. The ELU function is also similar to the rectified linear unit (ReLU), with a difference in output value for negative values of input. A three-layer network structure with one input layer, one hidden layer, and one output layer is adopted because of the limited computing power of the RPi 3 Model B+ module in the sensor [27]. No general guidelines exist for specifying the optimal number of nodes required in the hidden layer [34]. The number of nodes in the hidden layers can be estimated using Equation (2), as recommended by Fletcher and Goss [35]. The formula was confirmed by Huang and Foo [36] to provide the optimal network size, resulting in minimum error and a high correlation in the validation data set. There are three output nodes representing the forecasted water levels with lead periods of 1, 2, and 3 h.

$$N = 2n \tag{2}$$

where N is the number of nodes in the hidden layer and n is the number of incoming signals. The output from the neural network is calculated by propagating an input signal through each layer until the output layer outputs its values. It is a so-called feed-forward network. As mentioned above, the weights initially are random values and modified by reducing the differences between the output and a known output. The procedure repeatedly optimizes the weights until the value of the objective root mean square error (*RMSE*) function, shown in Equation (3), falls below a certain threshold. In this study, the threshold is 0.01.

$$RMSE = \sqrt{\frac{1}{K}\sum_{i=1}^{K=3}(P_i - O_i)^2} \tag{3}$$

where P_i is the predicted water level and O_i is the observed water level. K is the number of outputs and here refers to the forecasted water levels with three lead times. This learning procedure is called the backpropagation approach and was proposed by Rumelhart et al. [37]. It is a method for training the weights in a multilayer feed-forward neural network structure. A Python module Scikit-learn was applied for the ANN model computation [38].

Since the output of the developed ANN model is the water level, the selection of the input factors must be based on the characteristics and shifts of the outputs at a given location. The change in the time series water level is not only dependent on rainfall records in upstream watersheds and river inflows but also related to previous water levels based on river discharge conditions. Moreover, the length of the lag phase of each input factor is influenced by the distance between input and output locations, and it determines the length of the input sequence. In fact, the selection of input factors has a large impact on the accuracy and efficiency of ANN models. There is no global way to select the input factors for an ANN model [39]. Thus, parameter selection for edge computing is important to maximize the computing efficiency of ANNs. The efficiency of calculations must be optimized for the appropriate number of input factors. In this study, a cross-correlation analysis (cc^2), shown in Equation (4), one of the most widely used methods for factor selection, as discussed by Babel and Shinde [39], was carried out between the outputs (forecasted water levels at a given location) and input factors with a lag phase length.

$$cc^2 = \frac{\sum_{i=1}^{n-k}(X_i - \overline{X})(Y_{i+k} - \overline{Y})}{\sqrt{\sum_{i=1}^{n}(X_i - \overline{X})^2}\sqrt{\sum_{i=1}^{n}(Y - \overline{Y})^2}} \tag{4}$$

where n is the total number of time sequences in hours and k represents the time lag value. X and Y are the water level and a possible input factor, respectively. $\overline{X}$ and $\overline{Y}$ denote average values. Only the factors with a relatively high correlation value with the output were adopted in the proposed ANN models. In addition to the original inputs, two extra input factors were included in the cross-correlation analysis: water level variation (W_r) and the frequency of water level change (W_f) for consecutive records in a time interval (e.g., 1 h). The definitions of W_r and W_f are shown below:

$$W_{r,i} = X_{obs,i} - X_{obs,i-1} \tag{5}$$

$$W_{f,i} = W_{r,i} - W_{r,\,i-1} \tag{6}$$

Mathematically, W_r and W_f represent the first- and second-order differences of the water level sequence at a target location, respectively. Physically, W_r and W_f are the velocity and acceleration of the change water level, respectively. Zhong et al. [40] found that considering the first- and second-order differences in the water level sequence can improve the forecasting accuracy of ANN models. However, they used this information to identify the level of data fluctuations and then applied the Kalman filter algorithm for local optimization. Details of the selected factors were not discussed in their study. In contrast, this study is the first attempt to apply these variables as input factors for the proposed ANN models to perform water level forecasting. Details of the analysis are described in the Results and Discussion section.

4. Results and Discussion

The ANN models were integrated into sensors, and their performance was evaluated in real cases. The discussion of the results is divided into three parts: (1) data preparation, (2) development, and (3) application. The research flowchart of this process is shown in Figure 5.

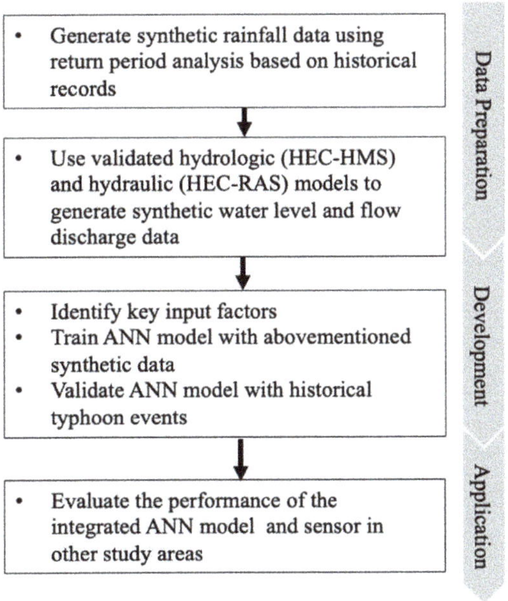

Figure 5. Research flowchart of the proposed ANN models.

4.1. Data Preparation

4.1.1. Generation of Synthetic Rainfall Data for Different Return Periods

Data quality and quantity are important for the accuracy of data-driven models (e.g., ANN models). The well-calibrated data from 2012 to 2017, including rainfall, flow discharge, and water stage, from the experimental watershed in the Yilan River Basin (Figure 1), were adopted. Following the research flowchart shown in Figure 5, a frequency analysis using rainfall data from five rainfall stations was conducted, and the magnitude of extreme events was related to the corresponding frequency of occurrence through the use of a probability distribution. To find the magnitude associated with a certain return period, the standard frequency factor method [41] is used, as follows:

$$X_T = \overline{X} + Ks \tag{7}$$

where X_T is the calculated rainfall value in a certain period, $\overline{X}$ is the mean rainfall value from historical data, K is the frequency factor, and s is the standard deviation of the historical data. K was selected for 2-, 5-, 10-, 25-, 50-, and 100-year return period events based on the Pearson III distribution [42]. The calculated cumulative rainfall for a 24-h rainfall duration is shown in Table 1. In terms of topography, the upper parts of the Yilan River Basin have mountain topography and steep slopes. There are wide flood plains from the lower reaches to the Pacific Ocean. The stations YR_R2 and YR_R4 are located in mountain and floodplain areas, respectively. As a result, YR_R2 and YR_R4 have the greatest and fewest values among all stations. The rainfall values are consistent with the variations in topography.

Table 1. Calculated 24-h rainfall values at five stations for different return periods.

Station ID	24-h Duration Rainfall for Different Return Periods in mm					
	2-yr	**5-yr**	**10-yr**	**25-yr**	**50-yr**	**100-yr**
YR_R1	208.96	264.35	298.96	340.15	369.35	397.30
YR_R2	205.90	283.71	336.73	403.20	451.81	499.36
YR_R3	191.88	256.75	305.44	369.67	415.85	466.46
YR_R4	178.11	220.21	242.81	267.33	283.37	298.00
YR_R5	263.98	332.60	369.57	408.09	433.36	456.17

Hydrographs specify the precipitation depth in 24 successive time intervals of 1 h duration over a total of 24 h. Such hydrographs are necessary inputs to hydrological and hydraulic models to generate flow discharge and water level data in the Yilan River Basin for different return periods. The details associated with hydrological and hydraulic models are discussed in the next section. The annual 24-h maximum rainfall value at each station from 2012 to 2017 was selected, and the average contribution (%) of each hour to the 24-h duration was calculated. These contributions were reordered in a time sequence with the maximum contribution occurring at the center of the 24-h duration and the remaining contributions arranged in descending order alternatively to the right and to the left of the center value to form a hyetrograph. The results are shown in Figure 6.

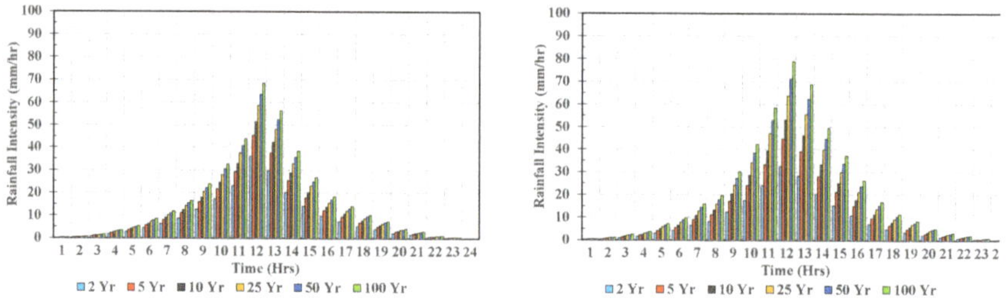

(a) (b)

Figure 6. *Cont.*

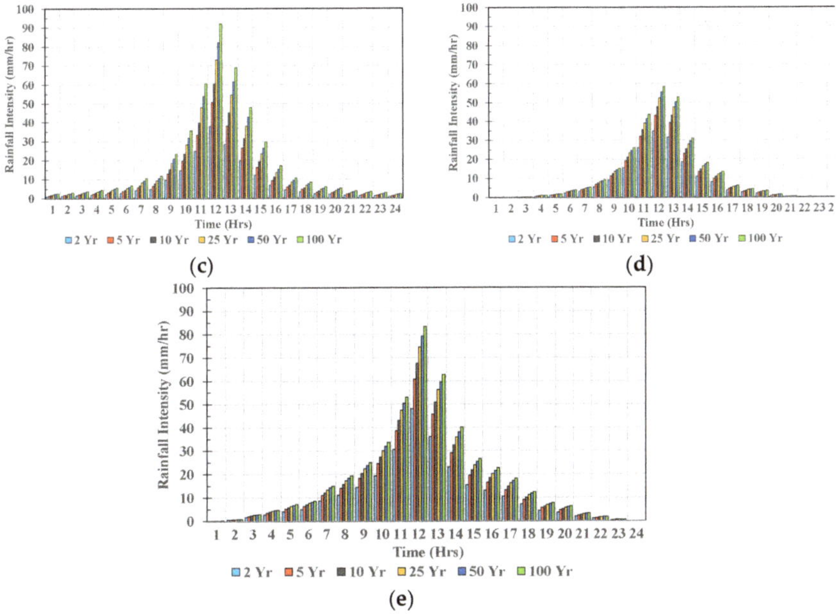

Figure 6. (**a–e**) The hourly rainfall distribution for different return periods in the Yilan River basin at YR_R1-YR_R5.

4.1.2. Generation of Synthetic Water Level and Flow Discharge Data

The abovementioned synthetic rainfall data were used with the hydrological model Hydrologic Modeling System (HEC-HMS) and the hydraulic model River Analysis System (HEC-RAS) to generate discharge and water level data for five return periods. HEC-HMS simulates rainfall runoff processes at the watershed level and includes different components, such as the runoff volume, baseflow, and channel flow. For more details, please refer to the Technical Reference Manual [43] and User's Manual [44]. In this study, an initial loss and a constant loss rate were subtracted from the precipitation depth, and the remaining depth was referred to as precipitation excess. Thereafter, excess precipitation was transformed to direct surface runoff through the SCS unit hydrograph (SCS-UH) method.

The total flow at YR_Q1 in the Yilan River Basin (Figure 1) was the sum of the direct runoff plus the base flow, and the base flow was obtained from an initial value multiplied by an exponential decay constant. The calculated total flow from the HEC-HMS model was then used as the upstream boundary condition for the downstream HEC-RAS model to calculate the variation in the water level downstream. To validate the performance of the HEC-HMS model, Typhoons Soulik (2012), Dujuan (2015), and Megi (2016) were considered. Table 2 shows the comparisons between the observations and simulations. Differences in peak discharge and time to peak discharge were below 15% and less than 2 h, respectively. Since the results met the relevant performance requirements, the calibrated model was then used to generate synthetic discharge values at YR_Q1 for further analysis. The inflow results associated with different return periods are shown in Figure 7.

Table 2. The validated performance of HEC-HMS for three typhoons.

Event	Soulik (2012)	Dujuan (2015)	Megi (2016)
Difference in peak discharge (%)	14.8	3.83	14.1
Difference in time to peak discharge (hour)	1	2	0

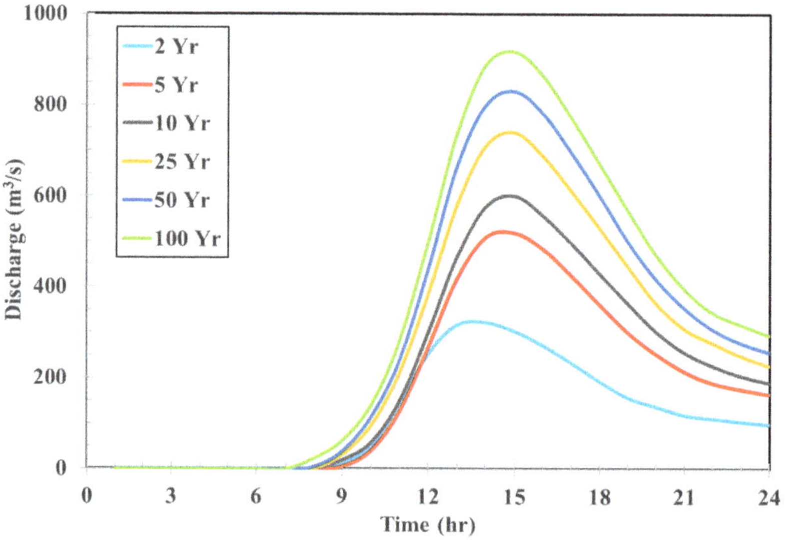

Figure 7. Synthetic inflow hydrograph at YR_Q1 in the Yilan River basin for different return periods.

There are four water level stations downstream of YR_Q1 (Figure 1). Among them, data from YR_S1, YR_S2, and YR_S3 were used as input data to train the ANN model. The HEC-RAS model was used to estimate water level variations at the abovementioned locations, and YR_S4 was used as the downstream boundary. HEC-RAS is a 1D river hydraulic model based on the Saint-Venant equations. These equations are approximated with the implicit Preissmann scheme and solved numerically using the Newton–Raphson iteration approach [45]. The downstream boundary condition was assumed to be the observed water levels during Typhoon Dujuan (2015). In comparison with observations, the performance was evaluated at YR_S2 in terms of temporal variations in water level, and the results are shown in Figure 8. The results demonstrate that differences in peak water level and time to peak water level were below 10% and zero hours, respectively. In conclusion, both the hydrological and hydraulic results confirm that the model parameters were well-tuned to generate the data needed for the development of the ANN model in the next section.

4.2. ANN Model Development

4.2.1. Correlation Analysis and Input Factor Selection

As described in Section 3.2, precipitation from YR_R1 to YR_R5, flow discharge at YR_Q1, and water levels from YR_S1 to YR_S3 were assumed to be correlated with the water level output at YR_S2. A correlation analysis between the targeted water level at the present time and the abovementioned variables from previous periods was performed using Equation (4). This model was considered the ANN_0 model. To include physical features such as the velocity and acceleration of water level variations, a correlation analysis between the first-order and second-order differences of the output and its values from previous periods was conducted. In this way, two more models were developed, named the ANN_1 and ANN_2 models. All of the correlation results are shown in Table 3. The variables with the highest correlation results with those in previous periods were selected as the model inputs. For example, for the ANN_0 model, the highest correlation results are 0.795 and 0.917 for YR_R1 at t−4 h and YR_S1 at t−1 h, respectively. As a result, four variables of YR_R1 and one variable of YR_S1 were selected for the ANN_0 model. However, in some cases, such as YR_R1 in the ANN_1 model, the correlation results 7 and 8 h earlier were 0.601 and 0.608, respectively. These values were different at three decimal digits. Other rainfall-related input factors, such as YR_R2, YR_R3, YR_R4, and YR_R5, were the variables 7 h earlier. To be consistent with other rainfall input factors and to increase computational efficiency, the variables 7 h earlier were selected for YR_R1. In addition, few variables were included, so the efficiency was increased considering the limited computing resources of the sensors. As a result, there were a total of 26, 46, and 46 input factors for the ANN_0, ANN_1, and ANN_2 models, respectively, and details of the input factor selection are listed in Table 4.

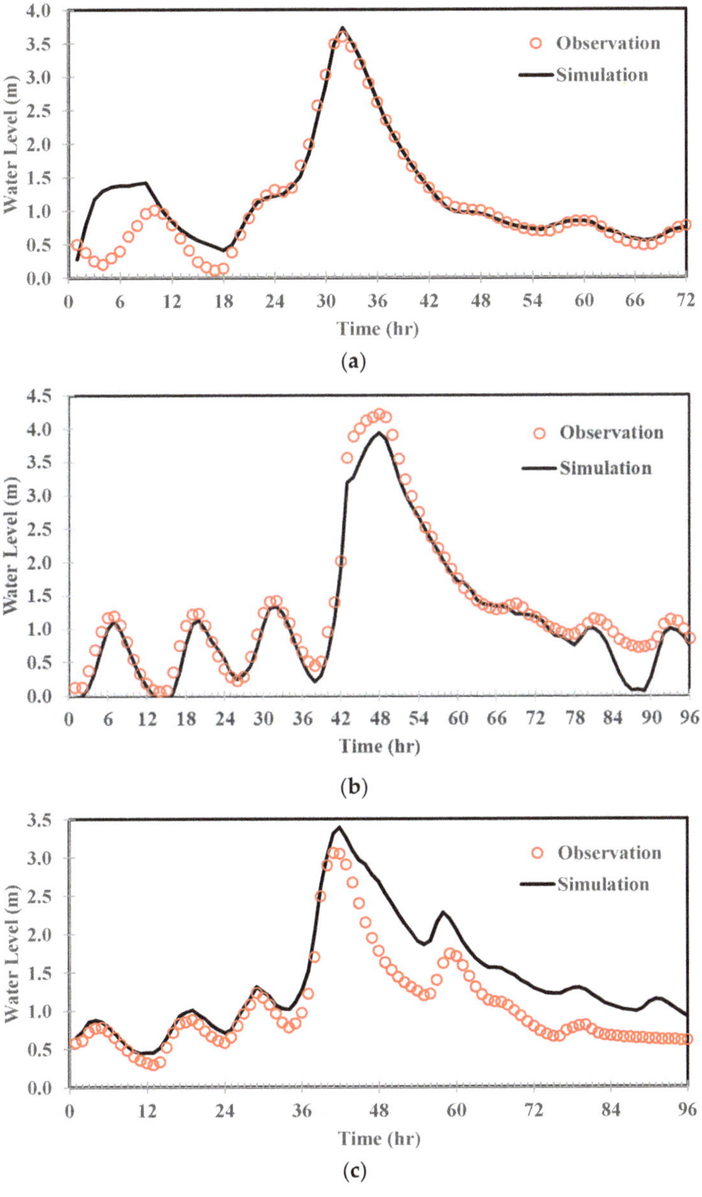

Figure 8. Comparison of the simulated and observed water levels at YR_R2 for (**a**) Typhoon Soulik; (**b**) Typhoon Dujuan; and (**c**) Typhoon Megi.

Table 3. Correlation matrix for output and input variables.

Model	Lag (Hour)	YR_R1	YR_R2	YR_R3	YR_R4	YR_R5	YR_Q1	YR_S1	YR_S2	YR_S3
ANN_0	1	0.586	0.595	0.534	0.538	0.576	0.863	0.917	0.923	0.887
	2	0.712	0.721	0.652	0.662	0.701	0.784	0.788	0.795	0.777
	3	0.782	0.791	0.710	0.725	0.767	0.661	0.625	0.639	0.652
	4	0.795	0.807	0.716	0.734	0.780	0.507	0.440	0.465	0.519
	5	0.762	0.775	0.678	0.697	0.742	0.336	0.243	0.278	0.376
ANN_1	1	−0.278	−0.281	−0.297	−0.306	−0.274	0.394	0.488	0.680	0.471
	2	−0.037	−0.046	−0.044	−0.045	−0.031	0.555	0.601	0.232	0.494
	3	0.177	0.171	0.173	0.183	0.182	0.645	0.643	0.054	0.462
	4	0.348	0.341	0.333	0.353	0.349	0.664	0.640	0.070	0.445
	5	0.473	0.467	0.442	0.470	0.472	0.624	0.612	0.138	0.460
	6	0.557	0.533	0.510	0.549	0.552	-	-	-	-
	7	0.601	0.595	0.542	0.585	0.589	-	-	-	-
	8	0.608	0.604	0.540	0.582	0.595	-	-	-	-
	9	0.570	0.571	0.499	0.539	0.559	-	-	-	-
ANN_2	1	−0.260	−0.264	−0.283	−0.291	−0.257	0.400	0.488	0.680	0.471
	2	−0.013	−0.022	−0.026	−0.024	−0.008	0.562	0.601	0.231	0.494
	3	0.205	0.198	0.195	0.207	0.209	0.651	0.643	0.054	0.462
	4	0.376	0.369	0.357	0.379	0.377	0.665	0.640	0.070	0.445
	5	0.499	0.494	0.465	0.498	0.497	0.618	0.612	0.138	0.460
	6	0.577	0.573	0.531	0.573	0.568	-	-	-	-
	7	0.609	0.604	0.557	0.599	0.595	-	-	-	-
	8	0.604	0.604	0.546	0.589	0.592	-	-	-	-
	9	0.556	0.556	0.493	0.527	0.541	-	-	-	-

Table 4. ANN models and their input factors.

Model Name	Input Combination	No. of Factors
ANN_0	YR_R1(t−1 . . . ,t−4), YR_R2(t−1 . . . ,t−4), YR_R3(t−1 . . . ,t−4), YR_R4(t−1 . . . ,t−4), YR_R5(t−1 . . . ,t−4), YR_Q1(t−1), YR_S1(t−1), YR_S2(t . . . , t−2), YR_S3(t−1)	26
ANN_1	YR_R1(t−1 . . . ,t−7), YR_R2(t−1 . . . ,t−7), YR_R3(t−1 . . . ,t−7), YR_R4(t−1 . . . ,t−7), YR_R5(t−1 . . . ,t−7), YR_Q1(t−1 . . . ,t−4), YR_S1(t−1 . . . ,t−3), YR_S2(t, t−1), YR_S3(t−1, t−2)	46
ANN_2	YR_R1(t−1 . . . ,t−7), YR_R2(t−1 . . . ,t−7), YR_R3(t−1 . . . ,t−7), YR_R4(t−1 . . . ,t−7), YR_R5(t−1 . . . ,t−7), YR_Q1(t−1 . . . ,t−4), YR_S1(t−1 . . . ,t−3), YR_S2(t, t−1), YR_S3(t−1, t−2)	46

4.2.2. Model Training and Testing

Random sampling was employed to split the input data from Section 4.1 into training and testing sets at an 80–20% ratio. For more details in terms of random sampling, a dataset included the input factors listed in Table 4. For example, there were 46 data needed in a dataset to train the model and produce water levels at t + 1, t + 2, and t + 3. Shown in Table 4, all data in the dataset were in a sequential order. The amount of dataset was depended on the data availability during the training process. For example, if a 24-h was available, there were 15 datasets available for training process. At each training, observed or synthetic water levels at t + 1, t + 2, t + 3 were used for performance evaluation. Two extra experiments were conducted. One involved using data from 2-, 5-, 10-, 25-, and 50-yr return periods for training and data from the maximum 100-yr return period for testing. Another involved using data from 5-, 10-, 25-, 50-, and 100-yr return periods for training and data from the minimum 2-yr return period for testing. The number of training data was fully prepared and the number of the data was constant, therefore, there was only one epoch done during this training process. The purpose of these experiments was to assess the ANN models and their forecasting capability beyond the training data range. The RMSE index (Equation (3)) was used to evaluate the model performance. The forecasting results with 1-, 2-, and 3-h lead times at location YR_R2 are shown in Table 5.

Table 5. RMSEs of different ANN models for the training and testing processes.

Model	Lead Time (Hours)	Cross-Validation RMSE (m)	Test for 100-yr Event RMSE (m)	Test for 2-yr Event RMSE (m)
ANN_0	1	0.3421	0.4532	0.5935
	2	0.4142	0.3192	0.5431
	3	0.7743	0.5878	0.6054
ANN_1	1	0.0553	0.1212	0.1065
	2	0.1085	0.1962	0.1129
	3	0.1655	0.2162	0.0987
ANN_2	1	0.1229	0.1204	0.1155
	2	0.0678	0.1029	0.1135
	3	0.0778	0.1253	0.1286

The results demonstrated that the worst performance among the three models for all three lead times was from the ANN_0 model; its RMSE results were 0.3421 m and 0.7743 m for 1- and 3-h lead times, respectively. The performance of the other two tests for all three models was comparable to that in the cross-validation test. This finding confirmed that the proposed ANN models have the capability to forecast data beyond the testing data range. In comparison, the ANN_1 and ANN_2 models yielded RMSEs that were all below 0.2 m. The ANN_2 model displayed better performance for the results with 2- and 3-h lead times than ANN_1. However, the performance of these two models deteriorated when the forecasting lead time was increased. According to the abovementioned results, the following tests were continuously implemented using the ANN_1 and ANN_2 models.

To test the performance of the proposed ANN models for operational purposes, three historical typhoon events, namely, Yutu (2018), Mangkhut (2018), and Maria (2018), were considered. Three typhoons were split into two typhoons for training and one typhoon for testing. The results are demonstrated in Table 6, and the naming convention is based on the names used in the test case. The performance of both models was fairly consistent. All RMSEs were below or close to 0.1 m regardless of the lead time. According to the individual results, the ANN_2 model performed slightly better than the ANN_1 model. A temporal comparison between observations and the simulations of both models is shown in Figure 9. The results demonstrated that both models agree fairly well with the observations for all three typhoons. It was interesting to find that performance did not deteriorate when the lead time was increased. In contrast, both models produced worse results with a 1-h lead time when the peak water level occurred during Typhoon Yutu in comparison with those results for 2- and 3-h lead times.

Table 6. Comparison of RMSEs for different ANN models and historical typhoon events.

Model	Lead Time (Hour)	Typhoon Yutu (2018) RMSE (m)	Typhoon Mangkhut (2018) RMSE (m)	Typhoon Maria (2018) RMSE (m)
ANN_1	1	0.0954	0.0751	0.0756
	2	0.0759	0.0729	0.0931
	3	0.1000	0.0611	0.1069
ANN_2	1	0.0977	0.0591	0.0742
	2	0.0508	0.0611	0.0893
	3	0.0530	0.0475	0.0912

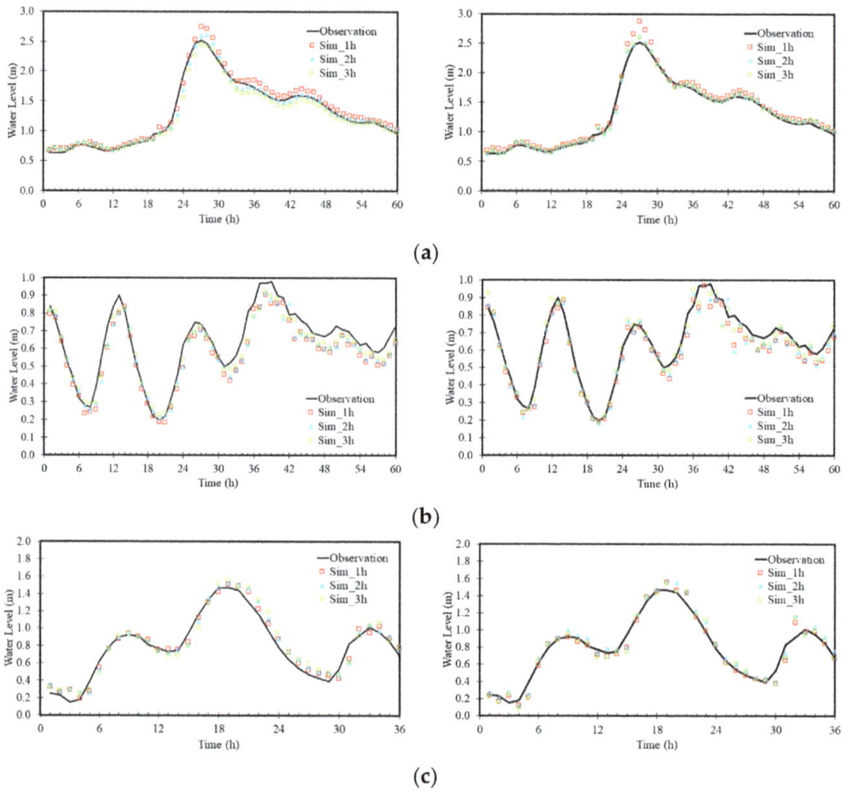

Figure 9. Comparison of simulated and observed water levels at YR_R2 for the ANN_1 model (**left**) and ANN_2 model (**right**) at Yutu (**a**), Mangkut (**b**), and Maria (**c**).

Additionally, the calculation times of the models were compared for different hardware configurations. The comparison was conducted with a hardware configuration that included an AMD Ryzen 94900 central processing unit, an NVIDIA GeForce RTX 2060 (PC) and an RPi 3B+ (the sensor mentioned in Section 3.1), among other components. Using Typhoon Yutu with the ANN_2 model as an example, the calculation time was 5 min if the model was run on the PC and 30 min if it was run on the sensor. The results for the PC and the sensor were consistent, but the calculation time when the model ran on the sensor was 6 times slower than when it ran on the PC. Therefore, calculation time is an issue that must be addressed in future investigations if the sensor is installed on site for real operation. In conclusion, all the results above confirmed the capability of the proposed ANN models to forecast water levels with up to a 3-h lead time. According to the comparison of model performance, the ANN_2 model can be continually applied for further applications and will be discussed in the next section.

4.3. Applications

The proposed ANN_2 model and integrated sensor were then applied to three other canals and rivers for real-world tests. The details of the geographic locations of these three study areas can be found in Figure 1. The same input factors as in Table 4 were selected, but the number of gages varied according to the number of gages installed in the study areas. For example, there is only one rainfall station near the Shimen Canal; therefore, the number of input factors decreased from 46 to 17. The list of the input factors for these three study areas is shown in Table 7. In addition to the RMSE shown in Equation (3), the coefficient of determination (R^2) described below was used to evaluate system performance in these real-world cases.

$$\begin{aligned} R^2 &= 1 - \frac{SS_{res}}{SS_{tot}} \\ SS_{res} &= \sum(P_i - O_i)^2 \\ SS_{tot} &= \sum(P_i - \overline{O})^2 \end{aligned} \tag{8}$$

where O_i and $\overline{O}$ are the hourly observations and mean of the observations, respectively, and P_i is the prediction. If the predictions exactly match the observations, $SS_{res} = 0$ and $R^2 = 1$. A detailed discussion for each case is given below. In the applications, the sensor was continually receiving data. If the sensor collected new data, the model was retraining with newly collected data. Therefore, a new epoch was completed. This process was repeated until the end of the experiment.

Table 7. ANN models and their input factors for various applications.

Model Name	Input Combination	No. of Factors
Shimen Canal model	SC_R1(t−1 . . . ,t−7), SC_Q1(t−1 . . . ,t−4), SC_S1(t−1 . . . ,t−3), SC_S2(t, t−1), SC_S3(t−1, t−2)	17
Toucian River model	TR_R1(t−1 . . . ,t−7), TR_R2(t−1 . . . ,t−7), TR_R3(t−1 . . . ,t−7), TR_R4(t−1 . . . ,t−7), TR_Q1(t−1 . . . ,t−4), TR_S1(t−1 . . . ,t−3), TR_S2(t, t−1), TR_S3(t−1, t−2)	39
Beinan River model	BR_R1(t−1 . . . ,t−7), BR_R2(t−1 . . . ,t−7), BR_R3(t−1 . . . ,t−7), BR_R4(t−1 . . . ,t−7), BR_Q1(t−1 . . . ,t−4), BR_S1(t−1 . . . ,t−3), BR_S2(t, t−1), BR_S3(t−1, t−2)	39

4.3.1. Shimen Canal

The distance between SC_R1 and SC_R3 is approximately 650 m and is shown in Figure 1. Three sensors were installed at SC_R1, SC_R2, and SC_R3. The experiment was performed on site during 24 June 2021, and 25 June 2021. There were a total of 200 observations collected by each sensor for an hour, and the average value was used for model input. Other data, such as discharge and precipitation data, were retrieved from local stations. The system started to produce water levels at SC_R2 with 1-, 2-, and 3-h lead times after the fifth hour of installation. The overall testing time was 35 h. The comparison between observations and simulations is shown in Figure 10. The errors, which were defined as the difference between observation and prediction, were within 0.075 m. The largest error of 0.075 m was found in Figure 10a with a 1-h lead time. One possible reason for the error was human interference. The canal is operated at a certain water level for the purpose of irrigation. This study did not include the factors of human operations, and the performance deteriorated once human inference was carried out. The RMSEs were between 0.02 and 0.03 m. According to the performance, the system was able to produce the variation in the water levels. However, because of manual operations such as gate control upstream of the canal, R^2 was only in the range of 0.3 to 0.45. The total computation time needed to train the proposed ANN_2 model in the sensor and produce water level forecasts using the observations was 8 min.

4.3.2. Toucian and Beinan Rivers

To avoid the impact of manual operations on system performance, the Toucian and Beinan Rivers were selected to test system performance. Unfortunately, the distance between the observed water surface and the installation of the sensor was beyond the range of the maximum measurement distance. Therefore, the following experiments were conducted by using the data retrieved from the Water Resources Agency directly. The evaluation period was from 3 June 2021, to 31 December 2021, for the Toucian River. Typhoon In-fa on July 24 and Typhoon Lupit on August 6 influenced this study area during this period. Figure 11 shows that the largest difference between observations and predictions at TR_S2 (see the location in Figure 1) was 1.3 m among all forecasts. This was the time when Typhoon In-fa had an impact on this area (solid circle in Figure 11). Similar to previous cases, the system started to produce forecasts the 5th hour after the experiment started. It was confirmed that having more data in the training process increased the accuracy of the ANN_2 model. The errors between observations and simulations were decreased to below 0.5 m for the second typhoon event (dashed circle in Figure 11) and thereafter. Finally, the overall R^2 and RMSEs were approximately 0.98 and 0.045 m, respectively.

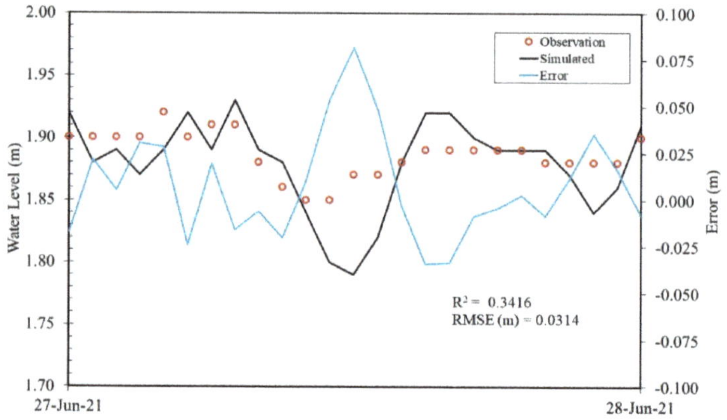

(a)

Figure 10. *Cont.*

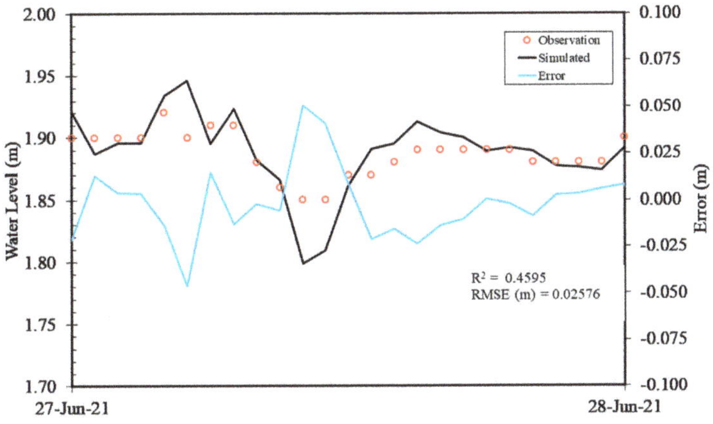

(**b**)

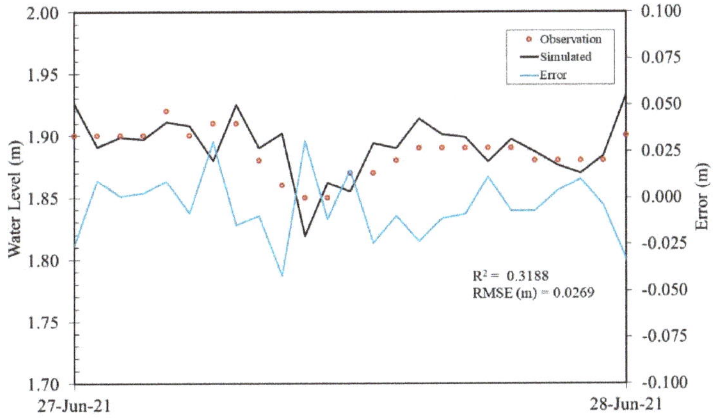

(**c**)

Figure 10. (**a–c**) Comparison of simulation and observed water levels at SC_S2 of Shimen canal for lead times t + 1 h, t + 2, and t + 3 h, respectively.

For the Beinan River, the evaluation period was from 1 July 2021, to 31 December 2021. Typhoon Lupit on August 6 and Typhoon Kompasu on October 14 influenced this study area during the period. Figure 12 shows that the greatest difference between the observations and predictions at BR_S2 (see the location in Figure 1) was below 1 m. The largest errors were found when the highest and lowest water levels were observed (solid and dashed circles in Figure 12), and extreme values such as these were not included in the training data. The overall R^2 and RMSEs were approximately 0.98 and 0.08 m, respectively. In conclusion, based on the above experiments, the proposed ANN_2 model and integrated sensor show excellent potential to perform edge computing locally and generate water level forecasts for real-time operation. The forecasting accuracy was influenced if the water levels were beyond the values in the training data set. Furthermore, the performance of the proposed system decreased if human interference occurred in the study area.

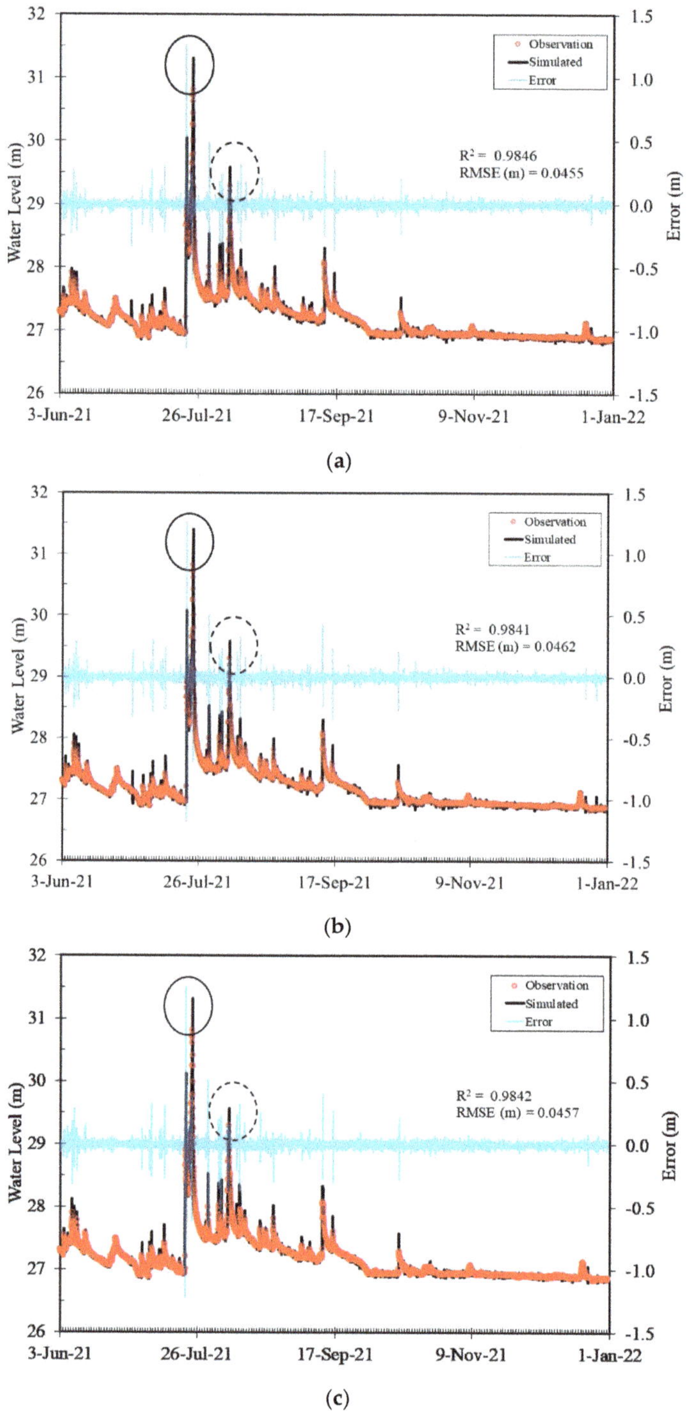

Figure 11. (**a**–**c**) Comparison of simulation and observed water levels at TR_S2 of the Touciaan River for lead times t + 1 h, t + 2, and t + 3 h, respectively.

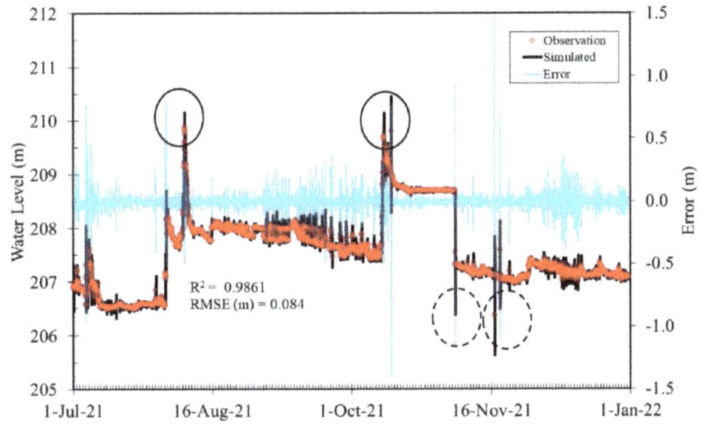

(**a**)

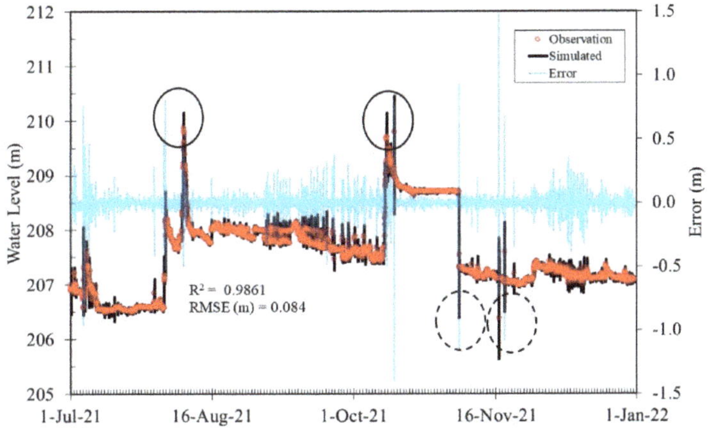

(**b**)

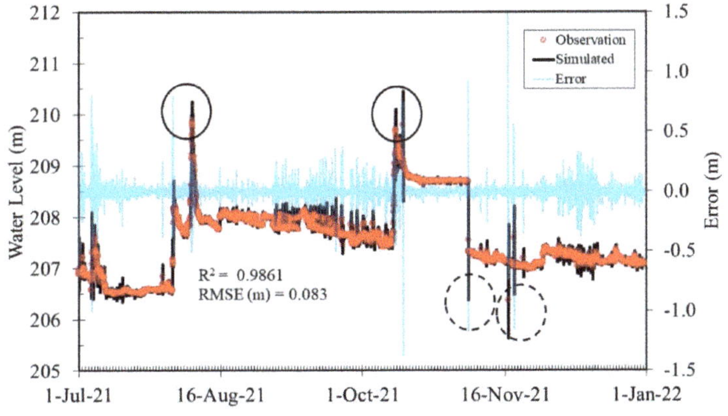

(**c**)

Figure 12. (**a**–**c**) Comparison of simulation and observed water levels at BR_S2 of the Beinan River for lead times t + 1 h, t + 2, and t + 3 h, respectively.

5. Conclusions

In this study, an ANN-based model was integrated into a Raspberry Pi-based sensor to implement edge computing for hourly river water level forecasting. The ANN model is capable of forecasting the river level with a high level of precision by only using previously observed water level, rainfall information, and flow discharge as inputs without the need for other hydrological and meteorological parameters. Edge computing is a form of computing that is conducted on site or near a targeted location, thus minimizing the need for data to be processed at a remote data center and increasing the efficiency of the emergency response. This study is a first attempt to combine real-time customized sensors and ANN algorithms in practice. Based on historical measured data from the Yilan River in Yilan County, synthetic upstream rainfall and discharge data were generated for six different return periods using the Pearson III probabilistic model and the HEC-HMS hydrological model with synthetic inflow data. The downstream water level data were obtained with the aid of the HEC-RAS hydraulic model. Different input combinations, including first-order difference and second-order difference water levels, were investigated to enhance the precision of the ANN model. The results demonstrated that the proposed ANN model has the capability to precisely forecast the future fluctuations in the water level of rivers in a short time and with a small number of inputs. The model was then embedded into the customized sensor to forecast the water level over different time horizons up to 3 h in advance. Finally, a comprehensive comparison between forecasts and observations was performed for three other rivers and canals. The findings revealed that the proposed water level sensor with the ANN model exhibited a high level of performance when it was applied to real events. Therefore, the integration proposed in this study is very promising and could be incorporated into a new generation of flood warning systems to prevent and mitigate the impacts of floods in downstream areas. However, the time required to train the ANN model and the system to produce results is over 30 min. Due to the limited computing power of the sensor, the amount of data required to train the model during real-time operation while maintaining high forecasting accuracy to speed up the computing process needs to be investigated further. In addition, different options of microcontroller units with more computing power will also be considered in future studies. Finally, in the current study, only an on-site experiment was performed because of the limitation of devices. More on-site experiments must be performed, and input factors of the ANN model regarding human interference should be included in future studies to extend the system application scope.

Author Contributions: C.-H.L. and T.-H.Y. developed the theoretical formalism, performed the analytic calculations and performed the numerical simulations. O.T.W. analyzed the data and produced figures and tables. C.-H.L., T.-H.Y. and O.T.W. contributed to the final version of the manuscript. All authors have read and agreed to the published version of the manuscript.

Funding: This study was supported by the National Science and Technology Council, Taiwan under Research Grant MOST 111-2625-M-A49-006.

Institutional Review Board Statement: Not applicable.

Informed Consent Statement: Informed consent was obtained from all subjects involved in the study.

Data Availability Statement: The experimental watershed data can be accessed in [23], and the data that support the findings of this study are available from the corresponding author, T.-H.Y., upon reasonable request.

Acknowledgments: The authors would like to thank the National Center for High-performance Computing (NCHC) for the experimental watershed data sets.

Conflicts of Interest: The authors declare no conflict of interest.

References

1. Centre for Research on the Epidemiology of Disasters (CRED). *2021 Disasters in Numbers*; CRED: Brussels, Belgium, 2021.
2. Okazawa, Y.; Yeh, P.J.-F.; Kanae, S.; Oki, T. Development of a global flood risk index based on natural and socio-economic factors. *Hydrol. Sci. J.* **2011**, *56*, 789–804. [CrossRef]
3. Yildirim, E.; Demir, I. An Integrated Flood Risk Assessment and Mitigation Framework: A Case Study for Middle Cedar River Basin, Iowa, US. *Int. J. Disaster Risk Reduct.* **2021**, *56*, 102113. [CrossRef]
4. United Nations Office for Disaster Risk Reduction. *Global Assessment Report on Global Disaster Risk Reduction GAR 2022-Our World at Risk: Transforming Governance for a Resilient Future*; United Nations Office for Disaster Risk Reduction: Geneva, Switzerland, 2022.
5. Kang, S.; David, D.S.K.; Yang, M.; Yu, Y.C.; Ham, S. Energy-Efficient Ultrasonic Water Level Detection System with Dual-Target Monitoring. *Sens. Basel* **2021**, *21*, 2241. [CrossRef] [PubMed]
6. Helmrich, A.M.; Ruddell, B.L.; Bessem, K.; Chester, M.V.; Chohan, N.; Doerry, E.; Eppinger, J.; Garcia, M.; Goodall, J.L.; Lowry, C.; et al. Opportunities for crowdsourcing in urban flood monitoring. *Environ. Model. Softw.* **2021**, *143*, 105124. [CrossRef]
7. Oo, Z.L.; Lai, T.W.; Moe, A. Real time water level monitoring for early warning system of flash floods using Internet of Things (IoT). In Proceedings of the 2019 Joint International Conference on Science, Technology and Innovation, Mandalay by IEEE, Mandalay, Myanmar, 16 September 2019; IEEE: New York, NY, USA, 2019.
8. Chari, K.S.; Thirupathi, M.; Hariveena, C. IoT-based Flood Monitoring and Alerting System using Raspberry Pi. *IOP Conf. Ser. Mater. Sci. Eng.* **2020**, *981*, 042078. [CrossRef]
9. Pandeya, B.; Uprety, M.; Paul, J.D.; Sharma, R.R.; Dugar, S.; Buytaert, W. Mitigating flood risk using low-cost sensors and citizen science: A proof-of-concept study from western Nepal. *J. Flood Risk Manag.* **2021**, *14*, e12675. [CrossRef]
10. Teixidó, P.; Gómez-Galán, J.A.; Gómez-Bravo, F.; Sánchez-Rodríguez, T.; Alcina, J.; Aponte, J. Low-Power Low-Cost Wireless Flood Sensor for Smart Home Systems. *Sensors* **2018**, *18*, 3817. [CrossRef] [PubMed]
11. Kadir, E.A.; Siswanto, A.; Rosa, S.L.; Syukur, A.; Irie, H.; Othman, M. Smart sensor node of WSNs for river water pollution monitoring system. In Proceedings of the 2019 International Conference on Advanced Communication Technologies and Networking (CommNet), Rabat, Morocco, 12–14 April 2019; pp. 1–5.
12. Aslanpour, M.S.; Toosi, A.N.; Cicconetti, C.; Javadi, B.; Sbarski, P.; Taibi, D.; Assuncao, M.; Gill, S.S.; Gaire, R.; Dustdar, S. Serverless edge computing: Vision and challenges. In Proceedings of the ACSW 21: 2021 Australasian Computer Science Week Multiconference, Dunedin, New Zealand, 1–5 February 2021; Association for Computing Machinery: New York, NY, USA, 2021; pp. 1–10.
13. Gokul, H.; Suresh, P.; Vignesh, B.H.; Kumaar, R.P.; Vijayaraghavan, V. Gait recovery system for parkinson's disease using machine learning on embedded platforms. In Proceedings of the 2020 IEEE International Systems Conference (SysCon), Montreal, QC, Canada, 24 August–20 September 2020; IEEE: New York, NY, USA, 2020; pp. 1–8.
14. Peruzzi, G.; Galli, A.; Pozzebon, A. A Novel Methodology to Remotely and Early Diagnose Sleep Bruxism by Leveraging on Audio Signals and Embedded Machine Learning. In Proceedings of the 2022 IEEE International Symposium on Measurements & Networking (M&N), Padua, Italy, 18–20 July 2022; IEEE: New York, NY, USA, 2022; pp. 1–6.
15. Xu, Y.; Nascimento, N.M.M.; de Sousa, P.H.F.; Nogueira, F.G.; Torrico, B.C.; Han, T.; Jia, C.; Rebouças Filho, P.P. Multi-sensor edge computing architecture for identification of failures short-circuits in wind turbine generators. *Appl. Soft Comput.* **2021**, *101*, 107053. [CrossRef]
16. Hao, S.; Hao, W.; Fu, J.; Jiang, F.; Zhang, Q. Landslide Monitoring and Early Warning System based on Edge Computing. *IOP Conf. Series Earth Environ. Sci.* **2021**, *861*, 042056. [CrossRef]
17. Hernández, D.; Cecilia, J.M.; Cano, J.-C.; Calafate, C.T. Flood Detection Using Real-Time Image Segmentation from Unmanned Aerial Vehicles on Edge-Computing Platform. *Remote Sens.* **2022**, *14*, 223. [CrossRef]
18. Esposito, M.; Palma, L.; Belli, A.; Sabbatini, L.; Pierleoni, P. Recent Advances in Internet of Things Solutions for Early Warning Systems: A Review. *Sensors* **2022**, *22*, 2124. [CrossRef] [PubMed]
19. Nevo, S.; Morin, E.; Gerzi Rosenthal, A.; Metzger, A.; Barshai, C.; Weitzner, D.; Voloshin, D.; Kratzert, F.; Elidan, G.; Dror, G.; et al. Flood forecasting with machine learning models in an operational framework. *Hydrol. Earth Syst. Sci.* **2022**, *26*, 4013–4032. [CrossRef]
20. Thrysøe, C.; Balstrøm, T.; Borup, M.; Löwe, R.; Jamali, B.; Arnbjerg-Nielsen, K. FloodStroem: A fast dynamic GIS-based urban flood and damage model. *J. Hydrol.* **2021**, *600*, 126521. [CrossRef]
21. Costabile, P.; Costanzo, C.; De Lorenzo, G.; Macchione, F. Is local flood hazard assessment in urban areas significantly influenced by the physical complexity of the hydrodynamic inundation model? *J. Hydrol.* **2020**, *580*, 124231. [CrossRef]
22. Zakaria, M.N.A.; Malek, M.A.; Zolkepli, M.; Ahmed, A.N. Application of artificial intelligence algorithms for hourly river level forecast: A case study of Muda River, Malaysia. *Alex. Eng. J.* **2021**, *60*, 4015–4028. [CrossRef]
23. Sit, M.; Demir, I. Decentralized flood forecasting using deep neural networks. *arXiv* **2019**, arXiv:1902.02308 2019.
24. Hussain, F.; Wu, R.-S.; Wang, J.-X. Comparative study of very short-term flood forecasting using physics-based numerical model and data-driven prediction model. *Nat. Hazards* **2021**, *107*, 249–284. [CrossRef]
25. Bande, S.; Shete, V.V. Smart flood disaster prediction system using IoT & neural networks. In Proceedings of the 2017 International Conference on Smart Technologies for Smart Nation (SmartTechCon), Bengaluru, India, 17–19 August 2017; IEEE: New York, NY, USA, 2017; pp. 189–194.

26. Abdullahi, S.I.; Habaebi, M.H.; Abd Malik, N. Intelligent flood disaster warning on the fly: IoT-based management platform using 2-class neural network to predict flood status. *Bull. Electr. Eng. Inform.* **2019**, *8*, 706–717. [CrossRef]
27. Alasali, F.; Tawalbeh, R.; Ghanem, Z.; Mohammad, F.; Alghazzawi, M. A Sustainable Early Warning System Using Rolling Forecasts Based on ANN and Golden Ratio Optimization Methods to Accurately Predict Real-Time Water Levels and Flash Flood. *Sensors* **2021**, *21*, 4598. [CrossRef]
28. Samikwa, E.; Voigt, T.; Eriksson, J. Flood Prediction Using IoT and Artificial Neural Networks with Edge Computing. In Proceedings of the 2020 International Conferences on Internet of Things (iThings) and IEEE Green Computing and Communications (GreenCom) and IEEE Cyber, Physical and Social Computing (CPSCom) and IEEE Smart Data (SmartData) and IEEE Congress on Cybermatics (Cybermatics), Rhodes, Greece, 2–6 November 2020; IEEE: New York, NY, USA, 2020; pp. 234–240.
29. Al Qundus, J.; Dabbour, K.; Gupta, S.; Meissonier, R.; Paschke, A. Wireless sensor network for AI-based flood disaster detection. *Ann. Oper. Res.* **2020**, 1–23. [CrossRef]
30. National Center for High-performance Computing (NCHC). Taiwan Experimental Watershed Platform. Available online: http://140.110.144.164/bg.php (accessed on 12 January 2022).
31. Prince, P.; Hill, A.; Covarrubias, E.P.; Doncaster, P.; Snaddon, J.L.; Rogers, A. Deploying Acoustic Detection Algorithms on Low-Cost, Open-Source Acoustic Sensors for Environmental Monitoring. *Sens. Basel* **2019**, *19*, 553. [CrossRef] [PubMed]
32. Acosta-Coll, M.; Ballester-Merelo, F.; Martinez-Peiró, M.; De la Hoz-Franco, E. Real-Time Early Warning System Design for Pluvial Flash Floods—A Review. *Sensors* **2018**, *18*, 2255. [CrossRef]
33. Septiana, Y. Design of prototype decision support system for flood detection based on ultrasonic sensor. In *MATEC Web of Conferences*; EDP Sciences: Les Ulis, France, 2018; Volume 197, p. 03017. [CrossRef]
34. Chen, L.-H.; Wang, T.-Y. Artificial neural networks to classify mean shifts from multivariate $\chi 2$ chart signals. *Comput. Ind. Eng.* **2004**, *47*, 195–205. [CrossRef]
35. Fletcher, D.; Goss, E. Forecasting with neural networks: An application using bankruptcy data. *Inf. Manag.* **1993**, *24*, 159–167. [CrossRef]
36. Huang, W.; Foo, S. Neural network modeling of salinity variation in Apalachicola River. *Water Res.* **2002**, *36*, 356–362. [CrossRef]
37. Rumelhart, D.E.; Hinton, G.E.; Williams, R.J. Learning representations by back-propagating errors. *Nature* **1986**, *323*, 533–536. [CrossRef]
38. Pedregosa, F.; Varoquaux, G.; Gramfort, G.; Michel, V.; Thirion, B.; Grisel, O.; Blondel, M.; Prettenhofer, P.; Weiss, R.; Dubourg, V.; et al. Scikit-learn: Machine learning in python. *J. Mach. Learn. Res.* **2011**, *12*, 2825–2830.
39. Babel, M.S.; Shinde, V.R. Identifying Prominent Explanatory Variables for Water Demand Prediction Using Artificial Neural Networks: A Case Study of Bangkok. *Water Resour. Manag.* **2010**, *25*, 1653–1676. [CrossRef]
40. Zhong, C.; Jiang, Z.; Chu, X.; Guo, T.; Wen, Q. Water level forecasting using a hybrid algorithm of artificial neural networks and local Kalman filtering. *Proc. Inst. Mech. Eng. Part M J. Eng. Marit. Environ.* **2017**, *233*, 174–185. [CrossRef]
41. Chow, V.T. A general formula for hydrologic frequency analysis. *Eos. Trans. Am. Geophys. Union* **1951**, *32*, 231–237. [CrossRef]
42. Chow, V.; Maidment, D.; Mays, L. *Applied Hydrology*; McGraw-Hill Book Company: New York, NY, USA, 1988.
43. USACE. *Hydrologic Modeling System HEC-HMS Technical Reference Manual CPD-74B*; Hydrologic Engineering Center: Davis, CA, USA, 2000.
44. USACE. *Hydrologic Modeling System HEC-HMS v35, User's Manual*; Army Corps of Engineers, Hydrologic Engineering Center (HEC): Davis, CA, USA, 2010.
45. USACE. *HEC-RAS River Analysis System Hydraulic Reference Manual v4.1*; US Army Corps of Engineers, Hydrologic Engineering Center (HEC): Davis, CA, USA, 2010.

sensors

MDPI

Systematic Review

E-Cardiac Care: A Comprehensive Systematic Literature Review

Umara Umar [1,*], Sanam Nayab [1], Rabia Irfan [1], Muazzam A. Khan [2] and Amna Umer [3]

[1] School of Electrical Engineering and Computer Science (SEECS), National University of Sciences and Technology (NUST), Islamabad 44800, Pakistan
[2] Department of Computer Sciences, Quaid i Azam University, Islamabad 45320, Pakistan
[3] Department of Computational Sciences, The University of Faisalabad (TUF), Faisalabad 38000, Pakistan
* Correspondence: uumar.msit19seecs@seecs.edu.pk

Abstract: The Internet of Things (IoT) is a complete ecosystem encompassing various communication technologies, sensors, hardware, and software. IoT cutting-edge technologies and Artificial Intelligence (AI) have enhanced the traditional healthcare system considerably. The conventional healthcare system faces many challenges, including avoidable long wait times, high costs, a conventional method of payment, unnecessary long travel to medical centers, and mandatory periodic doctor visits. A Smart healthcare system, Internet of Things (IoT), and AI are arguably the best-suited tailor-made solutions for all the flaws related to traditional healthcare systems. The primary goal of this study is to determine the impact of IoT, AI, various communication technologies, sensor networks, and disease detection/diagnosis in Cardiac healthcare through a systematic analysis of scholarly articles. Hence, a total of 104 fundamental studies are analyzed for the research questions purposefully defined for this systematic study. The review results show that deep learning emerges as a promising technology along with the combination of IoT in the domain of E-Cardiac care with enhanced accuracy and real-time clinical monitoring. This study also pins down the key benefits and significant challenges for E-Cardiology in the domains of IoT and AI. It further identifies the gaps and future research directions related to E-Cardiology, monitoring various Cardiac parameters, and diagnosis patterns.

Keywords: arrhythmia; artificial intelligence (AI); cardiac; communication technologies; Electrocardiogram (ECG); systematic literature review (SLR)

Citation: Umar, U.; Nayab, S.; Irfan, R.; Khan, M.A.; Umer, A. E-Cardiac Care: A Comprehensive Systematic Literature Review. *Sensors* **2022**, *22*, 8073. https://doi.org/10.3390/s22208073

Academic Editors: Andrei Velichko, Dmitry Korzun and Alexander Meigal

Received: 30 August 2022
Accepted: 4 October 2022
Published: 21 October 2022

1. Introduction

Following the available information as confirmed by the World Health Organization (WHO) [1], cardiovascular disease claims a large number of causalities across the globe [2] and is responsible for approximately 80% of sudden deaths. Moreover, in more than 15% of the deaths, cardiac arrhythmia is considered the chief reason. Thus, promoting cardiovascular health is vital and requires an overhaul of healthcare systems [3].

The rapidly expanding Internet of Things (IoT) [4] technology has the capability to monitor and control the critical human functions, irrespective of where the individual is located or what they are doing. Medical IoT (MIoT) is a cutting-edge technology that functions by exploiting the advantages of the Internet at a very affordable cost with minimum effort. The MIoT-based cardiac system guarantees monitoring the physical symptoms [5] of cardiac patients, such as temperature, Blood Pressure (BP), Oxygen Saturation (SPO2), Electrocardiogram (ECG), Heart Rate (HR) [6], and linked environmental parameters effectively and without any failure. The MIoT cardiac care framework is a customized paradigm that meets the requisite medical and safety standards of pervasive cardiac healthcare, including serious heart-related issues.

Various cardiac (heart) abnormalities can be detected through an Electrocardiogram (ECG) which is a medical testing platform that keeps track of electrical activity the heart generates as it contracts. An electrocardiograph is a device that records patient's ECG. An ECG is a valuable tool for identifying problems associated with heart rate or heart rhythm.

It offers assistance to the physician in determining whether a patient is having a heart attack or has had one in the past. An ECG is usually the first option for a cardiac test because of its proven dependability. An ECG is helpful to determine if one's pulse is difficult to feel (bradycardia), or it is too fast (tachycardia) to count accurately. An ECG can also show heart rhythm irregularities, i.e., arrhythmia. The main types of arrhythmia are mentioned in Table 1.

Table 1. Various Types of Arrhythmias.

Types of Arrhythmia	Explanation
Tachyarrhythmias	A fast heart rhythm with a rate of more than 100 beats per minute.
Bradyarrhythmias	Slow heart rhythms that may be caused by disease in the heart's conduction system.
Supraventricular arrhythmias	Arrhythmias that begin in the atria (the heart's upper chambers). "Supra" means above; "ventricular" refers to the lower chambers of the heart, or ventricles.
Ventricular arrhythmias	Arrhythmias that begin in the ventricles (the heart's lower chambers).

Similarly, atrial fibrillation, atrial flutter, and premature or extra beats are the other types of cardiac issues. Figure 1 shows waveforms for different arrhythmia types. Atrial fibrillation refers to a rapid, disorganized, and irregular heart rhythm., while atrial flutter is an atrial arrhythmia generated by a fast circuit in the atrium. Compared to atrial fibrillation, atrial flutter is typically more organized and regular.

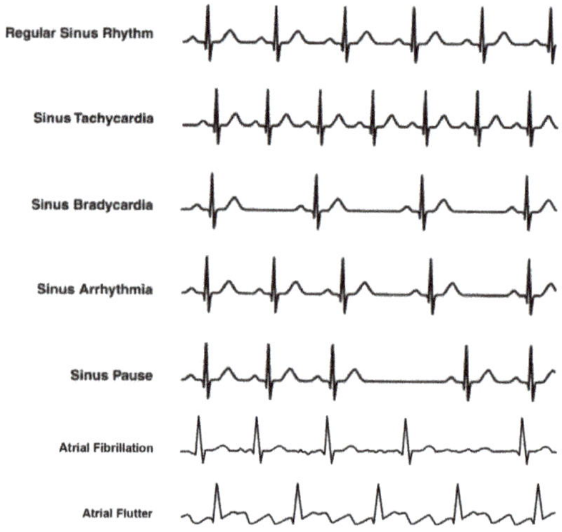

Figure 1. Types of arrhythmia.

A comprehensive review of E-Cardiology, which encompasses the Internet of Things, artificial intelligence, and cardiology could help understand the essential building blocks of an IoT-based cardiac care system and intelligent diagnosis of various cardiovascular diseases. It can also help to develop a complete picture of various hardware devices (sensors), AI techniques, and communication technologies adopted by the existing studies in the field of intelligent cardiac healthcare.

Following the introduction, Section 2 of this paper briefly discusses related works; Section 3 highlights the contributions made by this paper. Section 4 elaborates on the review methodology adopted for conducting the survey. Section 5 gives the outcomes of the selected studies with a detailed analysis of the research questions (RQs). This section is further divided into four subsections. Section 6 contains a discussion. Section 7 summarises the conclusions.

2. Related Works

This section presents a brief explanation of the related surveys in the field of IoT-based cardiac healthcare.

The primary goal of the study [7] was to collect the latest facts, figures, and evidence on the use of preprocessing techniques for heart disease classification. The review study also summarised the impact of the most frequently used preprocessing tasks and techniques and the performance in the field of cardiology. This review paper covered the literature from 2000 to June 2019.

A survey on IoT and AI in healthcare was presented by [8] for 2007 to February 2018. The paper highlighted the top application classifications, which included wearables, sensor networks, connectivity options, and disease detection and treatment. This review identified gaps and provided future research directions related to technology and design. However, this survey analysed only three online databases.

A review article on data mining techniques frequently used in the field of cardiology until 2015 was presented in [9]. The performance comparison of various data mining models in cardiology were also discussed in this review paper.

The authors in [10] presented a survey on the Internet of Things (IoT) for healthcare using mobile computing. This systematic study investigated how mobile computing assisted IoT in a healthcare environment. Moreover, the intention of this paper was to analyse the impact of mobile computing on IoT technology in Smart hospitals and the field of healthcare. This study covered the literature between 2011 and 2019.

Another study [11] proposed a substantial review of various IoT applications in a life-saving environment, as well as various other fields in Smart cities. It also contrasted IoT with M2M and highlighted some drawbacks of IoT technology. This review article covered 2013 to 2018 through the Scopus database.

Another study [12] presented literature on (IoT) technologies and several projects for healthcare in 2018. This paper provided a review of primary medical IoT sensors and an overview of state-of-the-art IoT infrastructure essential for healthcare. It focused on the latest IoT technologies for healthcare services, such as cloud computing, big data, RFID, WSN, Bluetooth, Wi-Fi, and other vital medical sensors. However, this study lacks a systematic review.

The study [13] highlighted various IoT applications and was presented in 2022. The study focused on IoT adoption in Pakistan and France in 2020. This systematic study highlighted the barriers and possibilities for the implementation of IoT applications. It also indicated the influence of COVID-19 on IoT adoption in the healthcare domain.

The [14] systematic review discussed telemedicine and healthcare IoT (HIoT). It covered 146 articles between 2015 and 2020. The articles were divided into five categories after a technical analysis. In addition to the benefits and limitations of the selected methods, a comprehensive comparison of evaluation techniques, tools, and metrics was also included. This study presented a summary of healthcare applications of IoT (HIoT).

The discussion so far is limited to only a particular aspect of Smart healthcare/E-Cardiology and does not genuinely attempt to cover the domain holistically. When we say "entire domain", it means AI-based IoT, which encompasses preprocessing techniques and also various communication technologies. According to the deficiencies of the existing review papers, we provide a comprehensive systematic literature review for the following reasons:

- The latest research articles need to be covered to assess the current state of the art.
- The present studies do not cover all the aspects of E-Cardiology.

The following section highlights the contributions made by this review study, thus bringing novelty to this systematic review study.

3. Contributions

1. This review paper highlights the influence of IoT, communication technologies, AI models, and preprocessing techniques in cardiac healthcare using our review protocol. Moreover, this study covers the complete and latest infrastructure for E-Cardiology, including its benefits and challenges. Thus, this systematic review covers almost all aspects of E-Cardiology which have not been discussed before in such a comprehensive way under one umbrella.
2. The study presents the systematic analysis of the most recent studies (2016 to 2021) to investigate our formulated research questions.
3. This paper incorporates monitoring of vital CCU parameters, ECG analysis, and classification of various heart disorders, thus giving a thorough picture of E-Cardiology.
4. This review study provides recommendations and future guidelines for researchers and cardiologists as well.

The next section discusses the research methodology adopted for our SLR.

4. Review Methodology

A systematic literature review (SLR) paradigm is followed in this paper for reviewing papers from the most reliable resources, as shown in Figure 2. Principally, the research work, applications, and monitoring/detection techniques provided by AI-aided MIoT in cardiac care are considered. The primary studies have been then passed through a quality assessment process for the study analysis to produce the best fit results.

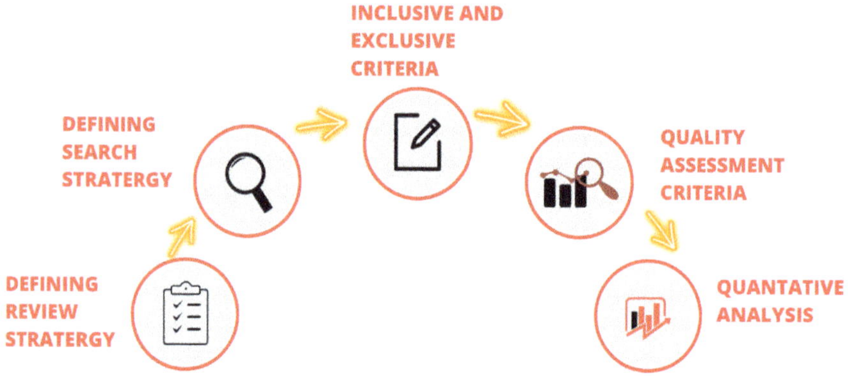
INCLUSIVE AND
EXCLUSIVE
CRITERIA
DEFINING
SEARCH
STRATERGY
QUALITY
ASSESSMENT
CRITERIA
DEFINING
REVIEW
STRATERGY
QUANTATIVE
ANALYSIS

Figure 2. SLR protocol outline.

The following subsections briefly describe the detail of each step involved in our review protocol.

4.1. *Defining Review Strategy*

The application of medical IoT in cardiac care is a compelling field of study for the researchers, so the primary focus of this SLR was to formulate the research questions exploring how medical IoT is affecting cardiac care and the significance of artificial intelligence in the diagnosis and detection of various heart diseases.

The review questions in Table 2 indicate how MIoT and AI are contributing to cardiac healthcare systems in Smart hospitals.

Table 2. Review questions and their motivation.

No.	Review Question	Motivation
RQ 1	What are the vital hardware components/sensors used in E-Cardiac architecture for different CCU parameters?	The main focus of this question is to identify different types of sensors and their features most often used in IoT-based Cardiac Healthcare.
RQ 2	What are the most important communication technologies used in E-Cardiac Care?	The question aims to find the most commonly used communication technologies in MIoT-based Cardiology.
RQ 3	Which pre-processing techniques are used in E-Cardiology along with the most widely used AI classifiers/models?	This question is designed to explore the current work in the field of medical IoT accompanied by artificial intelligence in cardiac healthcare and to identify various classification and preprocessing techniques used for predicting cardiovascular diseases.
RQ 4	What are the significant issues and challenges in the current E-Cardiology?	This question investigates major benefits, and current challenges of IoT-based cardiac healthcare system.

4.2. Defining Search Strategy

Once the research questions were designed, the next step was to indicate and state the search strategy to be followed precisely. Therefore, the primary literature mentioned in Appendix A (Table A1) was identified using three search strings which were used in the five digital databases, namely IEEE Xplore, ACM Digital Library, SpringerLink, ScienceDirect, and Google Scholar. These are the most popular online data resources in the domain of computer science and information technology. Second, these digital libraries were used as sources for previous systematic literature reviews related to computer science and E-Cardiology [15].

Our search span included the period of 2016 to 2021. The criteria used for the selection of search terms or keywords is mentioned below [16]:

- The important terms were extracted from the research questions.
- Synonyms and alternate spellings were identified for the key terms.
- Keywords were identified from various books and relevant research articles.
- For synonyms or alternating spellings, the Boolean operator OR was used.
- Boolean AND operator was used to interlink significant terms.

After the critical analysis of the key terms, three search strings were formed in order to extract the relevant information. These search strings were checked on each of the aforementioned databases by changing their patterns to retrieve the best relevant results. The three search strings are given in Table 3.

Table 3. Search strings used for data retrieval.

No.	Search String
1	(internet of things OR IoT OR IoT-based OR smart health) AND (cardiac OR heart OR CCU) AND (monitoring OR detection OR diagnosis OR disease OR parameters)
2	(intelligent OR artificial intelligence OR AI OR machine learning OR deep learning OR preprocessing OR reduction OR cleaning OR data mining) AND (cardiac OR heart OR ECG OR arrhythmia OR cardiovascular OR smart health OR healthcare OR smart healthcare OR cardiology) AND (technique OR methods OR classification OR algorithm)
3	(internet of things OR IoT OR IoT-based) AND (cardiac OR heart OR CCU OR smart health OR smart healthcare) AND (benefits OR advantages OR challenges OR issues OR disadvantages)

4.3. Inclusion and Exclusion Criteria

To identify and include studies relevant to answer the RQs, inclusion and exclusion criteria were developed as described in the section "Defining Review Strategy". To find the most appropriate publications, we defined the inclusion and exclusion criteria as mentioned in Table 4.

Table 4. Inclusion and exclusion criteria.

Inclusion Criteria	Exclusion Criteria
The papers published in English were chosen on priority.	The papers published in other languages were not selected.
The most recently published research papers, i.e., 2016 to 2021, were singled out for studies.	Gray literature was excluded from the study list.
Papers describing an overview of current approaches that implement modern tools and techniques in E-Cardiology were selected.	Papers not defining the topic appropriately were excluded.
The main aim was to target the primary studies such as original research papers.	Duplicated material was removed.

The authors evaluated each forthcoming paper to decide whether it should be included or excluded. The selection of papers was accomplished by following the three steps mentioned below.

The first step included the removal of duplicated and redundant papers; perusing the keywords, abstracts, and titles of research articles was the next step. Reading of full length research papers was carried out in the last step. Accordingly, the inclusion and exclusion criteria were implemented to their full effect. The articles that attracted difference of opinion were discussed and reviewed again by the authors, either using the full text or the partial text, until a consensus was achieved on an agreed-upon draft.

4.4. Quality Assessment Criteria

In this step, based upon the coherence and relevancy, we analyzed all the collected studies to address the defined research questions. A deep analysis of each paper was made, and based on our research questions, 134 papers were selected. Out of those 134 research papers, the papers having considerable citation count, appearing in good impact factor journals, and being delivered at highly ranked conferences were finally selected, thus leaving a total of 104 papers for the review, shown in Appendix A (Table A1).

4.5. Quantitative Analysis

The last step of our review protocol design was conducted to execute necessary statistical analysis on quantitative data. In this step, we quantitatively summarised and analyzed the results extracted from various sources such as conferences, journals, and book sections. Then, we carried out some quantitative statistical analysis of the findings to explore more about our research questions (RQs) and trends.

Figure 3 gives a thorough overview of our screening and assessment method for the statistical analysis of our literature. Five databases were chosen for the review, as illustrated in this figure. A total of 502 documents were chosen for review and analysis. The majority of papers were discovered to be duplicates. Thus, 203 records were eliminated before screening. Papers were removed for a few different reasons. Articles were chosen in the screening process based on a planned inclusion and exclusion strategy. Following the screening, 104 papers were chosen based on inclusion and exclusion standards.

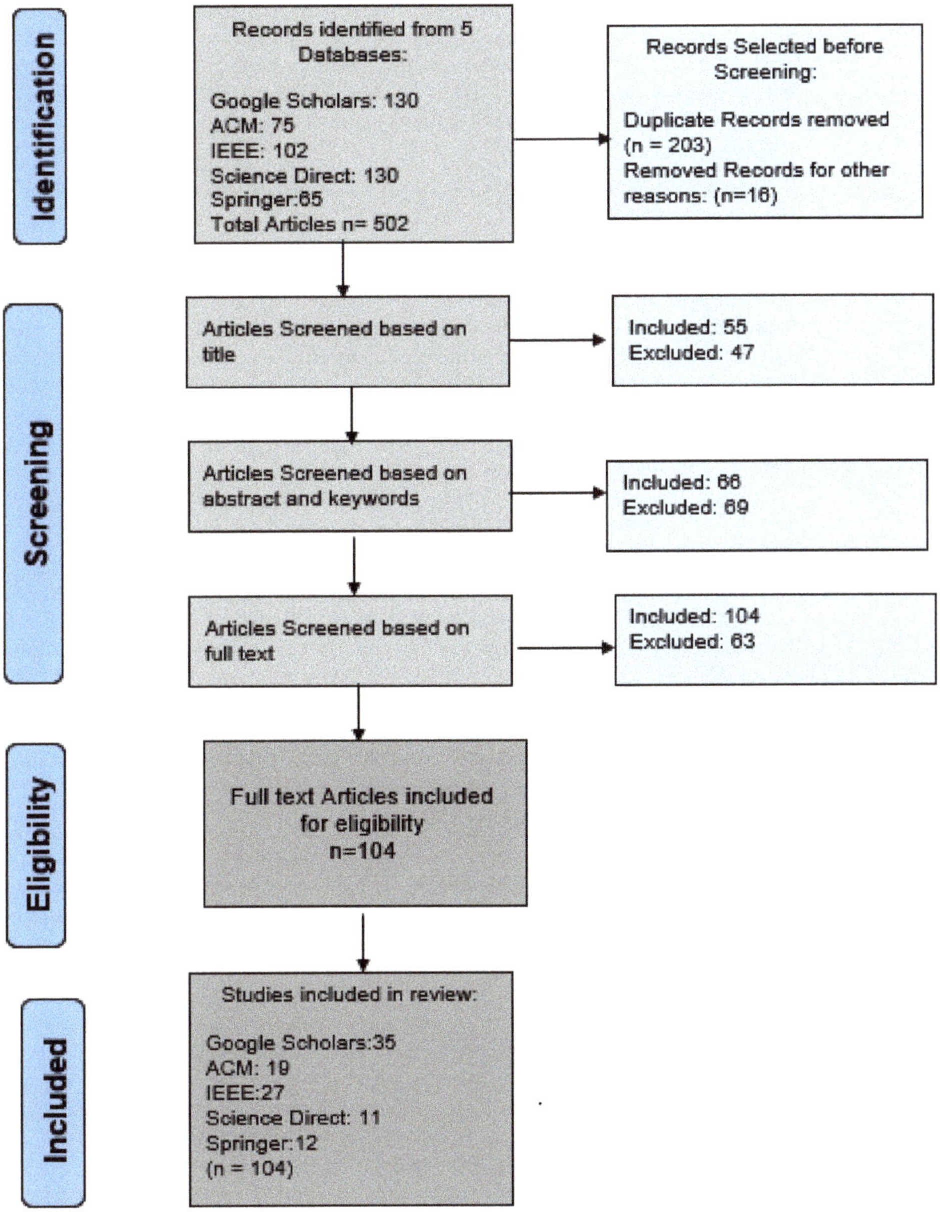

Figure 3. Flow diagram showing the screening process for the systematic review.

The next section highlights the "Outcomes" of this systematic review.

5. Outcomes

5.1. RQ 1: What Are the Vital Hardware Components/Sensors Used in E-Cardiac Architecture for Different CCU Parameters?

The cardiac healthcare monitoring system in an IoT sphere encompasses the various IoT sensory modules and technologies attached to the patient, receiving sensory data, and sending data to the cloud for further monitoring, processing, and decision making. In an IoT-based cardiac healthcare monitoring system, the sensors, such as heart rate/pulse sensor, temperature sensor, blood pressure sensor, blood oxygen sensor, and ECG sensor, obtain sensory parametric values from the patient, transmit data through specific communication technologies to the cloud, apply machine learning practices to the learned parametric values, and generate alerts to the specialist suggesting timely action when warranted.

(i) Heart Rate Sensory Unit

Heart rate monitoring plays a crucial role in patient cardiac abnormalities diagnosis, detection, and classification. Several cardiac ailments and disorders occur due to a patient's high or low heart rate. Normal beats per minute (bpm) are 60–100. Less than 60 bpm is considered to be low and greater than 100 is considered to be high bpm. We discovered comprehensive studies that used several types of heart beat sensors for bpm monitoring. The studies [17,18] used heart beat pulse sensors to measure patient heart rates in a real-time environment. In this article [19], the KY 093 module was used to obtain heart rate values. Using a MAX30100 pulse oximeter, the authors in [20] collected heart beat information. The publications [21–23] utlized an ECG module AD8232 to obtain the patients heart rate data in real time for monitoring purposes. Table 5 mentions recent studies on heart rate sensors. Each heart rate sensor has its own set of properties. This table shows some important characteristics of several heart beat sensor variants such as pins, type, operating voltage, low current supply, accuracy, and so on.

(ii) Temperature Sensory Unit

Body temperature is an essential parameter for the development of cardiac healthcare monitoring. Various analog and digital temperature sensors are available for determining body temperature. Temperature can be measured in celsius or fahrenheit. Temperatures above 37.5 or 38.3 celsius are considered high. The temperature sensor LM35 is referenced in [24–27] for health monitoring. The authors in [18,28] used an 18DS20 sensor for temperature monitoring in a real-time environment. Table 6 shows several of the temperature sensors, along with descriptions. The LM35 and 18DS20 sensors are the most widely employed temperature sensors in the research studies that we analysed.

(iii) Blood Pressure (BP) Sensory Unit

BP monitoring is a fundamental biological measure for the detection and diagnosis of cardiac incongruities and anomalies. BP values can be obtained using various sensory units and devices. Systolic and diastolic values are captured by BP sensors or devices to be examined by a physician. Normal BP is less than 120/80 mmHg, while low BP, called "hypotension", is below 90/60 mmHg, and high BP, called "hypertension", is above 140/90 mmHg. Our research discovered a publication on E-Cardiology that dealt with cardiac patients' BP. In 2017 [29], a digital BP monitor (OMRONHBP1300) was used to monitor and automatically detect cardiac arrhythmia. The paper published in 2019 [30] examined predicting cardiac ailments in E-Cardiology using ECG, cholesterol, and BP. The MPX10 BP sensor was utilised in the 2020 publication [27] for patient health monitoring. Table 7 shows lists of sensors and devices utilized in the past few years for BP monitoring of cardiac patients, along with their comparable attributes.

The multiple modules of BP sensors and devices used in past studies, as well as different sensors of other cardiac parameters, are shown in Table 7.

Table 5. Features of heart rate sensors/devices.

Heart Rate/ Pulse Rate Sensors	Features							
	Major Pins	INT	Type	Operating Voltage	BPM	Low Supply Current	Electrodes Configuration	Acc
Pulse Sensor [31]	GND, Vcc, Signal	N	IR LED (Analog)	3.3 V to 5.0 V	Y	N/A	N	N/A

Table 5. *Cont.*

Heart Rate/ Pulse Rate Sensors	Features							
	Major Pins	INT	Type	Operating Voltage	BPM	Low Supply Current	Electrodes Configuration	Acc
AD8232 [32]	GND, 3.3 V, Output, LO+, LO−, SDN	Y	IR LED (Analog)	3.6 V	Y	170 µA (typical)	Y	N/A
KY-039 [33]	GND, Vcc, Signal	N	IR LED (Analog)	5 V	Y	N/A	N	N/A
Holter Device [34]	3/5/12 Electrodes	Y	Digital Device	N/A	Y	N/A	Y	N/A
SpO2 Sensor device [35]	Fingertip Sensor	Y	IR LED (Analog)	N/A	Y	N/A	N	±2% for SPO2, ±2 bpm for Pulse Rate
MAX30100 Pulse Oximeter and Heart Sensor [36]	VIN, SCL, SDA, INTERRUPT, IRD, RD, GND	Y	Int IR LED, Photo Sensor	1.8 V and 3.3 V	Y	170 µA, (typical)	N	98.84% for SPO2, 97.11% for Heart Rate

Acc—accuracy; BPM—beats per minute; GND—ground; INT—integrated IR; LED—infrared light-emitting diode; IRD—IR LED to driver; LO—leads off; N/A—not applicable; N—no; RD—red LED to driver; SCL—serial clock; SDA—serial data; SDN—shutdown control input; V—voltage; VCC—voltage common collector; VIN—voltage input; Y—yes.

(iv) Oxygen Sensory Unit

Blood oxygen can be monitored using several IoT-based blood oxygen sensory units, such as pulse oximetry sensors, to obtain oxygen saturation levels along with a patient's heart rate. Ready-made wearable devices are also available to measure blood oxygen saturation levels. Blood oxygen is measured in percentage. The normal blood oxygen saturation is 90 to 100%. The study [37] describes a pervasive healthcare monitoring service system that uses an SpO2 device to measure oxygen saturation. The MAX30100 pulse oximeter has proven to be useful in measuring blood oxygen levels in cardiac patients [20]. Our findings and the literature on IoT-based cardiovascular healthcare monitoring used the sensors mentioned in Table 8 to measure oxygen saturation. This table lists several important and common features of oxygen saturation sensors and devices, such as addressed parameters, voltage, type, accuracy, pins, range, and so on. Table 8 shows that blood oxygen sensors/devices are used for cardiac patients in very few studies.

(v) ECG Unit

ECG is the most crucial biological parameter for monitoring, detecting, predicting, and classifying cardiac irregularities and variations in the human heart. The ECG AD8232 module was used in the studies [21,22,38–40] to monitor ECG and detect cardiac anomalies in cardiovascular patients. Heart abnormalities were detected with the use of the ECG AD8233 module [41]. In Table 9, recent papers published on multiple ECG sensors and devices are mentioned along with their necessary and comparable features. Low supply current, electrodes, the sampling rate, right leg drive shut down, single supply operation, high pass filter, output, operating temperature, pins, and other features of various ECG modules are considered as the most notable attributes.

Table 10 shows detailed and comprehensive literature analysed to find IoT-based cardiovascular sensors and devices used in previous studies from 2016 to 2021. This table demonstrates that the majority of research on ECG has been conducted using the ECG AD8232 module to detect anomalies in cardiac patients.

Table 6. Features of temperature sensors/devices.

Temperature Sensor	Features						
	Type	°C/°F or Both	Acc	Operating Voltage Range	Alarm Signaling	Major Pins	Measurement Range
LM35 [42]	Analog	°C	0.5 °C Acc guaranteeable at +25 °C	4 V to 30 V	N	VCC, VOUT, GND	Range is −55° to +150 °C
DS18B20 [43]	Digital	Both	±0.5 °C Acc from −10 °C to +85 °C	3.0 V to 5.5 V	Y	GND, DQ, VDD, NC	Range is 55 °C to +125 °C and 67 °F to +257 °F
MCP9700 [44]	Analog	°C	±4 °C (max.), 0 °C to +70 °C	2.3 V to 5.5 V	N	Vout, Vcc, GND, NC	Range is −40 °C to +125 °C
TMP100 [45]	Digital	°C	±1 °C (Typical) from −55 °C to 125 °C and ±2 °C (Max) from −55 °C to 125 °C	2.7 V to 5.5 V	Y	ADD0, ADD1, ALERT, GND, SCL, SDA, V+	Range is −55 and +125 °C

Acc—accuracy; ADD—address select; °C/°F —centigrade/fahrenheit; DQ—data in/out; GND—ground; N—no; NC—no connection; SDA—serial data; SDN—shutdown control; V—voltage; VCC—voltage common collector; VDD—power supply voltage; VOUT—output; Voltage Y—yes.

Table 7. Features of blood pressure sensors/devices.

BP Sensors	Features									
	Freq	Range	Major Pins	Pressure Hysteresis	Lin	Supply Voltage	Full Scale Span	RT	Offset Stability	Acc
MPX10 Series Pressure Sensor [46]	N/A	0–10 kPa	GND, Vs, +Vout, −Vout	±0.1 typical	Min −1.0, Max 1.0	3.0–6.0 Vs	Min 20 mV, Max 50 mV	1.0 ms	±0.5% VFSS	N/A
Omron HBP-1300 digital Device [47,48]	50/60 Hz	0 to 300 mmHg	Start/Stop, Mode, Last Reading (buttons)	N/A	N/A	100–240 V AC	N/A	N/A	N/A	Within ±3 mmHg
Typical BP Monitor Sensor [49]	N/A	0 to 258 mmHg	Tube, Pressure Cuff, Pressure Control Valve, Bulb	typical ±0.25%	typical ±0.25%	N/A	N/A	1.0 ms	N/A	±1 mmHg

Acc—accuracy; BP—blood pressure IR; kPa—kiloPascal's; LED—infrared light-emitting diode; mmHg—millimeters of mercury; ms—millisecond; N/A—not applicable; RT—response time; V—voltage; Vout—voltage output; Vs—power supply.

Table 8. Features of oxygen sensors/devices.

Oxygen Sensors (Oximeter)	Features								
	INT	**Addressed Parameters**	**Power Supply Voltage**	**Type**	**Acc SpO2**	**Acc PR**	**Major Pins**	**SpO2 Range**	**PR Range**
MAX30100 [36]	Y	HR, SpO2	1.8 V to 3.3 V	IR LED	99.62%	97.55%	VIN, SCL, SDA, interrupt, IRD, RD, GND	N/A	N/A
SpO2 Sensor Device [50]	Y	HR, SpO2	D.C. 3.4 V ~D.C.4.3 V	IR LED	±2% (80–100%); ±3% (70–79%)	±2% bpm	N/A	35 to 100%	25 to 250 bpm

Acc—accuracy; GND—ground; INT—integrated; IRD—IR led to driver; HR—heart rate; N/A—not applicable; PR—pulse rate; RD—red LED to driver; SDA—serial data; SDN—shutdown control; V—voltage; VIN—voltage input; Y—yes.

Table 9. Features of ECG sensor/devices.

ECG Sensors/Devices	Features										
	INT	**Single/Multi Lead**	**Low Supply Current**	**Elec**	**SR**	**Right Leg Drive Shut Down**	**Single Supply OPER**	**HPF**	**Out**	**OPER TEMP**	**Major Pins**
AD8232 [32]	Y	Single Lead	170 µA (typical)	2 or 3	360 HZ	N	2.0 V to 3.5 V	2 Poles	Rail to Rail	40 °C to +85 °C	GND, 3.3 V, OUT, LO−, LO+, ~SDN, RA, LA, RL
Holter Device [34]	Y	Multi Lead	N/A	3, 5 or 12	125 HZ	N/A	one AAA battery	N/A	ECG Signal Rec on Monitor	+10 °C to +40 °C	Multiple Leads
ADAS1000 [51]	Y	Multi Lead	N/A	5 or 6	800 HZ	N/A	3.15 V to 5.5 V	N/A	Monitor	−40 °C to +85 °C	64 lead LQFP [52], 56 lead LFCSP (Both has diff. pins)
AD8233 [53]	Y	Single Lead	50 A typical	2 or 3	N/A	Y	1.7 V to 3.5 V	2 Poles Adjustable HPF	Rail to Rail	−40 °C to +85 °C	20 pins (GND, VS+, REFIN, HP-SENSE, HP-DRIVE, SDN, AC/DC, FR, etc.
Shimmer 3 [54–57]	Y	Multi Lead	T60 µA Maximum	4	24 MHZ	N/A	450 mAh battery	N/A	On Windows PC and SQL	N/A	5 ECG pins, 5 EMG pins

AC/DC—alternating current/direct current; EMG—electromyography; FR—fast restore; GND—ground; HPF—high pass filter; HPSENSE—high pass sense; HPDRIVE—high-pass driver; HZ—hertz; INT—integrated; LA—left arm; LO—leads off; MHZ—megahertz; NA—not applicable; N—no; OPER TEMP—operation temperature; PC—personal computer; RA—right arm; REFIN—reference buffer input; RL—right leg; SDN—shutdown control input; SQL—structure query language sampling rate; V—voltage; Vs—power supply terminal; Y—yes.

Table 10. Sensors used in previous studies.

Year	Sensors Used						
	ECG Module	**Temp Sensor**	**BP Sensor**	**Pulse/ HB Sensor**	**Oxygen Sensor**	**Other Sensor /Device**	**Integrated Sensor**
2016 [17]	✗	MCP9700	✗	Pulse Sensor	✗	✗	✗
2016 [58]	✗	✗	✗	✗	✗	PCG Sensor	✗
2016 [59]	✗	✗	✗	✗	✗	✗	Wrist band for HB & BP (DNNS)
2016 [19]	✗	✗	✗	FingerTip-Optical Sensor for PPG	✗	✗	✗
2016 [60]	✗	✗	✗	✗	✗	Wearable Watch (PPG sensor)	✗
2016 [61]	Galilio Board plateform for ECG (UB-MMNS)	✗	✗	✗	✗	✗	✗
2017 [37]	Holter Devices		(UB-MNNS)	Holter Device, SpO2 Device (UB-MNNS)	SpO2 Sensor Device (DNNS)	✗	
2017 [62]	✗	✗	✗	Pulse Sensor	✗	✗	✗
2017 [19]	✗	18DS20	✗	KY-093	✗	✗	✗
2017 [29]	✗	✗	OMRONH--BP1300	PPG Sensor		External Defibillator	✗
2017 [63]	(UB-MNNS)	(UB-MNNS)	(UB–MNNS)	HB Sensor	✗	Alchol Sensor, EMG (MNNS)	✗
2017 [64]	Wearable SOC ECG (MNNS)	✗	✗	✗	✗	✗	✗
2018 [65]	✗	✗	✗	✗	✗	✗	MAX30100 (SpO2, HB)
2018 [66]	✗	✗	✗	Pulse Sensor	✗	✗	✗
2018 [18]	✗	✗	✗	Pulse Sensor	✗	✗	✗
2018 [38]	ECG Module AD8232	✗	✗	Pulse Sensor	✗	✗	✗
2018 [20]	ECG Module AD8232	✗	✗	MAX30100	MAX30100	✗	✗
2018 [24]	✗	LM35	(UB–MNNS)	HB Sensor	✗	✗	✗
2018 [67]	✗	✗	✗	✗	✗	✗	WWSN for ECG, BP, Respiratory
2019 [28]	✗	18DS20	✗	HB sensor	✗	✗	✗
2019 [25]	Pulse Sensor	LM35	✗	Pulse Sensor	✗	✗	✗
2019 [26]	✗	LM35	✗	Pulse Sensor	✗	✗	✗
2019 [40]	ECG Module AD8232	✗	✗	✗	✗	✗	✗

Table 10. Cont.

Year	Sensors Used						
	ECG Module	Temp Sensor	BP Sensor	Pulse/ HB Sensor	Oxygen Sensor	Other Sensor /Device	Integrated Sensor
2019 [21]	ECG Module AD8232	✗	✗	ECG Module AD8232	✗	✗	✗
2019 [68]	✗	✗	✗	✗	✗	Bio Sensors of hospital	✗
2019 [69]	✗	✗	✗	✗	✗	✗	Watch for HB, CL, bp, (DNNS)
2019 [30]	ECG AD8232 Module	✗	BP Cuff (UB-MNNS)	Heart Rate Monitor	✗	Near Infrared Sensor for CL	✗
2019 [70]	ECG AD8232 Module	✗	✗	✗	✗	✗	✗
2019 [71]	(UB-MNNS)	✗	✗	✗	✗	✗	✗
2020 [72]	(UB-MNNS)	✗	✗	✗	✗	✗	✗
2020 [73]	✗	(UB-MNNS)	(UB-MNNS)	Pulse Sensor	✗	✗	✗
2020 [74]	✗	✗	✗	HB sensor	✗	Alchohal Sensor (MNNS)	✗
2020 [75]	✗	✗	✗	✗	✗	✗	MD, AC, ENV Sensors (MNNS)
2020 [27]	ECG Module AD8232	LM35	MPX10	Pulse Sensor	Pulse Sensor	✗	✗
2020 [76]	3 Lead VCG signals (MNNS)	✗	✗	✗	✗	✗	✗
2020 [22]	ECG Module AD8232	✗	✗	ECG Module AD8232	✗	✗	✗
2020 [77]	ADAS1000	TMP100	✗	✗	✗	✗	✗
2020 [78]	Multiple ECG devices (MNNS)	✗	✗	✗	✗	✗	✗
2020 [79]	Shimmer3 ECG Unit	✗	✗	✗	✗	✗	✗
2020 [23]	ECG Module AD8232	✗	✗	ECG Module AD8232	✗	✗	✗
2021 [80]	✗	✗	(UB-MNNS)	(UB-MNNS)	✗	Glucose Sensor (MNNS)	✗
2021 [81]	Wearabale Smart ECG device (UB-DNNS)	✗	✗	✗	✗	✗	✗

Table 10. *Cont.*

Year	Sensors Used						
	ECG Module	Temp Sensor	BP Sensor	Pulse/ HB Sensor	Oxygen Sensor	Other Sensor /Device	Integrated Sensor
2021 [83]	Ready made ECG Device (UB-DNNS)	✗	✗	✗	✗	AllCheck Device	✗
2021 [82]	Self Made Device for ECG (NNS)	✗	✗	✗	✗	✗	✗
2021 [84]	Multiscale ECG from 3 Sensors (UB-MNNS)	✗	✗	Wearable HB Sensor (MNNS)	Respiratory Sensor (MNNS)	Optical Sensor (MNNS)	✗
2021 [41]	ECG Module AD8283	✗	✗	✗	✗	✗	✗

BP/bp—blood pressure; CL—cholesterol; DNNS—device name not specified; ECG—electrocardiogram; HB—heartbeat; HR—heart rate; INT—integrated; MNNS—module number not specified; PCG—phonocardiograph; PR—pulse rate; PPG—photoplethysmography; UB-DNNS—used but device name not specified UB-MNNS—used but module number not specified; ✗—The specified parameter is not addressed.

5.2. *RQ 2: What Are the Most Important Communication Technologies Used in E-Cardiac Care?*

Communication technologies and protocols can be defined as a set of rules, technologies, semantics, equipment, and programs used to transfer, process, communicate, and receive information. Communication technologies and protocols vary depending upon the technology and network type devised, developed, or utilized. Some of the protocols and communication technologies are discussed in this section. The publications mentioned in Table 11 address the communication technologies and protocols used in previous selected studies for the development of E-Cardiology, monitoring, detection, and classification. BL is a wireless technology for short-range communication and exchanging data between mobile and fixed devices. BL has a transmission power of 1 mw–100 mw and a 1 Mbps data rate. Its data transmission range is 30 feet. The wearable healthcare monitoring devices (wearable fitness watches and pulse oximeters) may have the BL features integrated. BL technology was also employed in previous research [19,39,41,58,66,73] for data transmission for E-Cardiology. In prior literature on E-Cardiology monitoring, BL technology was determined to be the most commonly used technology. Ethernet is a wired communication networking protocol that can be used in local area networks (LANs), metropolitan area networks (MANs), and wide area networks (WANs). Ethernet allows communication through data cables. The publications [58,83] used an Ethernet-wired technology for connectivity support between various hardware modules implemented for cardiovascular disease diagnosis. One existing research study found that Ethernet-wired communication is rarely used in E-Cardiology. GSM is a cell-based or mobile communication modem that works as a mobile communication system. GSM technology is also used in E-Cardiology to send SMS messages or dial calls. GPS, which helps people to find their position on Earth, consists of networks of satellites and receivers or devices that determine location.

The communication technologies and protocols used in E-Cardiology in previous research studies and findings are detailed in Table 11.

Table 11. Communication technologies used in previous studies.

Year	Communication Technologies Used														
	BT	ETH	GSM	GPS	GPRS	MQTT	SMS	SMPP	ZB	WIFI	TCP/IP	Sc. P	Cloud	SP/PC	Internet
2016 [17]	N	N	Y	Y	Y	N	Y	Y	N	Y	N	N	Y	Y	N
2016 [58]	Y	Y	N	N	N	N	N	N	N	Y	Y	Y	Y	Y	N
2016 [59]	Y	N	N	N	N	N	Y	N	N	Y	N	Y	Y	N	N
2016 [85]	N	N	N	N	N	N	Y	N	N	N	N	N	N	Y	N
2016 [60]	N	N	N	N	N	N	N	N	N	N	N	N	N	Y	N
2016 [61]	N	N	N	N	N	N	N	N	N	Y	N	N	N	Y	N
2017 [37]	Y	N	Y	N	Y	N	N	N	N	Y	N	N	N	Y	Y
2017 [62]	N	N	N	N	N	N	N	N	N	N	N	N	N	N	N
2017 [19]	Y	N	Y	N	N	N	Y	N	N	Y	Y	N	Y	Y	N
2017 [29]	N	N	Y	N	Y	N	N	N	N	Y	N	N	Y	Y	N
2017 [63]	N	N	N	N	N	N	N	N	N	Y	Y	N	Y	Y	N
2017 [64]	N	N	N	N	N	N	N	N	N	Y	N	Y	Y	Y	N
2017 [39]	Y	N	N	Y	N	N	N	N	N	Y	N	N	N	Y	N
2018 [65]	N	N	Y	Y	Y	N	Y	N	N	Y	N	N	Y	Y	N
2018 [66]	Y	N	N	N	N	N	Y	N	N	Y	N	Y	Y	Y	N
2018 [18]	N	N	N	N	N	N	N	N	N	Y	N	N	Y	Y	N
2018 [38]	N	N	Y	N	N	N	Y	N	N	Y	Y	N	Y	Y	N
2018 [20]	N	N	N	N	N	N	N	N	N	Y	Y	N	Y	Y	N
2018 [24]	N	N	N	N	N	N	N	N	N	Y	Y	N	N	N	N
2018 [67]	Y	N	Y	Y	Y	N	N	N	N	Y	N	N	N	Y	N
2019 [28]	N	N	N	N	N	N	Y	N	N	N	N	N	N	Y	N
2019 [25]	Y	N	N	N	N	N	N	N	N	N	N	N	N	Y	N
2019 [26]	N	N	N	N	N	N	N	N	N	Y	Y	Y	Y	N	N
2019 [40]	N	N	N	N	N	N	N	N	N	Y	N	Y	Y	Y	N
2019 [21]	Y	N	N	Y	N	N	N	N	N	N	N	N	N	Y	N
2019 [68]	N	N	N	N	N	N	N	N	N	Y	N	Y	Y	Y	N
2019 [69]	Y	N	N	N	N	N	N	N	N	Y	N	N	Y	Y	N
2019 [30]	Y	N	N	N	N	N	N	N	N	Y	N	Y	Y	Y	N
2019 [70]	N	N	N	N	N	N	Y	N	N	N	N	N	N	Y	N
2019 [71]	Y	N	N	N	N	N	N	N	N	N	N	N	Y	Y	N
2020 [72]	N	N	N	N	N	N	N	N	N	Y	N	N	N	N	N
2020 [86]	N	N	N	N	N	N	N	N	N	Y	N	N	N	Y	N
2020 [73]	Y	N	Y	Y	Y	N	N	N	N	Y	N	N	Y	Y	N
2020 [74]	N	N	Y	N	Y	N	Y	N	Y	N	N	N	N	N	N
2020 [75]	Y	N	N	N	N	N	N	N	N	Y	Y	Y	Y	Y	N
2020 [27]	N	N	N	N	N	N	N	N	Y	Y	N	N	N	Y	N
2020 [76]	N	N	N	N	N	N	N	N	N	N	N	N	N	N	N

Table 11. *Cont.*

Year	Communication Technologies Used														
	BT	ETH	GSM	GPS	GPRS	MQTT	SMS	SMPP	ZB	WIFI	TCP/IP	Sc. P	Cloud	SP/PC	Internet
2020 [22]	N	N	N	N	N	Y	N	N	N	Y	N	N	Y	Y	N
2020 [77]	Y	N	Y	N	Y	N	Y	N	N	Y	Y	Y	Y	Y	N
2020 [78]	N	N	N	N	N	N	N	N	N	Y	N	N	Y	Y	N
2020 [79]	N	N	N	N	N	N	N	N	N	Y	N	N	Y	Y	N
2020 [23]	Y	N	N	N	N	N	N	N	N	Y	Y	Y	Y	Y	N
2021 [80]	Y	N	N	N	N	N	N	N	N	Y	N	Y	Y	Y	N
2021 [81]	N	N	N	Y	N	N	N	N	N	N	N	N	N	N	N
2021 [82]	Y	N	N	N	N	N	N	N	N	N	Y	N	Y	Y	N
2021 [83]	N	Y	N	N	N	Y	N	N	N	Y	Y	Y	Y	Y	N
2021 [84]	N	N	N	Y	N	N	N	N	N	Y	N	N	N	N	N
2021 [41]	Y	N	N	N	N	N	N	N	N	Y	N	N	Y	Y	N

BT—Bluetooth; GSM—global system for mobile communications; GPS—global positioning system; GPRS—general packet radio service; MQTT—message queuing telemetry transport; N—No; Sc.P—security protocols; SMS—short message service; SMPP—short message peer-to-peer; SP/PC—Smart phone/personal computer; TCP/IP—transmission control protocol/Internet protocol; WIFI—wireless fidelity; Y—yes.

5.3. RQ 3: Which Pre-Processing Techniques Are Used in E-Cardiology, along with the Most Widely Used AI Classifiers/Models?

RQ 3 is divided into two subsections. The first subsection investigates and compares various AI Models for the classification and prediction of CVD. This part explores various studies that use different machine learning and deep learning models for CVD prediction. Our study also provides a comprehensive explanation about the algorithms and methodologies used for prediction and classification techniques and the different datasets and performance metrics that we used to evaluate the models. Furthermore, the data preprocessing techniques used with different classifiers are also indicated in the second subsection below.

5.3.1. AI Classifiers/Models and E-Cardiology

The prediction of CVD is a much discussed topic of research in the realm of healthcare. AI-based prediction systems can be of great help in detecting disease at an earlier stage which can reduce risk associated with disease progression. The concept of AI is not new in cardiac electrophysiology with automated ECG interpretation. It has existed in some form or other since the 1970s [87].

Artificial Intelligence (AI) is the reflection of human cognitive functions from the surroundings acquired by applying algorithms, pattern matching, cognitive computing, and deep learning to achieve specific objectives [88]. The ongoing progress in AI, primarily in the sub-domains of machine learning (ML) and deep learning (DL), have caught the attention of physicians hoping to develop newly integrated, dependable, and potent methods for ensuring standard healthcare in the critical field of cardiology.

Machine learning (ML) is a subset of AI to "teach" computers to analyze huge datasets in a quick, accurate, and efficient manner by using complex computing and statistical algorithms [89]. Supervised ML is more successful in predicting survival compared to the traditional clinical risk scores [90].

The study [91] proved that the accuracy of disease prediction can be increased by using an unsupervised type of ML for obstructive coronary artery disease in nuclear cardiology.

Deep learning (DL) is a supervised ML methodology that relies on neural networks and is known for the automated algorithms required to extract meaningful patterns from data collections [92]. In the medical context, the most widespread deep learning algorithms are artificial neural networks (ANN), multilayer perceptron (MLP), convolution neural networks (CNN/ConvNet), recurrent neural networks (RNN), radial basis function network (RBFN), deep belief networks, and deep neural networks (DNN) [88]. Compared with traditional supervised ML, the real strength of DL is that it is an effective, powerful, and flexible approach to representing complicated raw input data that does not demand manual feature engineering. For instance, while addressing the issue of automated ECG interpretation, early conventional supervised ML techniques depended on human-defined ECG features. In contrast, the modern DL model extracts patterns within raw ECGs to detect sinus rhythm and various other arrhythmias with a performance that equals the result of any cardiologist [93].

The significant areas of cardiac healthcare that can benefit from ML/DL techniques are prognosis, diagnosis, classification, treatment, and clinical workflow. Table 12 presents an overview of different AI algorithms extracted from the literature review on heart disease diagnosis/classification.

Table 12. Overview of common ai techniques used in E-Cardiology.

No.	AI Algorithm	Description	Strengths	Limitations
1	Principal Component Analysis (Unsupervised)	A method of dimensionality reduction which aims to compute principal components and makes data more compressible.	1. Compute principal components 2. Avoids data overfitting 3. High variance, improved visualization 4. Reduce Complexity	1. Low interpretability of principal components. 2. Dimensionality reduction may result in information loss.
2	K-Means Clustering (Unsupervised)	Generates k number of centroids that help to define clusters of data.	1. Ensures convergence 2. Can warm-start the positions of centroids 3. Easily adjusts to new examples 4. Assists the doctors in making more accurate diagnosis	1. Not suitable for data varying in size and density 2. Noise sensitive
3	Decision Tree (Supervised)	For classifying examples, a decision tree is an easy and simple representation.	1. Easy to interpret 2. Avoids over-fitting by pruning 3. Less sensitive to outliers 4. Requires less data cleaning	1. Instability 2. Relatively inaccurate
4	K-Nearest Neighbor (Supervised)	Saves all available cases and allocates new cases based on a similarity measure.	1. Easy to implement & understand 2. Used for both classification & regression problems	1. Significantly slow as the data size increase 2. Computationally expensive 3. Requires high memory
5	Naïve Bayes (Supervised)	An easy probabilistic classifiers based on Bayes' theorem.	1. Scalable 2. Fast 3. Used for real-time predictions 4. Not requires large amounts of data	1. Assumes attributes are mutually independent 2. Zero Frequency limitation
6	Random Forest (Supervised)	A set of decision trees, usually trained with the "bagging" technique. It performs classification as well as regression tasks.	1. Used for prediction 2. Resistant to noise and overfitting 3. Flexible, can handle large datasets easily	1. Can take up lots of memory 2. Not that interpretable
7	Support Vector Machine (Supervised)	Indicates hyperplane which separates classes, based on a similarity measure, can be used as a linear or nonlinear kernel.	1. Fast 2. Relatively memory efficient 3. Works well with clear margin of separation between classes	1. Difficult to interpret 2. Not suitable for large datasets 3. May need normalization & scaling
8	Logistic Regression (Supervised)	The logistic paradigm can be used to model the probability of a certain class or event happening.	1. Easy to implement and interpret 2. Efficient to train	1. Performs poorly with large no. of variables 2. Used to predict only discrete functions 3. Not capture interactions automatically
9	Backpropagation (Supervised)	Backpropagation is a widely used algorithm for training feedforward neural networks. It is a reliable tool for increasing the accuracy of predictions.	1. Fast 2. Simple 3. Easy to analyze 4. Flexible	1. Sensitive to noisy/complex data 2. Performance of backpropagation depends on input data
10	Deep Learning (ANN) (Supervised)	Multilayered processing technique that mimics human neuronal structure. Different types of ANN are CNN or ConvNet , MLP, RBFN, RNN, etc.	1. No feature engineering 2. Learn complex functions 3. Enhanced Accuracy 4. Scalabale Model	1. Requires extremely large datasets 2. Intensive computational power 3. Difficult to interpret 4. Significant processing time

A comparative analysis of different AI techniques frequently used in Smart cardiology for the prognosis/diagnosis of various CVDs is given in Table 13.

As suggested by WHO, by 2030 almost 23.6 million individuals will die from heart-related causes [94]. CVDs are the main cause, but they can be cured and prevented. To reduce the risk involved, analysis is fundamental. The difficult part is accurate diagnosis [95].

Table 14 summarises the most recent work performed in the field of artificial intelligence related to CVDs.

Table 13. Comparative analysis of various AI techniques used for prognosis/diagnosis of CVDs.

No.	AI Techniques Used in Smart Cardiology	Performance Metrics									
		Cl. Acc	Sensitivity	Specificity	Flexibility	Efficiency	Com. CPLX	Interpretability	Large Dataset Handling	Training Time	Noise Tolerance
1	DT	L	Y	Y	Y	Y	L	H	N	S	N
2	RF	H	-	-	Y	-	L	L	Y	F	N
3	NB	L	Y	-	Y	Y	L	H	Y	F	Y
4	PCA-KNN	H	Y	Y	-	-	-	L	-	F	N
5	SVM	H	Y	Y	Y	Y	H	L	N	S	N
6	LR	L	-	-	Y	Y	L	H	Y	F	N
7	BP	H	Y	Y	Y	-	-	H	Y	-	N
8	DL (ANN)	H	Y	Y	Y	Y	H	L	Y	S	Y

PCA-KNN—principal component analysis with K-nearest neighbor; NB—naïve Bayes; RF—random forest; SVM—support vector machine; LR—logistic regression; DL—deep learning; ANN—artificial neural networks; BP—backpropagation; Y—yes; S—slow; F—fast; L—low; H—high; N—no.

Table 14. Summary of AI-methodologies and data preprocessing techniques identified for E-Cardiology, from different studies.

Ref #	Year	Findings								
		AI Methodology	Prognosis/ Diagnosis Task	Types of CVDs	Cardiac Parameter/s	Cardiac Dataset	Preprocessing Task	Data Preprocessing Techniques	Accuracy %	Complexity
[94]	2016	DT	Coronary Heart Disease	N/A	N/A	UCI	N/A	N/A	86.7	M
[96]	2016	BBNN	Arrhythmia	5	ECG	MIT-BIH	Feature Extraction	Hermit Basis Function	97	H
[97]	2016	NN	Arrhythmia	5	ECG	MIT-BIH	Denoising Feature Extraction	DWT DWT + PCA DWT + ICA	98.91	H
[98]	2016	PSO tuned SVM	Arrhythmia	12	ECG	MIT-BIH	Feature Extraction	DOST	99.18	H
[99]	2016	NN	Arrhythmia	5	ECG	MITBIH	Feature Extraction	DOM	95	M
[100]	2016	RF	Arrhythmia	5	ECG	MIT-BIH	Feature Extraction	WPE	94.61	M
[61]	2016	SVM	Arrhythmia	2	ECG	CT	Feature Extraction	DWT	98.9	M
[101]	2016	Paired-CNN	Coronary Artery Calcification	N/A	CCTA	CT	Feature Extraction	ConvNet	Sens. = 71	H
[102]	2017	DL	Arrhythmia	N/A	ECG	MIT-BIH	Feature Extraction	AlexNet (DNN)	92	H
[103]	2017	SVM	Arrhythmia	4	ECG	MIT-BIH	Denoising Feature Extraction	Multiresolution DWT	98.39	M
[104]	2017	RBF-NN	Arrhythmia	6	ECG	MIT-BIH	Denoising Feature Extraction	DWT EMD Features	99.89	H
[102]	2017	DL	Arrhythmia	3	ECG	MIT-BIH	Feature Extraction	Transferred Deep Learning	92	H
[105]	2018	SVM	Arrhythmia	3	ECG	CUDB VFDB	Feature Extraction	FFT	95.9	M
[106]	2018	SVM	Arrhythmia	5	ECG	MIT-BIH	Denoising Normalization Feature Extraction	Daubechies wavelets min-max Normalization PCANet	97.77	M
[107]	2018	Twin LS-SVM	Arrhythmia	16	ECG	MIT-BIH	Feature Extraction	Composite Dictionary (DOST + DST + DCT)	99.21	H
[108]	2018	MPNN	Arrhythmia	3	ECG	MIT-BIH	Denoising Feature Extraction	Daubechies wavelet Multiresolution DWT MPNN	99.07	H
[109]	2018	DL	Arrhythmia	5	ECG	MIT-BIH	Normalization Feature Extraction	Z-score normalization CNN and LSTM	98.10	H
[110]	2018	DL	Arrhythmia	2	ECG	MIT-BIH	Feature Extraction	DNN	99.68	M
[111]	2018	DBN	Arrhythmia	5	ECG	MIT-BIH	N/A	N/A	95.57	H
[91]	2018	DNN	Arrhythmia	N/A	CCTA	CT	Feature Extraction	DNN	Sens. = 82.3	H
[71]	2019	CNN	Arrhythmia	4	ECG	CT MIT-BIH	Feature Extraction	CNN	94.96 95.73	M
[112]	2019	MPNN-BP	Heart Disease	5	ECG	UCI	N/A	N/A	97.5	H
[93]	2019	DNN	Arrhythmia	12	ECG	CT	Denoising Feature Extraction	DNN	ROC = 97 F1 = 83.7	H
[68]	2019	Hybrid Model	Heart Disease	8	ECG, HR, BP	CT	Data Cleaning Denoising Feature Selection	Numerical Cleaner Filter SFS	98	H

Table 14. *Cont.*

Ref #	Year	Findings								
		AI Methodology	Prognosis/ Diagnosis Task	Types of CVDs	Cardiac Parameter/s	Cardiac Dataset	Preprocessing Task	Data Preprocessing Techniques	Accuracy %	Complexity
[113]	2020	CNN-KCL	Myocarditis	N/A	ECG	ZAS	Outlier Anomaly K-means clustering	K-means clustering CNN	92.3	H
[114]	2020	CNN	Myocardial Infarction	N/A	ECG	PTB	Data Augmentation Segmentation Feature Extraction	CNN	99.02	H
[115]	2020	DNN	Arrhythmia	6	ECG	TNMG	N/A	N/A	F1 = 80 Spec. = 99	H
[72]	2020	TWSVM	Arrhythmia	16	ECG	CT MIT-BIH	Feature Extraction	DWT	95.68	H
[78]	2020	DHCAF MCHCNN	Arrhythmia	5	ECG, HR	CT MIT-BIH	Denoising Feature Extraction	Daubechies wavelet-4 HWT	91.4 93	H
[116]	2021	E-D CNN-SVM	Myocardial Infarction	N/A	ECHO	HMC-QU	Featuring Engineering	CNN	80.24	H
[117]	2021	RF, NB	Coronary Heart Disease	N/A	N/A	OR	N/A	N/A	83.85 (RF) 82.35 (NB)	M
[118]	2021	AI	Cardiac Amyloidosis	N/A	ECG	MC	Feature Extraction	DNN	90	N/A
[119]	2021	CNN	Heart Failure	N/A	N/A	CT	Feature Selection	LASSO Regression	97	H

H—high; M—medium; N/A—not available; DL—deep learning; MPNN-BP—multilayer perceptron neural network-backpropagation; RF—random forest; WPE—wavelet packet entropy; CNN—convolutional neural network; CL—K means clustering; ZAS—Z alizadeh; PTB—physikalisch technische bundesanstalt; NB—naive Bayes; FFT—fast fourier transform; DNN—deep neural network; SVM—support vector machine; NN—neural networks; BBNN—block-based neural network; MC—Mayo Clinic; HWT—haar wavelet transform; EMD—empirical mode decomposition; RBNN—radial basis function neural network; OCAD—obstructive coronary artery disease; DBN—deep belief networks; ROC—receiver operating characteristic curve; DHCAF—dynamic heartbeat classification; SFS—sequential forward transform; DOST—discrete orthogonal stockwell transform; DOM—difference operation method; CCTA—cardiac CT angiography; PSO—particle swarm optimization; CUDB—Creighton University database; VFDB—ventricular fibrillation database; LS—SVM-least square SVM; OR—online repository; DBN—deep belief networks; ROC—receiver operating characteristic curve; DWT—discrete wavelet transform; DHCAF—dynamic heartbeat classification with adjusted features; MCHCNN—multi-channel heartbeat convolutional neural network.

5.3.2. Data Preprocessing Techniques in E-Cardiology

This section identifies and evaluates studies that applied data preprocessing techniques in cardiac disease classification. Data Preprocessing (DP) in AI is a critical stage that enhances the quality of data to achieve meaningful insights and is the initial step in the development of an AI model. Conventionally, real-world data is not in an appropriate format and contains errors or outliers. It usually lacks specific attribute values/trends, thus resulting in an inadequate AI model. Data preprocessing solves this problem by cleaning and organizing raw data to tailor it to the needs of building and training AI models. Hence, data preprocessing in AI is a data mining approach that reshapes raw data into a readable format that is readily available for an AI model to meet the high standards of performance [120]. Consequently, the algorithm can easily interpret the data's features.There are four primary ways of data preprocessing, i.e., (1) data cleaning, (2) data integration and formatting, (3) data transformation, and (4) data reduction.

Different preporocessing techniques used in past studies for diagnosing heart disease and other types of arrhythmia are also mentioned in Table 14, along with AI models. This table also lists the task performed by the preprocessing technique.

5.4. RQ 4: What Are the Major Issues and Challenges in Current E-Cardiology?

After conducting comprehensive research, we identified some significant benefits and major challenges in the field of MIoT to answer our RQ 4. These challenges and benefits have been emphasized on the basis of studies conducted by different researchers in the domain of MIoT and E-Cardiology. Based upon selection and rejection criteria, only valid and reliable papers were selected, as mentioned earlier. We incorporated only the latest benefits and challenges that were found to be unique in the domain of IoT and AI regarding healthcare and cardiology. A pictorial representation of these benefits and challenges is shown in Figure 4.

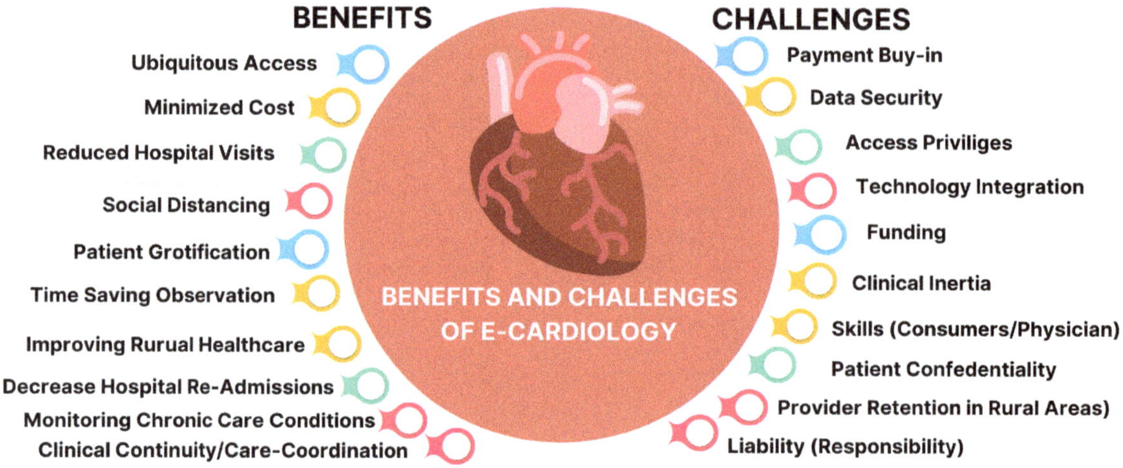

Figure 4. Benefits and challenges of E-Cardiology.

5.4.1. Benefits of E-Cardiology

Internet of Things (IoT) develops a linkage between "things", such as devices, gadgets, vehicles, and sensors. Likewise, the medical Internet of Things (MIoT)-based cardiovascular healthcare system monitors the physical symptoms [5] of cardiac patients at a very reasonable cost. These physical symptoms include temperature, blood pressure (BP), SPO2, and heartbeat, along with ECG [6] and associated numerical measurements. Significant benefits of IoT-based cardiology from various studies are noted in Table 15.

Table 15. Key issues and major benefits of IoT-based cardiology.

Ref #	Year	Findings		
		Key Challenges and Barriers of E-Cardiology with IoT	Data Related Issues	Benefits of IoT-Based E-Cardiology
[121]	2016	Security, Interoperability Unintended Behavior, Device Vulnerability	Privacy Consistency Integration	Cost Reduction Clinical Continuity Quality Life, Telemedicine
[122]	2016	Security, Interoperability Complexity, Scalability Device Vulnerability	Privacy	Cost Reduction Clinical Continuity Automation, Time Saving
[123]	2017	Security Energy Consumption Network Latency Intelligence in Medical Care System Predictability	Privacy Real-Time Processing	Cost Reduction Clinical Continuity, Automation, Time Saving, Quality Life, Telemedicine
[124]	2018	Security, Interoperability Energy Consumption Network Latency	Privacy	Ubiquitous Access, Quality Life Cost Reduction, Time Saving Reduced Hospital Visits
[11]	2019	Security, Interoperability Energy Consumption Internet Bandwidth	Privacy	N/A

Table 15. *Cont.*

Ref #	Year	Findings		
		Key Challenges and Barriers of E-Cardiology with IoT	**Data Related Issues**	**Benefits of IoT-Based E-Cardiology**
[125]	2019	Security Heterogeneity	Privacy, Reliability, Utility Validity, Generalizability Integrity, Objectivity, Data Overload, Completeness, Relevance	Personalized, Predictive, Participatory, Preventative, Persuasive, Perpetual, Programmable (7P)
[126]	2019	Security Unintended Behavior	Privacy, Confidentiality	Ubiquitous Access Cost Reduction Clinical Continuity Improved Accuracy Quality Life, Telemedicine
[127]	2019	Security Scalability	Privacy Data Overload	Ubiquitous Access Cost Reduction, Clinical Continuity Automation, Time Saving Quality Life Telemedicine
[128]	2019	Security Context-aware Computing Interoperability Energy Consumption	Privacy	N/A
[129]	2020	Unobtrusiveness Energy Consumption Quality of Service Scalabilty, Fixation Patient Indentification Body Impact on Signal Propagation	Reliability Integrity Data Protection Data Representation Accuracy	N/A
[130]	2020	Energy Consumption, Storage Patient's discomfort caused by Sensors	Privacy Data Overload Noise	Flexibility Clinical Continuity Remote Monitoring
[131]	2020	Security	Privacy Confidentiality Integrity, Data Loss Avallabilty Compromise	Remote Monitoring Cost Reduction, Time Saving Better Diagnostics Improved Clinical Infrastructure
[132]	2020	Security Mobility Heterogeneity Legal Aspects	Privacy	N/A
[133]	2021	Security, Scalability	N/A	Efficient, Cost Effective
[134]	2021	Security Scalability Interoperability, Energy Consumption, Low Latency Tolerance	Privacy Computational Intensity	Ubiquitous Access Time Saving, Cost Reduction Telemedicine, Quality Life Clinical Continuity Easy Usge

A comparison of some key factors in Smart cardiac care are shown in Table 16.

Artificial intelligence (AI) is another significant aspect of E-Cardiology. Until now, AI in cardiac electrophysiology has exhibited promising results. Primary advantages of AI-based cardiology are discussed in Table 17.

Table 16. Comparison of the existing evaluation factors in the Smart cardiac care.

Ref #	Year	Security	Privacy	Complexity	Integration	Reliability	System Predictability	Interoperability	Scalability	Heterogeneity	Energy Consumption	Network Latency
[122]	2016	✓	✓	✓	✓	✗	✗	✓	✗	✗	✗	✗
[121]	2016	✓	✓	✗	✓	✗	✗	✓	✗	✗	✗	✗
[135]	2017	✓	✗	✗	✗	✗	✓	✗	✗	✗	✓	✗
[123]	2017	✓	✓	✗	✗	✗	✓	✗	✗	✗	✓	✓
[124]	2018	✓	✓	✗	✗	✗	✗	✓	✗	✗	✓	✓
[11]	2019	✓	✓	✗	✗	✗	✗	✓	✗	✗	✓	✗
[126]	2019	✓	✓	✗	✗	✗	✗	✗	✗	✗	✗	✗
[127]	2019	✓	✓	✗	✗	✗	✗	✗	✓	✗	✗	✗
[125]	2019	✓	✓	✗	✓	✓	✗	✗	✗	✓	✗	✗

Table 16. *Cont.*

Ref #	Year	Security	Privacy	Complexity	Integration	Reliability	System Predictability	Interoperability	Scalability	Heterogeneity	Energy Consumption	Network Latency
[128]	2019	✓	✓	✗	✗	✗	✗	✓	✗	✗	✓	✗
[129]	2020	✗	✓	✗	✓	✓	✗	✗	✓	✗	✓	✗
[130]	2020	✗	✓	✗	✗	✗	✗	✗	✗	✗	✓	✗
[131]	2020	✓	✓	✗	✓	✗	✗	✗	✗	✗	✗	✗
[132]	2020	✓	✓	✗	✗	✗	✗	✗	✗	✓	✗	✗
[133]	2021	✗	✓	✗	✗	✗	✗	✗	✓	✗	✗	✗
[134]	2021	✓	✓	✓	✗	✗	✗	✓	✓	✗	✓	✓

✓—parameter mentioned; ✗—parameter not mentioned.

Table 17. Key challenges and primary benefits of AI-based cardiology.

Ref #	Year	Findings	
		Key Challenges and Barriers for E-Cardiology with AI	**Benefits of AI in E-Cardiology**
[136]	2016	Safety and transparency Algorithmic fairness and biases, Complexity Data privacy and information security Need for infrastructure, High quality data Public perceptions about AI, Informed consent	Better diagnosis, better services Improves quality of services Time saving Reduced treatment cost
[137]	2019	Fitting confounders accidentally versus actual signal, Generalizability, Algorithmic bias Possibility of adversarial attack Logistical challenges in deploying AI systems Robust and rigorous quality assurance Traditional reluctance to switch from existing model to AI model in healthcare Algorithmic accountability To develop a relation between physicians and human-centered AI tools	N/A
[138]	2019	Data privacy, Accountability Algorithmic bias Adaptability, Complexity	Improved healthcare Better diagnosis High accuracy
[139]	2019	Privacy and discrimination Dynamic information and consent Transparency and ownership	Speedy imaging, Increased efficiency Greater insight into predictive screening Decreased healthcare cost
[140]	2020	Respect for autonomy Beneficence Non-maleficence and justice	Lower cost Improved diagnosis and treatment
[141]	2021	Safety, Privacy and security threats Ethical challenges Regulatory and policy challenges Availability of quality data and Lack of data standardization Distribution shifts Upgrading hospital infrastructure	Disease prediction and diagnosis Better image interpretation Real-time monitoring
[142]	2021	Sometimes data reflects inherent biases and disparities Huge dataset requirement Patient's confidentiality Potential to be detrimental	Improved decision making Improved precision and predictability Intraoperative guidance via video

5.4.2. Challenges of E-Cardiology

Internet of Things (IoT) comes with various challenges as shown in Table 15. In addition to these challenges, ref. [129] proposed some other vital challenges, such as fixation of sensors, body impact on signal propagation, and synchronization, that may affect critical health services such as cardiac care. The MIoT-based healthcare systems are expected to produce a vast amount of data. Moreover, these sensors and devices are linked through networks, thus enabling real-time transmission of data. Therefore, hackers may attempt to target it. Moreover, the timely availability of medical data will affect the patient's life. Consequently, it is crucial to have real-time information with lower latency over the network [124].

Artificial intelligence (AI) has brought a revolution in the field of healthcare. It has especially made a great contribution in the domain of cardiac care, such as timely prediction and diagnosis of cardiovascular diseases (CVDs), ECG analysis, and arrhythmia classification. However, despite all these milestones, it carries some challenges. Table 17 describes critical issues and challenges of AI-based cardiology from different past studies.

It is hoped that these challenges can be met and that through MIoT and AI we can achieve new levels of technical and medical standards in the field of cardiac healthcare.

6. Discussion

Figure 5 shows the distribution of the selected studies (104 papers) according to our four research questions (RQs). The pie chart shows that 47 studies overlap RQ1 and RQ2, whereas 33 studies address RQ3 and 24 address RQ4.

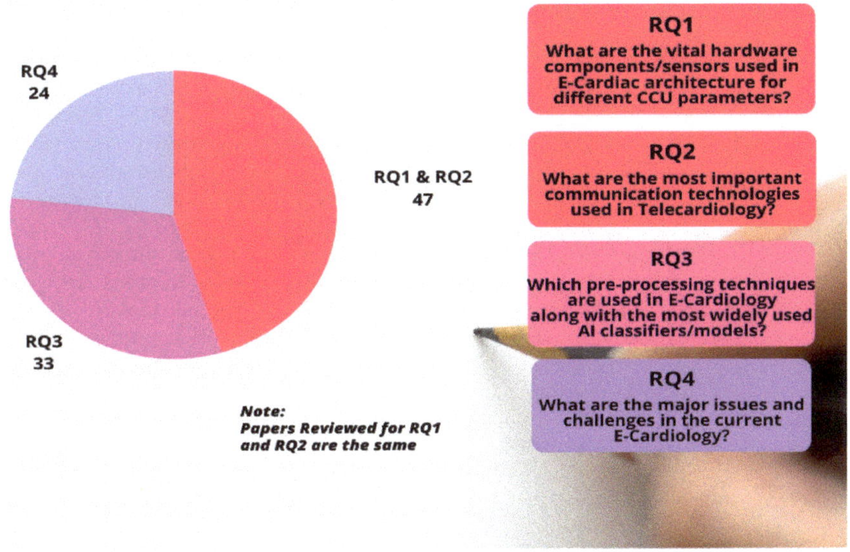

Figure 5. Statistical analysis of reviewed papers in terms of formulated RQs.

The outcomes of this systematic literature review suggest a noticeable increase in the research conducted in IoT using artificial intelligence in E-Cardiology. The research activities also incorporate monitoring CCU parameters, ECG analysis, and diagnosis/classification of various heart diseases. This extensive review study reveals that IoT sensors utilized for E-Cardiology are based upon analog sensors, digital sensors, and different wearable sensors or device modules. For fitness tracking and health monitoring activities, a variety of ready-made and wearable watches are also available. E-Cardiology patients can use a variety of wearable gadgets to track various cardiac healthcare characteristics. To establish expert E-Cardiology systems, several communication technologies and protocols for transmissions over a defined range need to be instituted and maintained. Our findings on communication technologies and protocols for the implementation of IoT-based cardiovascular healthcare monitoring and detection systems show that the following technologies provide viable tools to use in MIoT systems: Bluetooth (BL/BLE), ethernet, global system for mobile (GSM), global positioning system (GPS), global packet radio service (GPRS), message queuing telemetry transport (MQTT), short message service (SMS), email, zigbee, transmission control protocol/Internet protocol (TCP/IP), wireless fidelity (Wifi), security protocols, broadband/Internet, cloud, Smart cars, Smart phones/computers, etc. Our findings show that deep learning is often used in cardiac imaging procedures, particularly in echocardiography [88]. Furthermore, CNNs have been evaluated and found useful in calculating coronary artery calcium in cardiac CT angiography [101]. Though deep learning techniques are garnering attention in the field of Smart cardiology, we may infer that instead of depending on a particular AI model, hybrid techniques are expected to produce better results. From the results of our study, it may also be inferred that SVM was more frequently used in cardiac care than was deep learning. However, in recent years, deep learning has emerged as a more powerful and reliable tool for the detection and diagnosis of various heart diseases. It was also noted that data reduction appears to be a major concern of researchers when applying data mining/data preprocessing approaches to predict CVD. This literature review includes 24 studies devoted to major issues and challenges in E-Cardiology. These studies conclude that a major benefit of MIoT in cardiac healthcare is that it generates timely and accurate data, which results in better healthcare outcomes. One vital advantage of using ML techniques is the ability to fuse various types of data [143]. We also assessed the results and noted that mIoT devices do not possess the requisite data protocols and standards [131]. Therefore, many issues must be addressed to ensure IoT privacy and security [144,145], which is one of the major challenges of the IoT era. Moreover, the continuous monitoring of critical indicators requires reduced energy consumption and a longer battery life [146] to prevent a break of communication. This is also one of the significant challenges of MIoT. The medical data gathered using MIoT is seldom standardized and often fragmented. The data in legacy IT systems are usually generated with incompatible formats. Thus, the great challenge of interoperability needs to be addressed as well [124,147]. However, to move forward in the field of MIoT, fearing AI is no option.

Instead, we should work toward the smooth digitization of healthcare infrastructure [148]. Obviously, various benefits of AI cannot be implemented and utilized correctly without integrating AI into clinical decision making effectively and responsibly [149].

Figure 6 refers to the research work conducted based on the number of papers per annum. It shows the year-wise trends in publications in the field of E-Cardiology. It also indicates that the maximum number of papers selected for this survey was from 2019.

6.1. *Gaps, Future Recommendations*

In a future work, all the vital cardiac parameters can be combined with an intelligent cardiac care unit (CCU) to develop a complete picture of E-Cardiology. These parameters/indicators may be comprised of temperature, blood pressure, oxygen saturation, heart rate, and ECG analysis. In addition, in differentiating between normal and abnormal heartbeats, a Smart CCU can also be used to detect QRS complexes in electrocardiographic (ECG) signals to determine the presence of a cardiac malady and different arrhythmias. Integrated and wearable IoT solutions, which address all the necessary cardiac parameters of a heart patient, need to be implemented. The results and accuracy of the devices/sensors used in the development of an IOT-based cardiac system cannot be compromised. The implemented system must be tested, evaluated, and approved under the supervision of cardiologists. Advanced communication technologies, including secure network protocols, must be implemented. Data accessibility features, such as widespread data access, must be possible in a secure environment so that the data confidentiality and integrity are maintained. Ubiquitous access is also an important factor and can be achieved by storing the digital data on a cloud server.

6.2. *Limitations of the Review Study*

This review of literature has some limitations. First, many papers were conference proceedings; therefore some parameters remained inaccessible since their authors did not mention them in detail. Second, some of the studies on AI-based IoT architecture in cardiac healthcare could not be located even after following a comprehensive search protocol, such as gray literature and reports that were not published in the databases which we selected for review. Therefore, we suggest that an additional systematic study be conducted to cover the related literature from other important databases.

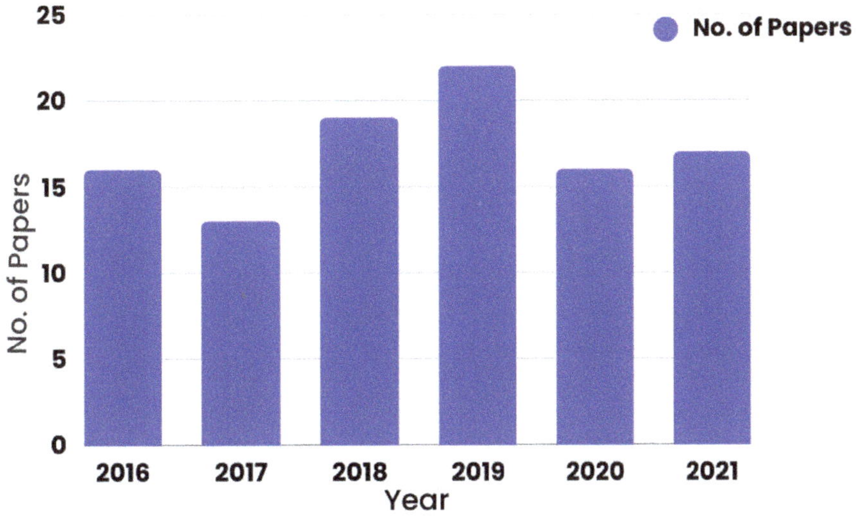

Figure 6. Year-wise trends in publications in the field of E-Cardiology.

7. Conclusions

This review study outlines a total of 104 primary studies from 2016 to 2021 based on our filtering process for supporting the proposed research. Quality assessment of the selected studies was conducted for the formulated research questions after a rigorous analysis.

This work mentions different sensors and communication technologies being used in cardiology. Moreover, this review study also describes various preprocessing techniques and AI algorithms used in the existing studies to diagnose and classify CVD and ECG analysis. This systematic review also provides comparative analysis of various existing techniques in the field of AI, medical sensors, and communication technologies. Finally, this study targets various advantages and issues indicated in the existing literature in the field of E-Cardiology. The interaction of MIoT and artificial intelligence makes cardiac healthcare more manageable by making various applications, services, communication protocols, third party APIs, and IoT sensors available. E-Cardiology guarantees more privacy and security to the IoT devices which are prone to hackers. Furthermore, AI-based diagnosis of various cardiovascular diseases in E-Cardiology helps save time, enabling cardiologists to focus more on treatment. This systematic work presents a review protocol to analyse how IoT applications assist cardiac healthcare and how various artificial intelligence (AI) models contribute to present and prospective research work of IoT in E-Cardiology. This study also indicates how different communication technologies bring privacy and security to IoT devices related to cardiac healthcare. The purpose of this paper is to highlight the influence of IoT, communication technologies, and AI techniques in cardiac healthcare in light of our systematic literature review protocol. Therefore, one can say that this systematic review covers the complete and latest infrastructure of E-Cardiology, along with its benefits and challenges which have not been examined before in such a comprehensive way.

Author Contributions: Conceptualization, R.I. and M.A.K.; methodology, R.I. and U.U.; validation, U.U. and S.N.; formal analysis, U.U. and S.N.; investigation, U.U. and S.N.; resources, R.I., U.U. and S.N.; writing—original draft preparation, U.U., S.N. and A.U.; writing—review and editing, R.I., U.U. and S.N.; visualization, A.U. and S.N.; supervision, R.I. All authors have read and agreed to the published version of the manuscript.

Funding: This research received no external funding.

Institutional Review Board Statement: Not applicable.

Informed Consent Statement: Not applicable.

Data Availability Statement: Not applicable.

Conflicts of Interest: The authors declare no conflict of interest.

Appendix A

Selected Literature

Summary of the selected literature consisting of 104 papers used in this systematic literature review is given in the Table A1.

Table A1. Selected Literature.

Sr.#	Ref#	Year	Paper Title
1	[17]	2016	Smart Real-Time Healthcare Monitoring and Tracking System using GSM/GPS Technologies
2	[58]	2016	Internet of Medical Things for Cardiac Monitoring: Paving The Way to 5G Mobile Networks
3	[59]	2016	IOT on Heart Attack Detection and Heart Rate Monitoring
4	[85]	2016	Heart Rate Monitoring System Using Finger Tip Through Arduino and Processing Software
5	[60]	2016	iCarMa: Inexpensive Cardiac Arrhythmia Management—An IoT Healthcare Analytics Solution
6	[94]	2016	Efficient Heart Disease Prediction System
7	[96]	2016	A new personalized ECG Signal Classification Algorithm using Block-based Neural Network and Particle Swarm Optimization
8	[97]	2016	Arrhythmia Recognition and Classification using Combined Linear and Nonlinear Features of ECG Signals
9	[98]	2016	Cardiac Arrhythmia Beat Classification Using DOST and PSO Tuned SVM
10	[99]	2016	High Performance Personalized Heartbeat Classification Model for Long-Term ECG Signal
11	[100]	2016	ECG Classification Using Wavelet Packet Entropy and Random Forests
12	[101]	2016	Automatic Coronary Artery Calcium Scoring in Cardiac CT Angiography using paired Convolutional Neural Networks
13	[61]	2016	ECG Signal Analysis and Arrhythmia Detection on IoT Wearable Medical Devices
14	[122]	2016	Study of IoT: Understanding IoT Architecture, Applications, Issues and Challenges
15	[121]	2016	Always Connected: The Security Challenges of the Healthcare Internet of Things
16	[136]	2016	Exploratory Study of Artificial Intelligence in Healthcare
17	[37]	2017	The IoT-based Heart Disease Monitoring System for Pervasive Healthcare Service
18	[62]	2017	Heartbeat Sensing and Heart Attack Detection using Internet of Things: IoT
19	[19]	2017	A Novel Cardiac Arrest Alerting System using IOT
20	[29]	2017	A Wearable Multiparameter Medical Monitoring And Alert System With First Aid
21	[63]	2017	Design And Implementation Of Low Cost Web Based Human Health Monitoring System Using Raspberry Pi 2
22	[64]	2017	Ultra-Low Power, Secure IoT Platform for Predicting Cardiovascular Diseases
23	[39]	2017	IOT Based Detection of Cardiac Arrythmia With Classification
24	[150]	2017	Student Research Abstract: A Novel IoT-based Wireless System to Monitor Heart Rate
25	[151]	2017	Cardiac Scan: A Non-contact and Continuous Heart-based User Authentication System
26	[102]	2017	Cardiac Arrhythmia Detection using Deep Learning
27	[103]	2017	Multiresolution Wavelet Transform based Feature Extraction and ECG Classification to Detect Cardiac Abnormalities
28	[104]	2017	ECG beat Classification using Empirical Mode Decomposition and Mixture of Features
29	[123]	2017	Internet of Medical Things (IOMT): Applications, Benefits and Future Challenges in Healthcare Domain
30	[152]	2018	Social Assistive Robot for Cardiac Rehabilitation: A Pilot Study with Patients with Angioplasty
31	[153]	2018	Impact of a Mobile Cycling Application on Cardiac Patients' Cycling Behavior and Enjoyment
32	[65]	2018	Pulse Oximetry and IOT based Cardiac Monitoring Integrated Alert System

Table A1. *Cont.*

Sr.#	Ref#	Year	Paper Title
33	[66]	2018	Detection of Cardiac Arrest Using Internet of Things
34	[18]	2018	Heart Attack Detection and Heart Rate Monitoring Using IoT
35	[38]	2018	IoT Based Continuous Monitoring of Cardiac Patients using Raspberry Pi
36	[20]	2018	Healthcare Monitoring System Based on Wireless Sensor Network for Cardiac Patients
37	[24]	2018	Heart Attack Detection By Heartbeat Sensing using Internet Of Things: IoT
38	[67]	2018	Real-Time Monitoring and Detection of "Heart Attack" Using Wireless Sensors and IoT
39	[105]	2018	Diagnosis of Shockable Rhythms for Automated External Defibrillators using a Reliable Support Vector Machine Classifier
40	[106]	2018	Automatic Recognition of Arrhythmia based on Principal Component Analysis Network and Linear Support Vector Machine
41	[107]	2018	Automated Recognition of Cardiac Arrhythmias using Sparse Decomposition over Composite Dictionary
42	[108]	2018	A Novel Adaptive Feature Extraction for Detection of Cardiac Arrhythmias using Hybrid technique MRDWT & MPNN Classifier from ECG Big Data
43	[109]	2018	Automated Diagnosis of Arrhythmia using Combination of CNN and LSTM Techniques with Variable Length Heart Beats
44	[110]	2018	A Deep Learning Approach for ECG-based Heartbeat Classification for Arrhythmia Detection
45	[111]	2018	A Novel Application of Deep Learning for Single-Lead ECG Classification
46	[91]	2018	Deep Learning for Prediction of Obstructive Disease From Fast Myocardial Perfusion SPECT A Multicenter Study
47	[124]	2018	Deploying Internet of Things in Healthcare: Benefits, Requirements, Challenges and Applications
48	[28]	2019	A Study on Heart Attack Detection by Heartbeat Monitoring Using IoT
49	[25]	2019	An Energy Efficient Wearable Smart IoT System to Predict Cardiac Arrest
50	[26]	2019	IoT Based Heart Attack Detection, Heart Rate and Temperature Monitor
51	[40]	2019	IoT based Diagnosing Myocardial Infarction through Firebase Web Application
52	[21]	2019	A Real-time Cardiac Monitoring using a Multisensory Smart IoT System
53	[68]	2019	An IoT based Efficient Hybrid Recommender System for Cardiovascular Disease
54	[69]	2019	Utilizing IoT Wearable Medical Device for Heart Disease Prediction using Higher Order Boltzmann Model: A Classification Approach
55	[30]	2019	The Cardiac Disease Predictor: IoT and ML Driven Healthcare System
56	[70]	2019	Machine Learning and IoT-based Cardiac Arrhythmia Diagnosis using Statistical and Dynamic Features of ECG
57	[71]	2019	Artificial Intelligence of Things Wearable System for Cardiac Disease Detection
58	[112]	2019	Neural Network Based Intelligent System for Predicting Heart Disease
59	[93]	2019	Cardiologist-level Arrhythmia Detection and Classification in ambulatory Electrocardiograms using a Deep Neural Network
60	[126]	2019	IoT Healthcare: Benefits, Issues and Challenges
61	[127]	2019	IoT, an Emerging Technology for Next Generation Medical Devices in Support of Cardiac Health Care—A Comprehensive Review
62	[11]	2019	IoT Technology, Applications and Challenges: A Contemporary Survey
63	[128]	2019	Internet of Things applications: A Systematic Review
64	[125]	2019	Smart Healthcare in the Era of Internet-of-Things
65	[130]	2019	Challenges and opportunities in IoT Healthcare Systems: A Systematic Review
66	[138]	2019	AI in Healthcare: Ethical and Privacy Challenges
67	[137]	2019	Key Challenges for Delivering Clinical Impact with Artificial Intelligence
68	[139]	2019	Healthcare uses of Artificial Intelligence: Challenges and Opportunities for Growth
69	[149]	2019	Artificial Intelligence in Clinical Decision Support: Challenges for Evaluating AI and Practical Implications
70	[72]	2020	An Efficient IoT-Based Platform for Remote Real-Time Cardiac Activity Monitoring
71	[86]	2020	IOT Based Heart Attack Detection & Heart Rate Monitoring System

Table A1. *Cont.*

Sr.#	Ref#	Year	Paper Title
72	[73]	2020	Remote Health and Monitoring, Heart Attack Detection and Location Tracking System with IoT
73	[74]	2020	IOT Based Heart Attack and Alcohol Detection in Smart Transportation and Accident
74	[75]	2020	HealthFog: An Ensemble Deep Learning based Smart Healthcare System for Automatic Diagnosis of Heart Diseases in Integrated IoT and Fog Computing Environments
75	[27]	2020	IoT based Health Care Monitoring Kit
76	[76]	2020	Automated Detection of Posterior Myocardial Infarction From VCG Signals Using Stationary Wavelet Transform Based Features
77	[22]	2020	IoT Based Real-Time Remote Patient Monitoring System
78	[77]	2020	Design, Fabrication, and Testing of an IoT Healthcare Cardiac Monitoring Device
79	[78]	2020	A Framework for Cardiac Arrhythmia Detection from IoT-based ECGs
80	[79]	2020	SAREF4health: Towards IoT Standard-based Ontology-Driven Cardiac E-health Systems
81	[23]	2020	An IoT Patient Monitoring Based on Fog Computing and Data Mining: Cardiac Arrhythmia Usecase
82	[113]	2020	CNN-KCL: Automatic Myocarditis Diagnosis using Convolutional Neural Network Combined with K-means Clustering
83	[114]	2020	Detection of Myocardial Infarction Based on Novel Deep Transfer Learning Methods for Urban Healthcare in Smart Cities
84	[115]	2020	Automatic Diagnosis of the 12-lead ECG using a Deep Neural Network
85	[129]	2020	Internet of Things Based Distributed Healthcare Systems: A Review
86	[131]	2020	IoT-Enabled Healthcare: Benefits, Issues and Challenges
87	[132]	2020	A Comprehensive Review on the Emerging IoT Cloud based Technologies for Smart Healthcare
88	[140]	2020	Ethical Challenges of Integrating AI into Healthcare
89	[80]	2021	Monitoring Patients to Prevent Myocardial Infarction using Internet of Things Technology
90	[81]	2021	Filtering the ECG Signal towards Heart Attack Detection using Motion Artifact Removal Technique
91	[82]	2021	Artificial-Intelligence-Enhanced Mobile System for Cardiovascular Health Management
92	[83]	2021	AMBtalk: A Cardiovascular IoT Device for Ambulance Applications
93	[84]	2021	Predicting Cardiovascular Events with Deep Learning Approach in the Context of the Internet of Things
94	[41]	2021	IoT Based Wearable Monitoring Structure for detecting Abnormal Heart
95	[154]	2021	An Advanced Patient Health Monitoring System
96	[155]	2021	Development of Smart Health Monitoring System using Internet of Things
97	[116]	2021	Early Detection of Myocardial Infarction in Low-Quality Echocardiography
98	[119]	2021	Prediction of Heart Disease Using Deep Convolutional Neural Networks
99	[117]	2021	AI-Based Smart Prediction of Clinical Disease Using Random Forest Classifier and Naive Bayes
100	[118]	2021	Artificial Intelligence Enhanced Electrocardiogram for the Early Detection of Cardiac Amyloidosis
101	[133]	2021	IOT in Healthcare: Challenges, Benefits, Applications and Opportunities
102	[134]	2021	A Survey on IoT Smart Healthcare: Emerging Technologies, Applications, Challenges, and Future Trends
103	[141]	2021	Secure and Robust Machine Learning for Healthcare: A Survey
104	[142]	2021	AI in Healthcare: Medical and Socio-Economic Benefits and Challenges

References

1. WHO: The Top 10 Causes of Death. Available online: http://www.who.int/mediacentre/factsheets/fs310/en/index.html (accessed on 10 April 2020).
2. Available online: https://www.who.int/news-room/fact-sheets/detail/cardiovasculardiseases-(cvds) (accessed on 11 November 2020).
3. Umar, U.; Khan, M.A.; Irfan, R.; Ahmad, J. IoT-based Cardiac Healthcare System for Ubiquitous Healthcare Service. In Proceedings of the 2021 International Congress of Advanced Technology and Engineering (ICOTEN), Taiz, Yemen, 4–5 July 2021; IEEE: New York, NY, USA, 2021; pp. 1–6.
4. Internet of Things: Internet of Things. Available online: https://www.en.wikipedia.ord/wiki/internetofthings (accessed on 10 April 2020).

5. Bao, J.; Shou, X.; Wang, H.; Yang, H. Study on heartbeat information acquired from pressure cushion based on body sensor network. In Proceedings of the 2013 IEEE International Conference on Green Computing and Communications and IEEE Internet of Things and IEEE Cyber, Physical and Social Computing, Beijing, China, 20–23 August 2013; pp. 1103–1108.
6. Lin, C.-T.; Chuang, C.-H.; Huang, C.-S.; Tsai, S.-F.; Lu, S.-W.; Chen, Y.-H.; Ko, L.-W. Wireless and wearable eeg system for evaluating driver vigilance. *IEEE Trans. Biomed. Circuits Syst.* **2014**, *8*, 165–176. [PubMed]
7. Benhar, H.; Idri, A.; Fernandez-Aleman, J. Data preprocessing for heart disease classification: A systematic literature review. *Comput. Methods Programs Biomed.* **2020**, *195*, 105635. [CrossRef] [PubMed]
8. Shah, R.; Chircu, A. Iot and ai in healthcare: A systematic literature review. *Issues Inf. Syst.* **2018**, *19*, 33–41.
9. Kadi, I.; Idri, A.; Fernandez-Aleman, J. Knowledge discovery in cardiology: A systematic literature review. *Int. J. Med. Inform.* **2017**, *97*, 12–32. [CrossRef] [PubMed]
10. Shah, N.; Ali, Y.; Ullah, N.; García-Magariño, I. Internet of things for healthcare using effects of mobile computing: A systematic literature review. *Wirel. Commun. Mob. Comput.* **2019**, *2019*, 5931315.
11. Balaji, S.; Nathani, K.; Santhakumar, R. Iot technology, applications and challenges: A contemporary survey. *Wirel. Pers. Commun.* **2019**, *108*, 363–388. [CrossRef]
12. AbdElnapi, N.M.M.; Omran, N.F.; Ali, A.A.; Omara, F.A. A survey of internet of things technologies and projects for healthcare services. In Proceedings of the 2018 International Conference on Innovative Trends in Computer Engineering (ITCE), Aswan, Egypt, 19–21 February 2018; pp. 48–55.
13. Al-rawashdeh, M.; Keikhosrokiani, P.; Belaton, B.; Alawida, M.; Zwiri, A. IoT Adoption and Application for Smart Healthcare: A Systematic Review. *Sensors* **2022**, *22*, 5377. [CrossRef]
14. Kashani, O.H.; Madanipour, M.; Nikravan, M.; Asghari, P.; Mahdipour, E. A systematic review of IoT in healthcare: Applications, techniques, and trends. *J. Netw. Comput. Appl.* **2021**, *192*, 103164. [CrossRef]
15. Esfandiari, N.; Babavalian, M.R.; Moghadam, A.-M.E.; Tabar, V.K. Knowledge discovery in medicine: Current issue and future trend. *Expert Syst. Appl.* **2014**, *41*, 4434–4463. [CrossRef]
16. Wohlin, C. Guidelines for snowballing in systematic literature studies and a replication in software engineering. In Proceedings of the 18th International Conference on Evaluation and Assessment in Software Engineering, London, UK, 13–14 May 2014; pp. 1–10.
17. Aziz, K.; Tarapiah, S.; Ismail, S.H.; Atalla, S. Smart real-time healthcare monitoring and tracking system using gsm/gps technologies. In Proceedings of the 2016 3rd MEC International Conference on Big Data and Smart City (ICBDSC), Muscat, Oman, 15–16 March 2016; pp. 1–7.
18. Patel, N.; Patel, P.; Patel, N. Heart attack detection and heart rate monitoring using iot. *Int. J. Innov. Adv. Comput. Sci. (IJIACS)* **2018**, *7*, 611–615.
19. Ajay, H.; Rao, A.; Balavanan, M.; Lalit, R. A novel cardiac arrest alerting system using iot. *Int. J. Sci. Technol. Eng.* **2017**, *3*, 78–83.
20. Gogate, U.; Bakal, J. Healthcare monitoring system based on wireless sensor network for cardiac patients. *Biomed. Pharmacol.* **2018**, *11*, 1681. [CrossRef]
21. Majumder, A.J.; Elsaadany, M.; Izaguirre, J.A.; Ucci, D.R. A realtime cardiac monitoring using a multisensory smart iot system. In Proceedings of the 2019 IEEE 43rd Annual Computer Software and Applications Conference (COMPSAC), Milwaukee, WI, USA, 15–19 July 2019; Volume 2, pp. 281–287.
22. Yew, H.T.; Ng, M.F.; Ping, S.Z.; Chung, S.K.; Chekima, A.; Dargham, J.A. Iot based real-time remote patient monitoring system. In Proceedings of the 2020 16th IEEE International Colloquium on Signal Processing & Its Applications (CSPA), Langkawi Island, Malaysia, 28–29 February 2020; pp. 176–179.
23. Moghadas, E.; Rezazadeh, J.; Farahbakhsh, R. An iot patient monitoring based on fog computing and data mining: Cardiac arrhythmia usecase. *Internet Things* **2020**, *11*, 100251. [CrossRef]
24. Gurjar, A.; Sarnaik, N.A. Heart attack detection by heartbeat sensing using Internet of Things: IoT. *Int. Res. J. Eng. Technol.* **2018**, *5*, 3332–3335.
25. Majumder, A.; ElSaadany, Y.A.; Young, R.; Ucci, D.R. An energy efficient wearable smart iot system to predict cardiac arrest. *Adv.-Hum. Interact.* **2019**, *2019*, 1507465. [CrossRef]
26. Vaishnave, A.K.; Jenisha, S.T.; Tamil Selvi, S. IoT Based Heart Attack Detection, Heart Rate and Temperature Monitor. *Int. Res. J. Multidiscip. Technovat.* **2019**, *1*, 61–70.
27. Acharya, A.D.; Patil, S.N. Iot based health care monitoring kit. In Proceedings of the 2020 Fourth International Conference on Computing Methodologies and Communication (ICCMC), Erode, India, 11–13 March 2020; pp. 363–368.
28. Shivakumar, E.; Hiremani, N. A Study on Heart Attack Detection by Heartbeat Monitoring Using Iot. *Int. Res. J. Eng. Technol.* **2019**, *6*, 4016–4020.
29. Manimaraboopathy, M.; Vijayalakshmi, S.; Hemavathy, D.; Priya, A. A wearable multiparameter medical monitoring and alert system with first aid. *Int. J. Smart Sens. Intell. Syst.* **2017**, *10*, 446. [CrossRef]
30. Tabassum, S.; Zaman, M.I.U.; Ullah, M.S.; Rahaman, A.; Nahar, S.; Islam, A.M. The cardiac disease predictor: Iot and ml driven healthcare system. In Proceedings of the 2019 4th International Conference on Electrical Information and Communication Technology (EICT), Khulna, Bangladesh, 20–22 December 2019; pp. 1–6.
31. Available online: https://bit.ly/3Eo4lEG (accessed on 11 September 2021).
32. Available online: https://bit.ly/3nALDTK (accessed on 11 September 2021).

33. Available online: https://datasheetspdf.com/datasheet/KY-039.html (accessed on 11 September 2021).
34. Available online: https://iss.jaxa.jp/en/kiboexp/pm/holter/holter.pdf (accessed on 11 September 2021).
35. Available online: https://www.amazon.com/oximeter-fingertip-saturation-batteries-GreyWhite/dp/B081JQJVPD (accessed on 11 September 2021).
36. Available online: https://datasheets.maximintegrated.com/en/ds/MAX30100.pdf (accessed on 11 September 2021).
37. Li, C.; Hu, X.; Zhang, L. The iot-based heart disease monitoring system for pervasive healthcare service. *Procedia Comput. Sci.* **2017**, *112*, 2328–2334. [CrossRef]
38. Mathivanan, M.; Balamurugan, M.; Nandini; Reddy, M. Iot basedcontinuous monitoring of cardiac patients using raspberry pi. *AIP Conf. Proc.* **2018**, *2039*, 020025.
39. Shah, J.; Danve, S. Iot Based Detection of Cardiac Arrythmia with Classification. In Proceedings of the International Conference on Emerging Trends in Engineering, Technology, Science and Management (ICETETSM-17), Delhi, India, 11 June 2017.
40. Sharma, A.K.; Saini, L.M. Iot based diagnosing myocardial infarction through firebase web application. In Proceedings of the 2019 3rd International Conference on Electronics, Communication and Aerospace Technology (ICECA), Coimbatore, India, 12–14 June 2019; pp. 190–195.
41. Kora, P.; Rajani, A.; Chinnaiah, M.; Swaraja, K.; Meenakshi, K. Iot based wearable monitoring structure for detecting abnormal heart. In Proceedings of the 2021 International Conference on Sustainable Energy and Future Electric Transportation (SEFET), Hyderabad, India, 21–23 January 2021; pp. 1–4.
42. Available online: https://pdf1.alldatasheet.com/datasheetpdf/view/517588/TI1/LM35.html (accessed on 11 September 2021).
43. Available online: https://www.alldatasheet.com/datasheetpdf/pdf/58557/DALLAS/DS18B20.html (accessed on 11 September 2021).
44. Available online: https://pdf1.alldatasheet.com/datasheetpdf/view/109863/MICROCHIP/MCP9700.html (accessed on 11 September 2021).
45. Available online: https://www.ti.com/lit/gpn/tmp100 (accessed on 11 September 2021).
46. Available online: https://www.nxp.com/docs/en/data-sheet/MPX10.pdf (accessed on 11 September 2021).
47. Available online: https://bit.ly/3GrPBXl (accessed on 11 September 2021).
48. Available online: https://www.hospitalsstore.com/omron-hbp-1300-digital-automaticblood-pressure-monitor/ (accessed on 11 September 2021).
49. Available online: https://www.vernier.com/product/blood-pressure-sensor/ (accessed on 11 September 2021).
50. Available online: https://bit.ly/3CgUslm (accessed on 11 September 2021).
51. Available online: https://bit.ly/3Gq1YmP (accessed on 11 September 2021).
52. Available online: https://www.alldatasheet.com/datasheetpdf/pdf/1007828/AD/ADAS1000-1BCPZ.html (accessed on 11 September 2021).
53. Available online: https://pdf1.alldatasheet.com/datasheetpdf/view/902688/AD/AD8233.html (accessed on 11 September 2021).
54. Available online: https://www.shimmersensing.com/products/shimmer3-ecgsensorspecifications-tab (accessed on 11 September 2021).
55. Available online: http://www.shimmersensing.com/products/ecg-development-kit (accessed on 11 September 2021).
56. Available online: https://bit.ly/2ZujQvT (accessed on 11 September 2021).
57. Available online: http://www.shimmersensing.com/products/ecg-developmentkitdownload-tab (accessed on 11 September 2021).
58. Jusak, J.; Pratikno, H.; Putra, V.H. Internet of medical things for cardiac monitoring: Paving the way to 5 g mobile networks. In Proceedings of the 2016 IEEE International Conference on Communication, Networks and Satellite (COMNETSAT), Surabaya, Indonesia, 8–10 December 2016; pp. 75–79.
59. Manisha, M.; Neeraja, K.; Sindhura, V.; Ramaya, P. Iot on heart attack detection and heart rate monitoring. *Int. J. Innov. Eng. Technol. (IJIET)* **2016**, *196*.
60. Puri, C.; Ukil, A.; Bandyopadhyay, S.; Singh, R.; Pal, A.; Mandana, K. Icarma: Inexpensive cardiac arrhythmia management—An iot healthcare analytics solution. In Proceedings of the First Workshop on IoT-Enabled Healthcare and Wellness Technologies and Systems, Singapore, 30 June 2016; pp. 3–8.
61. Azariadi, D.; Tsoutsouras, V.; Xydis, S.; Soudris, D. Ecg signal analysis and arrhythmia detection on iot wearable medical devices. In Proceedings of the 2016 5th International Conference on Modern Circuits and Systems Technologies (MOCAST), Thessaloniki, Greece, 12–14 May 2016; pp. 1–4.
62. Sidheeque, A.; Kumar, A.; Balamurugan, R.; Deepak, K.; Sathish, K. Heartbeat sensing and heart attack detection using internet of things: Iot. *Int. J. Eng. Sci. Comput.* **2017**, *7*, 6662–6666.
63. Kirankumar, C.; Prabhakaran, M. Design and implementation of low cost web based human health monitoring system using raspberry pi 2. In Proceedings of the 2017 IEEE International Conference on Electrical, Instrumentation and Communication Engineering (ICEICE), Karur, India, 27–28 April 2017; pp. 1–5.
64. Yasin, M.; Tekeste, T.; Saleh, H.; Mohammad, B.; Sinanoglu, O.; Ismail, M. Ultra-low power, secure iot platform for predicting cardiovascular diseases. *IEEE Trans. Circuits Syst. I Regul. Pap.* **2017**, *64*, 2624–2637. [CrossRef]
65. Murali, D.; Rao, D.R.; Rao, S.R.; Ananda, M. Pulse oximetry and iot based cardiac monitoring integrated alert system. In Proceedings of the 2018 International Conference on Advances in Computing, Communications and Informatics (ICACCI), Bengaluru, India, 19–22 September 2018; pp. 2237–2243.

66. Hemalatha, V.; Poykasi, K.; Sangeetha, P.; Gomathi, P. Detection of cardiac arrest using internet of things. *Int. J. Sci. Res. Comput. Sci.* **2018**, *3*, 793–801.
67. Geethalakshmi, T.S.T. Real-time monitoring and detection of "heart attack" using wireless sensors and iot. In Proceedings of the 2010 Fourth International Conference on Sensor Technologies and Applications, Venice, Italy, 18–25 July 2010.
68. Jabeen, F.; Maqsood, M.; Ghazanfar, M.A.; Aadil, F.; Khan, S.; Khan, M.F.; Mehmood, I. An iot based efficient hybrid recommender system for cardiovascular disease. *Peer-Netw. Appl.* **2019**, *12*, 1263–1276. [CrossRef]
69. Al-Makhadmeh, Z.; Tolba, A. Utilizing iot wearable medical device for heart disease prediction using higher order boltzmann model: A classification approach. *Measurement* **2019**, *147*, 106815. [CrossRef]
70. Devi, R.L.; Kalaivani, V. Machine learning and iot-based cardiac arrhythmia diagnosis using statistical and dynamic features of ecg. *J. Supercomput.* **2020**, *76*, 6533–6544. [CrossRef]
71. Lin, Y.-J.; Chuang, C.-W.; Yen, C.-Y.; Huang, S.-H.; Huang, P.-W.; Chen, J.-Y.; Lee, S.-Y. Artificial intelligence of things wearable system for cardiac disease detection. In Proceedings of the 2019 IEEE International Conference on Artificial Intelligence Circuits and Systems (AICAS), Hsinchu, Taiwan, 18–20 March 2019; pp. 67–70.
72. Raj, S. An efficient iot-based platform for remote real-time cardiac activity monitoring. *IEEE Trans. Consum. Electron.* **2020**, *66*, 106–114. [CrossRef]
73. Lokesh, S.; Pon Nandhakuamr, S.; Ranjith, R. Remote health and monitoring, heart attack detection and location tracking system with iot. *Hindusthan J. Inf. Commun. Mod. Comput.* **2020**, *1*, 1–5.
74. Kumari, K.V.R.; Sarma, G. Iot Based Heart Attack and Alcohol Detection in Smart Transportation and Accident Prevention for Vehicle Drivers. *Int. J. Recent Dev. Sci. Technol.* **2020**, *4*, 179–185.
75. Tuli, S.; Basumatary, N.; Gill, S.S.; Kahani, M.; Arya, R.C.; Wander, G.S.; Buyya, R. Healthfog: An ensemble deep learning based smart healthcare system for automatic diagnosis of heart diseases in integrated iot and fog computing environments. *Future Gener. Syst.* **2020**, *104*, 187–200. [CrossRef]
76. Prabhakararao, E.; Dandapat, S. Automated detection of posterior myocardial infarction from vcg signals using stationary wavelet transform based features. *IEEE Sens. Lett.* **2020**, *4*, 1–4. [CrossRef]
77. Zagan, I.; Gaitan, V.G.; Petrariu, A.-I.; Iuga, N.; Brezulianu, A. Design, fabrication, and testing of an iot healthcare cardiac monitoring device. *Computers* **2020**, *9*, 15. [CrossRef]
78. He, J.; Rong, J.; Sun, L.; Wang, H.; Zhang, Y.; Ma, J. A framework for cardiac arrhythmia detection from iot-based ecgs. *World Wide Web* **2020**, *23*, 2835–2850. [CrossRef]
79. Moreira, J.; Pires, L.F.; van Sinderen, M.; Daniele, L.; GirodGenet, M. Saref4health: Towards iot standard-based ontology-driven cardiac e-health systems. *Appl. Ontol.* **2020**, *15*, 385–410. [CrossRef]
80. Akhoondan, F.; Hamidi, H.; Broumandnia, A. Monitoring patients to prevent myocardial infarction using internet of things technology. *J. Community Health Res.* **2021**, *10*, 52–59. [CrossRef]
81. Selvaraj, S.; Ramya, P.; Priya, R.; Ramya, C. Filtering the ecg signal towards heart attack detection using motion artifact removal technique. In Proceedings of the 2021 Third International Conference on Intelligent Communication Technologies and Virtual Mobile Networks (ICICV), Tirunelveli, India, 4–6 February 2021; pp. 185–188.
82. Fu, Z.; Hong, S.; Zhang, R.; Du, S. Artificial-intelligence-enhanced mobile system for cardiovascular health management. *Sensors* **2021**, *21*, 773. [CrossRef]
83. Chen, W.-L.; Lin, Y.-B.; Chang, T.C.-Y.; Lin, Y.-R. Ambtalk: A cardiovascular iot device for ambulance applications. *Sensors* **2021**, *21*, 2781. [CrossRef] [PubMed]
84. Dami, S.; Yahaghizadeh, M. Predicting cardiovascular events with deep learning approach in the context of the internet of things. *Neural Comput. Appl.* **2021**, *33*, 7979–7996. [CrossRef]
85. Mallick, B.; Patro, A.K. Heart rate monitoring system using finger tip through arduino and processing software. *Int. J. Sci. Eng. Technol. Res. (IJSETR)* **2016**, *5*, 84–89.
86. Giri, S.; Kumar, U.; Sharma, V.; Kumar, S.; Kumari, S.; Rawani, R.K.; Pande, P.; Bhadra, B. Iot based heart attack detection & heart rate monitoring system. In Proceedings of the International Conference on Recent Trends in Artificial Intelligence, Iot, Smart Cities & Application (ICAISC 2020), Jharkhand, India, 16 July 2020.
87. Nygards, M.-E.; Hulting, J. An automated system for ecg monitoring. *Comput. Biomed. Res.* **1979**, *12*, 181–202. [CrossRef]
88. Romiti, S.; Vinciguerra, M.; Saade, W.; Cortajarena, I.A.; Greco, E. Artificial intelligence (AI) and cardiovascular diseases: An unexpected alliance. *Cardiol. Res. Pract.* **2020**, *2020*, 4972346. [CrossRef]
89. Alsharqi, M.; Woodward, W.; Mumith, J.; Markham, D.; Upton, R.; Leeson, P. Artificial intelligence and echocardiography. *Echo Res. Pract.* **2018**, *5*, R115–R125. [CrossRef] [PubMed]
90. Samad, M.D.; Ulloa, A.; Wehner, G.J.; Jing, L.; Hartzel, D.; Good, C.W.; Williams, B.A.; Haggerty, C.M.; Fornwalt, B.K. Predicting survival from large echocardiography and electronic health record datasets: Optimization with machine learning. *JACC Cardiovasc. Imaging* **2019**, *12*, 681–689. [CrossRef] [PubMed]
91. Betancur, J.; Commandeur, F.; Motlagh, M.; Sharir, T.; Einstein, A.J.; Bokhari, S.; Fish, M.B.; Ruddy, T.D.; Kaufmann, P.; Sinusas, A.J.; et al. Deep learning for prediction of obstructive disease from fast myocardial perfusion spect: A multicenter study. *JACC Cardiovasc. Imaging* **2018**, *11*, 1654–1663. [CrossRef] [PubMed]
92. Seetharam, K.; Kagiyama, N.; Sengupta, P.P. Application of mobile health, telemedicine and artificial intelligence to echocardiography. *Echo Res. Pract.* **2019**, *6*, R41–R52. [CrossRef] [PubMed]

93. Hannun, A.Y.; Rajpurkar, P.; Haghpanahi, M.; Tison, G.H.; Bourn, C.; Turakhia, M.P.; Ng, A.Y. Cardiologist-level arrhythmia detection and classification in ambulatory electrocardiograms using a deep neural network. *Nat. Med.* **2019**, *25*, 65–69. [CrossRef]
94. Saxena, K.; Sharma, R. Efficient heart disease prediction system. *Procedia Comput. Sci.* **2016**, *85*, 962–969.
95. Learning, M. Heart disease diagnosis and prediction using machine learning and data mining techniques: A review. *Adv. Comput. Sci. Technol.* **2017**, *10*, 2137–2159.
96. Shadmand, S.; Mashoufi, B. A new personalized ecg signal classification algorithm using block-based neural network and particle swarm optimization. *Biomed. Signal Process. Control* **2016**, *25*, 12–23. [CrossRef]
97. Elhaj, F.A.; Salim, N.; Harris, A.R.; Swee, T.T.; Ahmed, T. Arrhythmia recognition and classification using combined linear and nonlinear features of ecg signals. *Comput. Methods Programs Biomed.* **2016**, *127*, 52–63. [CrossRef]
98. Raj, S.; Ray, K.C.; Shankar, O. Cardiac arrhythmia beat classification using dost and pso tuned svm. *Comput. Methods Programs Biomed.* **2016**, *136*, 163–177. [CrossRef] [PubMed]
99. Li, P.; Wang, Y.; He, J.; Wang, L.; Tian, Y.; Zhou, T.-S.; Li, T.; Li, J.-S. High-performance personalized heartbeat classification model for long-term ecg signal. *IEEE Trans. Biomed. Eng.* **2016**, *64*, 78–86. [PubMed]
100. Li, T.; Zhou, M. Ecg classification using wavelet packet entropy and random forests. *Entropy* **2016**, *18*, 285. [CrossRef]
101. Wolterink, J.M.; Leiner, T.; de Vos, B.D.; van Hamersvelt, R.W.; Viergever, M.A.; Isgum, I. Automatic coronary artery calcium scoring in cardiac ct angiography using paired convolutional neural networks. *Med. Image Anal.* **2016**, *34*, 123–136. [CrossRef] [PubMed]
102. Isin, A.; Ozdalili, S. Cardiac arrhythmia detection using deep learning. *Procedia Comput. Sci.* **2017**, *120*, 268–275. [CrossRef]
103. Sahoo, S.; Kanungo, B.; Behera, S.; Sabut, S. Multiresolution wavelet transform based feature extraction and ecg classification to detect cardiac abnormalities. *Measurement* **2017**, *108*, 55–66. [CrossRef]
104. Sahoo, S.; Mohanty, M.; Behera, S.; Sabut, S.K. Ecg beat classification using empirical mode decomposition and mixture of features. *J. Med. Eng. Technol.* **2017**, *41*, 652–661. [CrossRef]
105. Nguyen, M.T.; Shahzad, A.; van Nguyen, B.; Kim, K. Diagnosis of shockable rhythms for automated external defibrillators using a reliable support vector machine classifier. *Biomed. Signal Process. Control* **2018**, *44*, 258–269. [CrossRef]
106. Yang, W.; Si, Y.; Wang, D.; Guo, B. Automatic recognition of arrhythmia based on principal component analysis network and linear support vector machine. *Comput. Biol. Med.* **2018**, *101*, 22–32. [CrossRef]
107. Raj, S.; Ray, K.C. Automated recognition of cardiac arrhythmias using sparse decomposition over composite dictionary. *Comput. Methods Programs Biomed.* **2018**, *165*, 175–186. [CrossRef] [PubMed]
108. Rai, H.M.; Chatterjee, K. A novel adaptive feature extraction for detection of cardiac arrhythmias using hybrid technique mrdwt & mpnn classifier from ecg big data. *Big Data Res.* **2018**, *12*, 13–22.
109. Oh, S.L.; Ng, E.Y.; Tan, R.S.; Acharya, U.R. Automated diagnosis of arrhythmia using combination of cnn and lstm techniques with variable length heart beats. *Comput. Biol. Med.* **2018**, *102*, 278–287. [CrossRef] [PubMed]
110. Sannino, G.; de Pietro, G. A deep learning approach for ecg-based heartbeat classification for arrhythmia detection. *Future Gener. Comput. Syst.* **2018**, *86*, 446–455. [CrossRef]
111. Mathews, S.M.; Kambhamettu, C.; Barner, K.E. A novel application of deep learning for single-lead ecg classification. *Comput. Biol. Med.* **2018**, *99*, 53–62. [CrossRef]
112. Subhadra, K.; Vikas, B. Neural network based intelligent system for predicting heart disease. *Int. J. Innov. Technol. Explor. Eng.* **2019**, *8*, 484–487.
113. Sharifrazi, D.; Alizadehsani, R.; Joloudari, J.H.; Shamshirband, S.; Hussain, S.; Sani, Z.A.; Hasanzadeh, F.; Shoaibi, A.; Dehzangi, A.; Alinejad-Rokny, H. Cnn-kcl: Automatic myocarditis diagnosis using convolutional neural network combined with k-means clustering. *Preprints* **2020**, 2020070650. [CrossRef]
114. Alghamdi, A.; Hammad, M.; Ugail, H.; Abdel-Raheem, A.; Muhammad, K.; Khalifa, H.S.; El-Latif, A.; Ahmed, A. Detection of myocardial infarction based on novel deep transfer learning methods for urban healthcare in smart cities. *Multimed. Tools Appl.* **2020**, 1–22. [CrossRef]
115. Ribeiro, A.H.; Ribeiro, M.H.; Paixao, G.M.; Oliveira, D.M.; Gomes, P.R.; Canazart, J.A.; Ferreira, M.P.; Andersson, C.R.; Macfarlane, P.W.; Meira, W., Jr.; et al. Automatic diagnosis of the 12-lead ecg using a deep neural network. *Nat. Commun.* **2020**, *11*, 1760. [CrossRef]
116. Degerli, A.; Zabihi, M.; Kiranyaz, S.; Hamid, T.; Mazhar, R.; Hamila, R.; Gabbouj, M. Early detection of myocardial infarction in lowquality echocardiography. *IEEE Access* **2021**, *9*, 34442–34453. [CrossRef]
117. Jackins, V.; Vimal, S.; Kaliappan, M.; Lee, M.Y. Ai-based smart prediction of clinical disease using random forest classifier and naive bayes. *J. Supercomput.* **2021**, *77*, 5198–5219. [CrossRef]
118. Grogan, M.; Lopez-Jimenez, F.; Cohen-Shelly, M.; Dispenzieri, A.; Attia, Z.I.; Ezzedine, O.F.A.; Lin, G.; Kapa, S.; Borgeson, D.D.; Friedman, P.A.; et al. Artificial intelligence-enhanced electrocardiogram for the early detection of cardiac amyloidosis. In *Mayo Clinic Proceedings*; Elsevier: Amsterdam, The Netherlands, 2021.
119. Mehmood, A.; Iqbal, M.; Mehmood, Z.; Irtaza, A.; Nawaz, M.; Nazir, T.; Masood, M. Prediction of heart disease using deep convolutional neural networks. *Arab. J. Sci. Eng.* **2021**, *46*, 3409–3422. [CrossRef]
120. Available online: https://www.upgrad.com/blog/data-preprocessing-in-machine-learning (accessed on 25 December 2021).
121. Williams, P.A.; McCauley, V. Always connected: The security challenges of the healthcare internet of things. In Proceedings of the 2016 IEEE 3rd World Forum on Internet of Things (WF-IoT), Reston, VA, USA, 12–14 December 2016; pp. 30–35.

122. Soumyalatha, S.G.H. Study of iot: Understanding iot architecture, applications, issues and challenges. In Proceedings of the 1st International Conference on Innovations in Computing & Networking (ICICN16), Bengaluru, India, 12–13 May 2016.
123. Joyia, G.J.; Liaqat, R.M.; Farooq, A.; Rehman, S. Internet of medical things (IOMT): Applications, benefits and future challenges in healthcare domain. *J. Commun.* **2017**, *12*, 240–247. [CrossRef]
124. Shehabat, I.M.; Al-Hussein, N. Deploying internet of things in healthcare: Benefits, requirements, challenges and applications. *J. Commun.* **2018**, *13*, 574–580. [CrossRef]
125. Zhu, H.; Wu, C.K.; Koo, C.H.; Tsang, Y.T.; Liu, Y.; Chi, H.R.; Tsang, K.-F. Smart healthcare in the era of internet-of-things. *IEEE Consum. Electron. Mag.* **2019**, *8*, 26–30. [CrossRef]
126. de Michele, R.; Furini, M. Iot healthcare: Benefits, issues and challenges. In Proceedings of the 5th EAI International Conference on Smart Objects and Technologies for Social Good, Valencia, Spain, 25–27 September 2019; pp. 160–164.
127. Pavithr, K.; Saravanan, G. Iot, an emerging technology for next generation medical devices in support of cardiac health care—A comprehensive review. *Int. Res. J. Multidiscip. Technovat.* **2019**, *1*, 35–40. [CrossRef]
128. Asghari, P.; Rahmani, A.M.; Javadi, H.H.S. Internet of things applications: A systematic review. *Comput. Netw.* **2019**, *148*, 241–261. [CrossRef]
129. Birje, M.N.; Hanji, S.S. Internet of things based distributed healthcare systems: A review. *J. Data Inf. Manag.* **2020**, *2*, 149–165. [CrossRef]
130. Selvaraj, S.; Sundaravaradhan, S. Challenges and opportunities in iot healthcare systems: A systematic review. *SN Appl. Sci.* **2020**, *2*, 1–8. [CrossRef]
131. Al-Shargabi, B.; Abuarqoub, S. Iot-enabled healthcare: Benefits, issues and challenges. In Proceedings of the 4th International Conference on Future Networks and Distributed Systems (ICFNDS), St. Petersburg, Russia, 26–27 November 2020; pp. 1–5. [CrossRef]
132. Isravel, D.P.; Silas, S. A comprehensive review on the emerging iot-cloud based technologies for smart healthcare. In Proceedings of the 2020 6th International Conference on Advanced Computing and Communication Systems (ICACCS), Coimbatore, India, 6–7 March 2020; pp. 606–611.
133. Trayush, T.; Bathla, R.; Saini, S.; Shukla, V.K. Iot in healthcare: Challenges, benefits, applications, and opportunities. In Proceedings of the 2021 International Conference on Advance Computing and Innovative Technologies in Engineering (ICACITE), Greater Noida, India, 30–31 December 2021; pp. 107–111.
134. Tunc, M.A.; Gures, E.; Shayea, I. A survey on iot smart healthcare: Emerging technologies, applications, challenges, and future trends. *arXiv* **2021**, arXiv:2109.02042.
135. Tsoutsouras, V.; Azariadi, D.; Koliogewrgi, K.; Xydis, S.; Soudris, D. Software design and optimization of ecg signal analysis and diagnosis for embedded iot devices. In *Components and Services for IoT Platforms*; Springer International Publishing: Cham, Switzerland, 2017; pp. 299–322.
136. Alugubelli, R. Exploratory study of artificial intelligence in healthcare. *Int. J. Innov. Eng. Res. Technol.* **2016**, *3*, 1–10.
137. Kelly, C.J.; Karthikesalingam, A.; Suleyman, M.; Corrado, G.; King, D. Key challenges for delivering clinical impact with artificial intelligence. *BMC Med.* **2019**, *17*, 1–9. [CrossRef]
138. Bartoletti, I. Ai in healthcare: Ethical and privacy challenges. In Proceedings of the Conference on Artificial Intelligence in Medicine in Europe, Poznan, Poland, 26–29 June 2019; Springer International Publishing: Cham, Switzerland, 2019; pp. 7–10.
139. Racine, E.; Boehlen, W.; Sample, M. Healthcare uses of artificial intelligence: Challenges and opportunities for growth. In *Healthcare Management Forum*; SAGE Publications: Los Angeles, CA, USA, 2019; Volume 32, pp. 272–275.
140. Lehmann, L.S. Ethical challenges of integrating ai into healthcare. In *Artificial Intelligence in Medicine*; Springer International Publishing: Cham, Switzerland, 2020; pp. 1–5.
141. Qayyum, A.; Qadir, J.; Bilal, M.; Al-Fuqaha, A. Secure and robust machine learning for healthcare: A survey. *IEEE Rev. Biomed. Eng.* **2020**, *14*, 156–180. [CrossRef] [PubMed]
142. Shaheen, M.Y. AI in Healthcare: Medical and Socio-Economic Benefits and Challenges. *Sci. Prepr.* **2021**. [CrossRef]
143. Feeny, A.K.; Chung, M.K.; Madabhushi, A.; Attia, Z.I.; Cikes, M.; Firouznia, M.; Friedman, P.A.; Kalscheur, M.M.; Kapa, S.; Narayan, S.M.; et al. Artificial intelligence and machine learning in arrhythmias and cardiac electrophysiology. *Circ. Arrhythmia Electrophysiol.* **2020**, *13*, 007952. [CrossRef] [PubMed]
144. Hammoudeh, M.; Epiphaniou, G.; Belguith, S.; Unal, D.; Adebisi, B.; Baker, T.; Kayes, A.; Watters, P. A service-oriented approach for sensing in the internet of things: Intelligent transportation systems and privacy use cases. *IEEE Sens. J.* **2020**, *21*, 15753–15761. [CrossRef]
145. Abuarqoub, A. D-fap: Dual-factor authentication protocol for mobile cloud connected devices. *J. Sens. Actuator Netw.* **2020**, *9*, 1. [CrossRef]
146. Baig, M.M.; GholamHosseini, H.; Connolly, M.J. Mobile healthcare applications: System design review, critical issues and challenges. *Australas. Phys. Eng. Sci. Med.* **2015**, *38*, 23–38. [CrossRef]
147. Chen, H.; Chiang, R.H.; Storey, V.C. Business intelligence and analytics: From big data to big impact. *Mis Q.* **2012**, 1165–1188. [CrossRef]
148. Jiang, F.; Jiang, Y.; Zhi, H.; Dong, Y.; Li, H.; Ma, S.; Wang, Y.; Dong, Q.; Shen, H.; Wang, Y. Artificial intelligence in healthcare: Past, present and future. *Stroke Vasc. Neurol.* **2017**, *2*, 230–243. [CrossRef]

149. Magrabi, F.; Ammenwerth, E.; McNair, J.B.; de Keizer, N.F.; Hypponen, H.; Anen, P.N.; Rigby, M.; Scott, P.J.; Vehko, T.; Wong, Z.S.-Y.; et al. Artificial intelligence in clinical decision support: Challenges for evaluating ai and practical implications. *Yearb. Med. Inform.* **2019**, *28*, 128–134. [CrossRef]
150. ElSaadany, M. A Novel Iot-Based Wireless System to Monitor Heart Rate. Ph.D. Thesis, Miami University, Oxford, OH, USA, 2017.
151. Lin, F.; Song, C.; Zhuang, Y.; Xu, W.; Li, C.; Ren, K. Cardiac scan: A non-contact and continuous heart-based user authentication system. In Proceedings of the 23rd Annual International Conference on Mobile Computing and Networking, Salt Lake City, UT, USA, 16–20 October 2017; pp. 315–328.
152. Casas, J.; Irfan, B.; Senft, E.; Gutierrez, L.; Rincon-Roncancio, M.; Munera, M.; Belpaeme, T.; Cifuentes, C.A. Social assistive robot for cardiac rehabilitation: A pilot study with patients with angioplasty. In Proceedings of the Companion of the 2018 ACM/IEEE International Conference on Human-Robot Interaction, Chicago, IL, USA, 5–8 March 2018; pp. 79–80.
153. Geurts, E.; Hansen, D.; Dendale, P.; Coninx, K. Impact of a mobile cycling application on cardiac patients' cycling behavior and enjoyment. In Proceedings of the 11th PErvasive Technologies Related to Assistive Environments Conference, Corfu, Greece, 26–29 June 2018; pp. 257–264.
154. El-kenawy, E.-S.M.; Eid, M.; Ibrahim, A. An advanced patient health monitoring system. *J. Comput. Sci. Inf. Syst.* **2021**, *17*, 1–7.
155. Savaridass, M.P.; Ikram, N.; Deepika, R.; Aarnika, R. Development of smart health monitoring system using internet of things. *Mater. Today Proc.* **2021**, *45*, 986–989. [CrossRef]

sensors

MDPI

Review

Deep Learning for LiDAR Point Cloud Classification in Remote Sensing

Ahmed Diab [1], Rasha Kashef [2,*] and Ahmed Shaker [1,*]

[1] Department of Civil Engineering, Toronto Metropolitan University, Toronto, ON M5B 2K3, Canada
[2] Electrical, Computer, and Biomedical Engineering, Toronto Metropolitan University, Toronto, ON M5B 2K3, Canada
* Correspondence: rkashef@ryerson.ca (R.K.); ahmed.shaker@ryerson.ca (A.S.)

Abstract: Point clouds are one of the most widely used data formats produced by depth sensors. There is a lot of research into feature extraction from unordered and irregular point cloud data. Deep learning in computer vision achieves great performance for data classification and segmentation of 3D data points as point clouds. Various research has been conducted on point clouds and remote sensing tasks using deep learning (DL) methods. However, there is a research gap in providing a road map of existing work, including limitations and challenges. This paper focuses on introducing the state-of-the-art DL models, categorized by the structure of the data they consume. The models' performance is collected, and results are provided for benchmarking on the most used datasets. Additionally, we summarize the current benchmark 3D datasets publicly available for DL training and testing. In our comparative study, we can conclude that convolutional neural networks (CNNs) achieve the best performance in various remote-sensing applications while being light-weighted models, namely Dynamic Graph CNN (DGCNN) and ConvPoint.

Keywords: point clouds; deep learning; remote sensing

Citation: Diab, A.; Kashef, R.; Shaker, A. Deep Learning for LiDAR Point Cloud Classification in Remote Sensing. *Sensors* **2022**, *22*, 7868. https://doi.org/10.3390/s22207868

Academic Editors: Andrei Velichko, Dmitry Korzun and Alexander Meigal

Received: 12 September 2022
Accepted: 9 October 2022
Published: 16 October 2022

1. Introduction

The light detection and ranging (LiDAR) mapping generate precise spatial information about the shape and surface components of the Earth. Advancements in LiDAR mapping systems and their technologies have been proven to examine natural and manmade environments across various scales with higher accuracy, precision, and flexibility [1]. LiDAR Remote sensing provides an accurate 3D representation of scanned areas with many features that provide great performance for various applications. Such applications include Digital Elevation Model (DEM), Digital Surface Model (DSM), and Digital Terrain Model (DTM) generation, which, combined with intensity data, achieve excellent performance in urban land cover classification [2]. Some other urban applications include pavement crack detection [3], collapsed building detection [4], road markings and fixtures extraction and classification [5], cultural heritage classification [6], and change detection [7]. Because LiDAR is sensitive to variations in vertical vegetation structure, it makes it very effective for natural resources [8] and forest applications [7], such as tree species classification [9]. Additionally, full-waveform LiDAR adds more advantages to using LiDAR in forestry applications [10].

Various deep learning models have been developed with outstanding performance for data classification on point cloud datasets in multiple applications. Existing deep learning methods for point cloud classifications involve architectures based on the traditional neural network, the Multi-Layer Perceptron (MLP). These models are called PointNet-Based as they build on the pioneering work of PointNet [11]. PointNet is a great performer that is very lightweight but suffers from local information loss. Global features are features of a scene, object, or image that describe it as a whole, compared to local features that are extracted at different points and represent patches of the scene or image [12]. PointNet++ [13]

mitigates the loss by building a feature aggregation pyramid to learn hierarchically, similar to how a traditional Convolutional network learns. One of the biggest challenges of using LiDAR point clouds in deep learning is the unstructured shapes of the point cloud data; a convolutional kernel that works on uniform grid-structured data cannot be directly applied to the raw point cloud. A convolutional neural network can better capture spatial features, which performs better than a traditional neural network while being more lightweight than most handcrafted models. The convolutional neural network is structured as a convolution layer, non-linearity, e.g., Rectified linear unit (ReLU), and pooling layers to distil features from low-level to high-level [14]. Applying CNNs on point clouds involves the 2D projection of the point cloud to obtain images that can then be fed into traditional convolution layers in a convolutional neural network. Another approach is resampling or restructuring the point cloud into uniform volumetric grids using occupancy functions and 3D convolutional layers to create the CNN or to design novel convolutional layers that can operate on pointsets and the custom convolution operation to build the CNN.

This paper provides a roadmap for current DL deep learning models for LiDAR point cloud classifications in remote sensing. Existing deep learning methods can be classified as projection-based and point-based models. Each category enjoys specific characteristics; however, they show some limitations. Thus, this paper summarizes the significant subcategories: 2D projection, Multiview projection, voxelization, Convolutional-based networks, and graph convolutional networks. Additionally, we cover some examples that encompass most of the fundamentals within each subcategory. Remote sensing applications require different datasets or workflows; thus, we cover some examples from remote sensing that employ or build upon computer vision models. Our comparative analysis shows that DGCNN and ConvPoint have shown the best performance in various remote-sensing applications while being light-weighted models. The rest of this paper can be organized as Section 2 focuses on LiDAR point cloud data and processing overview, Section 3 introduces the primary computer vision deep learning models that are often used to classify 3D data, and Section 4 presents Point cloud computing tasks that are common in remote sensing applications, Section 5 introduces the benchmark 3D datasets used in training and testing of deep learning models grouped as objects, indoor, arial scanned, mobile scanned, and terrestrial scanned datasets, Section 6 shows the evaluation metrics commonly used to measure and benchmark model performance; Section 7 provides a comparative analysis of existing models on different datasets for different classification tasks. Finally, Section 8 concludes the paper.

2. LiDAR Point Clouds

A typical LiDAR system in remote sensing uses a laser, Global Positioning System (GPS) and an Inertial Measurement Unit (IMU) to approximate the heights of objects on the ground. Discrete LiDAR data are generated; each point represents high energy points along with rebounded energy. Discrete LiDAR points contain each point's x, y, and z values. The z value is used to obtain height. The LiDAR data can estimate surface structures with various methods [15]. The raw LiDAR data are delivered as points, known as point clouds, that can be further processed to create Digital Elevation Models (DEMs) or Triangulated Irregular Networks (TINs) [1]. Point data are commonly stored in LAS (LASer) format, regarded as an industry standard that contains information in a binary file specific to the LiDAR nature of data without being complex [15]. The LiDAR data can also contain other information such as the intensity of the rebounds, the point classification (if applicable), number of returns, time, and source of each point [1,15]. LiDAR scanners use a laser pulse to measure the distance from the sensor using the time for the laser pulse to return in the case of time-of-flight sensors (Figure 1a) [16] or using the triangulation angle on the optical sensor for triangulation-based scanners (Figure 1b) [17]. The LiDAR scanners then generate an [x, y, z] position relative to the sensor's locations based on the distance from the sensor and the degrees of rotation of the sensor, such as pitch, roll, and yaw [18]. Most LiDAR sensors also measure the intensity of the return signal, which can be used to differentiate between different surface types with different reflectivity [1]. Additionally, the sensor is often paired with a GPS and an IMU to capture data required for georeferencing and mapping of the point cloud.

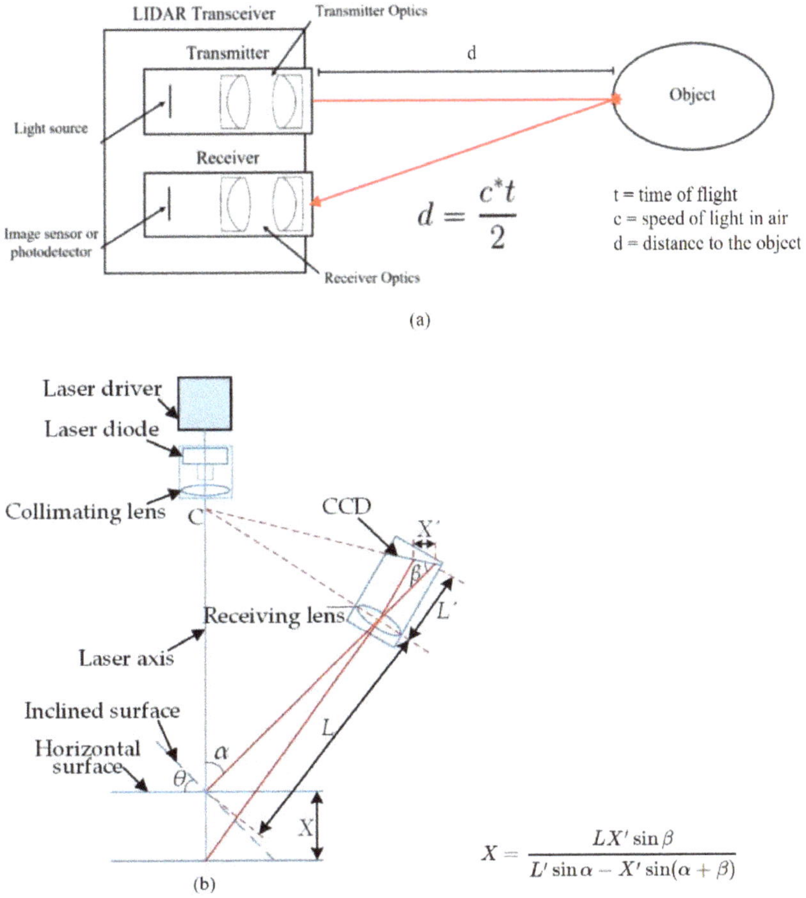

$$d = \frac{c^* t}{2}$$

$$X = \frac{LX' \sin\beta}{L' \sin\alpha - X' \sin(\alpha+\beta)}$$

Figure 1. Time of Flight LiDAR sensor calculation (**a**) [16] and triangulation-based LiDAR calculation (**b**) [17].

For supervised classification, a significant challenge when working on LiDAR point clouds is the variation in density inherent in the nature of the data. The density of similar objects is also varied, as it depends on the speed of the vehicle mounting the sensor. Some areas will be too dense and expensive to process, requiring some form of downsampling. Other regions of a point cloud will have few or no points present. Additionally, for LiDAR point clouds that include intensity values, the intensity of the same object could be affected by different conditions and result in the same object having slightly different intensities [18].

3. Point Cloud Computing

Remote sensing data go through multiple processing steps to generate information that can be consumed for production. Over the past few years, deep learning has been applied to almost all remote sensing data processing aspects. Most notably, classification and segmentation tasks. Regarding remote sensing 3D LiDAR point clouds, there is limited interest in whole scene classification and more in semantic classification or segmentation tasks. Some other examples of deep learning tasks tackled by deep learning include change detection, registration, fusion, and completion.

Traditionally, deep learning classification describes classifying an entire scene or an object as belonging to a specific class as a whole. One example of classification tasks that use 3D point clouds in remote sensing is the classification of tree species or roof types previously segmented. However, remote sensing classification tasks involve semantic classification and segmentation rather than aiming to identify an entire scene or object to a single class. A significant example of semantic classification is Land use/Land cover classification of Terrestrial and Arial Laser scanned (TLS/ALS) data. Segmentation divides and assigns the data into different target classes and is split into three types, semantic, instance, and panoptic segmentation [19]. Semantic segmentation assigns every point/pixel from the input data to one of the target classes without distinguishing different objects; for example, all tree points will be labelled trees. Instance segmentation involves identifying and labelling objects belonging to target classes while distinguishing them from each other, such as tree1, tree2, etc. Panoptic segmentation classifies every point/pixel in the input as part of a class while distinguishing separate objects of a class from each other [19].

The most common application of image fusion in LiDAR remote sensing is the fusion of 3D point clouds and RGB images to train a deep learning model for classification and segmentation tasks [20–22]. The features extracted from both types of data are used to enhance the performance of each class in the application of each class. Registration is the process of matching and aligning two or more images or point clouds in the case of LiDAR data obtained from different viewpoints and/or using different sensors; one example is illustrated in [23], which achieves state-of-the-art performance. Completion is the process of filling in missing information from datasets that could result from the limitations of the sensors, conditions at the time of data capture, or the method of capture. For far-away distances, the spatial resolution of a LiDAR sensor is lower, sometimes resulting in finer details, such as road markings, signs, poles, etc., showing up incomplete. One example of completion can be found in [5]. Most completion tasks on LiDAR point clouds are done before training a classification model to improve performance and robustness.

4. Deep Learning Models

Advances have been made to produce DL models that are lightweight and efficient. Feature learning models on 3D point clouds can be categorized as projection-based and point-based models. This section briefly discusses models used as backbones or improved for newer networks.

4.1. Projection-Based Methods

Some projection-based models create 2D projections from 3D point clouds and use traditional 2D feature learning. This process primarily depends on projection direction (X, Y or Z—default: Z) and other aspects such as the grid (size, scale, shape). Other projection models create volumetric grids or voxels through 3D feature extraction layers.

- 2D Convolutional Neural Networks

U-Net [24]: builds on a fully convolutional model and extends it to work with few training data while providing better performance. The U-Net architecture consists of repeated two unpadded 3×3 convolutions followed by ReLU and downsampling 2×2 max pooling with stride 2. For each convolution step, the number of feature channels is doubled. In the deconvolution steps, the features are upsampled and followed by a 2×2 convolution that halves the number of channels. The resulting feature map goes through cropping and two 3×3 convolutions followed by a ReLU. The cropping is necessary because of the border pixels lost after every convolution. Finally, a 1×1 convolution is applied to label pixels and generate segmentation results.

DeepLab [25]: employs atrous convolution [25,26] to change the scope of convolution and extract global features while also allowing larger networks without extra parameters. DeepLab proposes Atrous Spatial Pyramid Pooling (ASPP) to segment at different scales by applying the same filters at different sampling rates and field-of-views, then the outputs are added together. To overcome the toll downsampling and max pooling operations in deep convolutional neural networks (DCNNs), DeepLab implements the fully connected Conditional Random Field (CRF) from [27], which is trained separately from the rest of the network. Iterations DeepLabV3 [28] and DeepLabV3+ [29] improve the performance of DeepLab. Unlike [25], DeepLabV3 [28] performs batch normalization within ASPP. Additionally, global average pooling is applied to the last feature map. The resulting image-level features are fed into a 1×1 convolution with 256 filters, then multiplied to the desired spatial dimension. DeepLabV3 abandons the CRF and replaces it with concatenating and aggregating the resulting features and passing them through another 1×1 convolution with 256 filters before computing the final logits. DeepLabV3+ [29] uses a decoder module to refine segmentation results, especially around object boundaries. Depth-wise separable convolutions are applied to ASPP pooling and decoder modules resulting in a faster and more robust network.

VGGNet [30] evaluates the effect of increasing the network depth of a convolutional network using very small 3×3 convolution filters. It improves the classification performance compared to previous state-of-the-art models by pushing the depth to 16–19 weight layers. ResNet [31] adopts residual learning to every stacked layer in the convolutional network. The shortcut connections are added without increasing parameter or computation complexity. The residual learning allows deep networks with performance gain over shallower networks.

- Multiview representation

MVCNN [32] tackles 3D feature learning using traditional image-focused networks by making 2D renders of the 3D object from different angles and passing it through a standard CNN. MVCNN generates 80 views of the 3D object by placing 20 virtual "cameras" pointed at the object's centroid, then generates 4 renders per camera at 0-, 90-, 180-, and 270-degree rotation along the axis through the camera and object center. After each image is passed through the first CNN, the outputs are aggregated at a view-pooling layer which performs element-wise maximum operation across the different input views before passing through the remaining section of the network, i.e., the second CNN.

- Volumetric grid representation

VoxNet [33] uses occupancy grids to efficiently estimate occupied, free, and unknown space provided by ranging measurements. Small ($32 \times 32 \times 32$ voxels) dense voxels are used to optimize GPU usage. VoxNet uses a more basic 3D CNN to extract and learn features, consisting of 5 of two convolution layers, a convolution and pooling layer, and two fully connected layers. The model can perform object classification in real-time while achieving state-of-the-art performance. VoxelNet [34] introduces a multi-layer voxel feature encoding (VFE) that enables inter-point interaction within a voxel. The point cloud is divided into equally spaced voxels encoded using the stacked VFE layers, allowing complex local 3D information learning. VoxelNet works on object detection using a Region Proposal Network (RPN) at the final stage to create bounding boxes.

4.2. Point-Based Methods

Point-based methods consume unstructured and unordered point clouds. Some of the models covered in this section are used as backbones or parts of a larger architecture, while others are adapted for remote sensing tasks with minimal modifications.

- PointNets

PointNet [11] directly consumes point cloud data for feature extraction. The network provides a unified approach to 3D recognition that can be applied for various tasks such as object classification, instance segmentation, and semantic segmentation. PointNet uses Multi-Layer Perceptrons (MLPs) combined with a joint alignment network. To hold invariance under geometric transformations, the input is passed through a T-Net module [11], where it is multiplied by an affine transformation matrix. PointNet provides great performance while remaining lightweight and computationally efficient. PointNet cannot produce local features of neighbouring points; PointNet++ [13] introduces a class pyramid feature aggregation scheme. The scheme comprises three stacked layers: the sampling layer, the grouping layer, and the PointNet layer. This allows PointNet++ to extract features in a hierarchical fashion similar to traditional image learning, reducing local information loss. PointASNL [35] is an end-to-end network that effectively deals with noisy point clouds. The two primary components of the model are the adaptive sampling (AS) and the local-nonlocal (L-NL) modules. Initially, the AS module reweighs neighbour points surrounding the initial sampled points from the farthest point sampling and then adaptively adjusts the sampled points beyond the point cloud. The L-NL module captures the neighbour and long-range dependencies of the sampled point. Self-Organizing Network (SO-Net) [36] generates a Self-Organizing Map (SOM) to simulate point cloud spatial distribution. The SOM retrieves hierarchical features from individual points and SOM nodes. A Point-to-node search is performed on the output of the SOM for each point. Each point is normalized, and features are learned through a series of fully connected layers. Node feature extraction is done through channel-wise max-pooling the point features. Final learned features are extracted using a batch of fully connected layers referred to as a small PointNet.

- (Graph) Convolutional Point Networks

ConvPoint [37] proposes continuous convolution kernels to allow arbitrary point cloud sizes. Points {q} are selected iteratively from the input point cloud {p} until the target number of points is reached through a score-based process. Using a kd-tree built on the input point cloud, K-nearest neighbour search from {p} is performed on points in {q}. A convolution operation is performed for each subset, generating the output features. Operations detailed by ConvPoint are successfully adapted for classification, part segmentation, and semantic segmentation tasks. ConvPoint can produce significant performance with time- and cost-efficient. Dynamic Graph CNN (DGCNN) [38] generates local neighbourhood graphs and applies convolution on the edges connecting neighbour point pairs. Unlike traditional graph CNNs, DGCNN uses a dynamic graph where the set of k-nearest neighbours for a point change between layers in the network and is calculated from the sequence of embeddings. The EdgeConv block introduced by DGCNN computes edge features for each input point and applies an MLP followed by channel-wise symmetric aggregation. Taylor Gaussian mixture model (GMM) network (TGNet) [39] is composed of units named TGConv that perform convolution operations parametrized by a family of filters on irregular point sets. The filters are products of geometric features expressed by Gaussian weighted Taylor kernels and local point features extracted from local coordinates. TGConv features are aggregated using parametric pooling to generate feature vectors for each point. TGNet uses a CRF at the output layer to improve segmentation results.

5. Benchmark Datasets

Advancements in Deep learning on point clouds have attracted more and more attention, especially in the last few years. Several publicly available datasets were also released, which helped further support research on DL development. An increasing number of methods have been introduced to deal with various challenges related to point cloud processing, including 3D shape classification, 3D object detection and tracking, 3D point cloud segmentation, 3D point cloud registration, 6-DOF pose estimation, and 3D reconstruction [18]. Table 1 briefly overviews some of the most commonly used publicly available point cloud datasets. Outdoor datasets are classified based on acquisition technique, Aerial, Mobile, or Terrestrial Laser scanned data or ALS, MLS, and TLS, respectively. The remaining datasets in this paper are indoor laser-scanned datasets and datasets of object scans. While ModelNet40 and S3DIS are not LiDAR scanned datasets, they are included as we found that they are the most commonly tested datasets for their respective tasks in remote sensing classifications. ModelNet40 dataset consists of CAD files; most point cloud network testing uses a point cloud sampled from the 3D object files. The models that used the ModelNet40 dataset outlined later in the paper are tested on the dataset by sampling the objects into a point cloud and then applying the model. Similarly, S3DIS, while not LiDAR data, is a point cloud and the models tested on it are suitable for point clouds obtained from LiDAR scans.

Table 1. Benchmark datasets for training and testing deep learning on 3D point clouds.

Dataset	Data Type	Data Format	Points/Objects	No. of Classes	Density
ModelNet40 [40]	3D CAD	OFF Files	127,915 Models	40	N/A
ISPRS 3D Vaihingen [41]	ALS LiDAR	x, y, z, reflectance, return count	780.9 K pts	9	4–8 pts/m^2
Hessigheim 3D [42]	ALS LiDAR	x, y, z, intensity, return count	59.4 M training pts, 14.5 M validation pts	11	800 pts/m^2
2019 IEEE GRSS Data fusion contest [43]	ALS LiDAR	x, y, z, intensity, return count	83.7 M training pts, 83.7 M validation pts	6	Very dense
AHN(3) [44]	ALS LiDAR	x, y, z, intensity, return count, additional normalization, and location data	190.3 M pts	5	20 pts/m^2
RoofN3D [45]	ALS LiDAR	multipoints, multipolygons	118.1 K roofs	3	4.72 pts/m^2
semanticKITTI [46]	MLS LiDAR	x, y, z, reflectance, GPS data	4.549 K pts	25 (28)	Sparse
S3DIS [47]	Indoor Structured-light 3D scanner	x, y, z, r, g, b	215.0 M pts	12	35,800 pts/m^2
Paris-Lille-3D [48]	MLS LiDAR	x, y, z, reflectance, additional position data	143.1 M pts	10 coarse (50 total)	1000–2000 pts/m^2
Toronto3D [49]	MLS LiDAR	x, y, z, r, g, b, intensity, additional position data	78.3 M pts	8	1000 pts/m^2
ArCH [50]	TLS LiDAR, TLS+ALS LiDAR	x, y, z, r, g, b, normalized coordinates	102.1 M training pts, 34.0 M testing pts	6–9 depending on the scene	subsampled differently depending on the scene
Semantic3D [51]	TLS LiDAR	x, y, z, intensity, r, g, b	4.0 B pts	8	Very dense
3D Forest [52]	TLS LiDAR	x, y, z, intensity	467.2 K pts	4	15–40 pts/m^2

6. Performance Metrics

Various evaluation metrics have been used for segmentation, detection, and classification. The summary of the evaluation metrics [53] is shown in Table 2. Metrics for segmentation, detection, and classification are the intersection over union (IoU), mean IoU, and overall accuracy (OA) [53]. Detection and classification results are mainly analyzed using precision, recall and F1-score, which takes the true positives (TP), false positives (FP), and false negatives (FN) for calculation.

Table 2. Performance Evaluation Metrics.

Metric	Formula	
IoU	$IoU_i = \frac{c_{ii}}{c_{ii}+\sum_{j\neq i} c_{ij}+\sum_{k\neq i} c_{ki}}$	Where *cij* is ground truth class, *i* predicted as *j*
mIoU	$mIoU = \frac{\sum_{i=1}^{N} IoU_i}{N}$	Where N is the number of classes
OA	$OA = \frac{\sum_{i=1}^{N} c_{ii}}{\sum_{j=1}^{N} \sum_{k=1}^{N} c_{jk}}$	
Precision	$Precision = \frac{TP}{TP+FP}$	
Recall	$Recall = \frac{TP}{TP+FN}$	
F_1 score	$F_1 = \frac{2TP}{2TP+FP+FN}$	
Average precision (AP)	$AP = \frac{1}{11} \sum_{r\in\{0,1,\ldots,1\}} max_{:\geq r} p()$	
Kappa coefficient	$K = \frac{N\sum_{i=1}^{k} x_{ii} - \sum_{i=1}^{k}(x_{i+} \times x_{+i})}{N^2 - \sum_{i=1}^{k}(x_{i+} \times x_{+i})}$	

7. Comparative Analysis

The datasets ModelNet40, S3DIS, and Toronto3D provide an overview of benchmarks used for different classification tasks: object classification, indoor scene classification, and urban outdoor classification. Table 3 shows the performance comparison for the current 3D object classification, indoor scene segmentation, and outdoor urban semantic segmentation models using various evaluation metrics. The best-performing configuration for each model was selected. For example, using a higher sampled point cloud in ModelNet40 tests can produce better performance. Therefore, if the authors tested the models using different point counts, the best set of results is used. The results outlined in the table are obtained from the testing by each model's respective author(s) except for the ConvPoint results on Toronto3D, which we tested for this paper. From Table 3, we can see that DGCNN and ConvPoint achieve the best performance on most datasets while being lightweight relative to models with similar performance. Additionally, these two models have been tested on multiple different tasks and different types of datasets. The major limitation of ConvPoint is that the convolutional layer introduced is a scale agnostic, i.e., the object's size is important for scans and provides valuable information. DGCNN could be further improved by adjusting the implementation details to improve the computational efficiency of the model.

Most remote sensing papers use one of the previously outlined computer vision models. The model is deployed directly for the application dataset or modified and attached to post and/or preprocess pipelines. To further test the performance of the ConvPoint model in this paper, we have also experimentally trained ConvPoint on Toronto3D using labels such as L001, L003, and L004 and used L002 for testing. The training was run using batch size 8, block size 8, and #of points 8192 for 100 Epochs. The testing results are marked with a (*) in Table 4. Table 4 includes some applications categorized according to their dataset, performance, and remote sensing deployment. We can conclude that both DGCNN and ConvPoint have shown promising results across the different applications in remote sensing.

Table 3. Comparative Analysis of Deployed Models.

ModelNet40 Object Classification										
Method	**OA**			**Class Average Accuracy**						
PointNet [11]	89.2			86.2						
PointNet++ [13]	91.9			-						
ConvPoint [37]	92.5			89.6						
DGCNN [38]	93.5			90.7						
MVCNN [32]	90.1			79.5						
FKAConv [54]	92.5			89.5						
VoxNet [33]	83.0			-						
SO-Net [36]	93.4			90.8						
PointASNL [35]	93.2			-						
S3DIS Indoor Semantic segmentation										
Method	**OA**			**mIOU**						
PointNet [11]	78.62			47.71						
ConvPoint/Fusion [37]	85.2/88.8			62.6/68.2						
DGCNN [38]	84.1			56.1						
PointASNL [35]	-			68.7						
TGNet [39]	88.5			57.8						
FKAConv [54]	-			68.4						
Toronto3D Urban MLS Semantic segmentation										
Method	**OA**	**mIoU**	**Road**	**Road mrk.**	**Natural**	**Bldg**	**Util. line**	**Pole**	**Car**	**Fence**
PointNet++ [13]	84.88	41.81	89.27	0.00	69.00	54.10	43.70	23.30	52.00	3.00
DGCNN [38]	94.24	61.79	93.88	0.00	91.25	80.39	62.40	62.32	88.26	15.81
TGNet [39]	94.08	61.34	93.54	0.00	90.83	81.57	65.26	62.98	88.73	7.85
MSAAN [55]	95.90	75.00	96.10	59.90	94.40	85.40	85.80	77.00	83.70	17.70
ConvPoint * [37]	96.07	74.82	97.07	54.83	93.55	90.60	82.9	76.19	92.93	12.42
[56]	93.6	70.8	92.2	53.8	92.8	86.0	72.2	72.5	75.7	21.2

Table 4. Overview of some deep learning contributions focused on remote sensing data.

Paper	**Category**	**Architecture(s) Based on/ Proposed**	**Test Dataset**	**Performance** [1]	**Application**
[5]	2D Projection	CNN, cGAN	TUM MLS 2016	85.04 *	Road marking extraction, classification, and completion
[57]	2D Projection	1D CNN, 2D CNN, LSTM DNN	ISPRS 3D Vaihingen	79.4 *	ALS Point cloud classification
[56]	2D projection Point CNN	3D Convolution U-Net	Toronto3D	70.8 ^	MLS Point cloud semantic segmentation
[58]	Multi-view Projection	MVCNN	RoofN3D	99 * Saddleback 96 * Two-sided Hip 83 * Pyramid	Roof Classification
[59]	Voxelization	Clustering, Voxelization, 3D CNN	ISPRS 3D Vaihingen	79.60 *	ALS Point cloud classification

Table 4. *Cont.*

Paper	Category	Architecture(s) Based on/ Proposed	Test Dataset	Performance [1]	Application
[60]	Voxelization, 2D projection	DenseNet201	ISPRS 3D Vaihingen	83.62 *	ALS Point cloud classification
[61]	PointNet/MLP/FCL	PointNet++, Joint Manifold Learning, Global Graph-based	ISPRS 3D Vaihingen AHN3	66.2 * 83.7 *	ALS Point cloud classification
[62]	PointNet/MLP/FCL	PointNet++	Proprietary	95.4 ~	TLS Forest Point cloud Semantic Segmentation
[21]	PointNet/MLP/FCL	MSSCN, MLP, Spatial Aggregation Network	S3DIS ScanNet	89.8 ~ 86.3 ~	Point Cloud Semantic Segmentation
[55]	PointNet/MLP/FCL	MSAAN, RandLA-Net	CSPC (scene-2, scene-5) Toronto3D	64.5 ^, 61.8 ^, 75.0 ^	Point Cloud Semantic Segmentation
[63]	PointNet/MLP/FCL	PointNet T-Nets, FWNet, 1D CNN	ZORZI et al. 2019	76 *	Full-Waveform LiDAR Semantic Segmentation
[64]	Point CNN	Dconv, CNN, U-Net	ISPRS 3D Vaihingen	70.7 *	ALS Point cloud classification
[65]	Point CNN	ConvPoint, CNN	Saint-Jean NB (provincial website) Montreal QC (CMM)	96.6 ^ 69.9 ^	ALS Point cloud classification
[66]	Voxelization 3D CNN	3D CNN, DQN	ISPRS 3D Vaihingen	98.0 ~	Point cloud classification and reconstruction
[67]	Graph/Point CNN	Graph attention CNN	ISPRS 3D Vaihingen	71.5 *	ALS Point cloud classification
[68]	Graph/Point CNN	DGCNN	AHN3	89.7 *	ALS Point cloud classification
[6]	Graph/Point CNN	DGCNN	ArCH	81.4 *	Cultural Heritage point cloud segmentation

[1] f1-Score is denoted by *, mIOU is denoted by ^ and OA is denoted by ~.

8. Conclusions and Future Directions

Recent work on the advances of deep learning on LiDAR 3D point cloud processing was analyzed and summarized. An overview of the different model types and the state-of-the-art and/or fundamental models of each type was provided. Additionally, the performance of the models was provided on datasets for different classification tasks. The strongest performing models were trending towards 3D Graph CNNs and 3D CNNs [69,70] that work directly on the raw point cloud data. These models can provide state-of-the-art performance and remain computationally lightweight. Finally, different applications of remote sensing that deploy deep learning models were overviewed. One major challenge when comparing the remote sensing models was the lack of standardized test datasets and the frequent use of proprietary datasets. Notable test datasets available are Toronto3D, Paris-Lille 3D, ISPRS 3D, and S3dIS. Future Directions would involve expanding the application of the state-of-the-art methods in autonomous driving [71,72].

Author Contributions: Conceptualization, A.D., R.K. and A.S.; methodology, A.D., R.K. and A.S.; software, A.D., R.K. and A.S.; validation, A.D., R.K. and A.S.; formal analysis, A.D., R.K. and A.S.; investigation, A.D., R.K. and A.S.; resources, A.D., R.K. and A.S.; data curation, A.D., R.K. and A.S.; writing—original draft preparation, A.D., R.K. and A.S.; writing—review and editing, A.D., R.K. and A.S.; visualization, A.D., R.K. and A.S.; supervision, R.K. and A.S.; project administration, R.K. and A.S.; funding acquisition, R.K. and A.S.; All authors have read and agreed to the published version of the manuscript.

Funding: This research was funded by the Natural Sciences and Engineering Research Council of Canada (NSERC), grant number [RGPIN-2020-05857], and Smart Campus Integrated Platform Development Alliance project with FuseForward. The APC was funded by Toronto Metropolitan University.

Institutional Review Board Statement: Not applicable.

Informed Consent Statement: Not applicable.

Data Availability Statement: Not applicable.

Acknowledgments: We acknowledge the support of the Natural Sciences and Engineering Research Council of Canada (NSERC), [funding reference number RGPIN-2020-05857], and Smart Campus Integrated Platform Development Alliance project with FuseForward.

Conflicts of Interest: The authors declare no conflict of interest.

References

1. Carter, J.; Schmid, K.; Waters, K.; Betzhold, L.; Hadley, B.; Mataosky, R.; Halleran, J. Lidar 101: An Introduction to Lidar Technology, Data, and Applications. (NOAA) Coastal Services Center. Available online: https://coast.noaa.gov/data/digitalcoast/pdf/lidar-101.pdf (accessed on 13 April 2022).
2. Yan, W.Y.; Shaker, A.; El-Ashmawy, N. Urban land cover classification using airborne LiDAR data: A review. *Remote Sens. Environ.* **2015**, *158*, 295–310. [CrossRef]
3. Zhong, M.; Sui, L.; Wang, Z.; Hu, D. Pavement Crack Detection from Mobile Laser Scanning Point Clouds Using a Time Grid. *Sensors* **2020**, *20*, 4198. [CrossRef]
4. Xiu, H.; Shinohara, T.; Matsuoka, M.; Inoguchi, M.; Kawabe, K.; Horie, K. Collapsed Building Detection Using 3D Point Clouds and Deep Learning. *Remote Sens.* **2020**, *12*, 4057. [CrossRef]
5. Wen, C.; Sun, X.; Li, J.; Wang, C.; Guo, Y.; Habib, A. A deep learning framework for road marking extraction, classification and completion from mobile laser scanning point clouds. *ISPRS J. Photogramm. Remote Sens.* **2018**, *147*, 178–192. [CrossRef]
6. Pierdicca, R.; Paolanti, M.; Matrone, F.; Martini, M.; Morbidoni, C.; Malinverni, E.S.; Frontoni, E.; Lingua, A.M. Point Cloud Semantic Segmentation Using a Deep Learning Framework for Cultural Heritage. *Remote Sens.* **2020**, *12*, 1005. [CrossRef]
7. Dong, P.; Chen, Q. *LiDAR Remote Sensing and Applications*; CRC Press Taylor & Francis Group: Boca Raton, FL, USA, 2018.
8. Evans, J.S.; Hudak, A.T.; Faux, R.; Smith, A.M.S. Discrete Return Lidar in Natural Resources: Recommendations for Project Planning, Data Processing, and Deliverables. *Remote Sens.* **2009**, *1*, 776–794. [CrossRef]
9. Michałowska, M.; Rapiński, J. A Review of Tree Species Classification Based on Airborne LiDAR Data and Applied Classifiers. *Remote Sens.* **2021**, *13*, 353. [CrossRef]
10. Pirotti, F. Analysis of full-waveform LiDAR data for forestry applications: A review of investigations and methods. *iForest-Biogeosci. For.* **2011**, *4*, 100–106. [CrossRef]
11. Qi, C.R.; Su, H.; Mo, K.; Guibas, L.J. Pointnet: Deep learning on point sets for 3d classification and segmentation. In Proceedings of the IEEE Conference on Computer Vision and Pattern Recognition, Honolulu, HI, USA, 21–26 July 2017; pp. 652–660.
12. Lisin, D.A.; Mattar, M.A.; Blaschko, M.B.; Benfield, M.C.; Learned-Mille, E.G. Combining Local and Global Image Features for Object Class Recognition. In Proceedings of the Conference on Computer Vision and Pattern Recognition (CVPR'05)-Workshops, San Diego, CA, USA, 20–26 June 2005.
13. Qi, C.R.; Yi, L.; Su, H.; Guibas, L.J. Pointnet++: Deep hierarchical feature learning on point sets in a metric space. *Adv. Neural Inf. Process. Syst.* **2017**, *30*.
14. Liu, W.; Sun, J.; Li, W.; Hu, T.; Wang, P. Deep Learning on Point Clouds and Its Application: A Survey. *Sensors* **2019**, *19*, 4188. [CrossRef] [PubMed]
15. Wasser, L.A. The Basics of LiDAR—Light Detection and Ranging—Remote Sensing. NSF NEON | Open Data to Understand our Ecosystems, 22 October 2020. Available online: https://www.neonscience.org/resources/learning-hub/tutorials/lidar-basics (accessed on 1 September 2022).
16. Varshney, V. LiDAR: The Eyes of an Autonomous Vehicle. Available online: https://medium.com/swlh/lidar-the-eyes-of-an-autonomous-vehicle-82c6252d1101 (accessed on 15 August 2022).
17. Dong, Z.; Sun, X.; Chen, C.; Sun, M. A Fast and On-Machine Measuring System Using the Laser Displacement Sensor for the Contour Parameters of the Drill Pipe Thread. *Sensors* **2018**, *18*, 1192. [CrossRef]

18. Ioannidou, A.; Chatzilari, E.; Nikolopoulos, S.; Kompatsiaris, I. Deep learning advances in computer vision with 3D data: A survey. *ACM Comput. Surv.* **2017**, *50*, 1–38. [CrossRef]
19. Kirillov, A.; He, K.; Girshick, R.; Rother, C.; Dollar, P. Panoptic Segmentation. In Proceedings of the Computer Vision and Pattern Recognition (CVPR), 15–20 June 2019; pp. 9404–9413.
20. Zhang, R.; Li, G.; Li, M.; Wang, L. Fusion of images and point clouds for the semantic segmentation of large-scale 3D scenes based on deep learning. *ISPRS J. Photogramm. Remote Sens.* **2018**, *143*, 85–96. [CrossRef]
21. Du, J.; Jiang, Z.; Huang, S.; Wang, Z.; Su, J.; Su, S.; Wu, Y.; Cai, G. Point Cloud Semantic Segmentation Network Based on Multi-Scale Feature Fusion. *Sensors* **2021**, *21*, 1625. [CrossRef] [PubMed]
22. Yoo, J.H.; Kim, Y.; Kim, J.; Choi, J.W. 3D-CVF: Generating Joint Camera and LiDAR Features Using Cross-view Spatial Feature Fusion for 3D Object Detection. In *European Conference on Computer Vision*; Springer: Cham, Switzerland, 2020; pp. 720–736.
23. Zhang, Z.; Chen, G.; Wang, X.; Shu, M. DDRNet: Fast point cloud registration network for large-scale scenes. *ISPRS J. Photogramm. Remote Sens.* **2021**, *175*, 184–198. [CrossRef]
24. Ronneberger, O.; Fischer, P.; Brox, T. U-Net: Convolutional Networks for Biomedical Image Segmentation. In *Lecture Notes in Computer Science*; Springer: Cham, Switzerland, 2015.
25. Chen, L.-C.; Papandreou, G.; Kokkinos, I.; Murphy, K.; Yuille, A.L. DeepLab: Semantic Image Segmentation with Deep Convolutional Nets, Atrous Convolution, and Fully Connected CRFs. *IEEE Trans. Pattern Anal. Mach. Intell.* **2018**, *40*, 834–848. [CrossRef]
26. Holschneider, M.; Kronland-Martinet, R.; Morlet, J.; Tchamitchian, P. *A Real-Time Algorithm for Signal Analysis with the Help of the Wavelet Transform*; Wavelets: Berlin/Heidelberg, Germany, 1990.
27. Krähenbühl, P.; Koltun, V. Efficient inference in fully connected crfs with gaussian edge potentials. *Adv. Neural Inf. Process. Syst.* **2011**, *24*.
28. Chen, L.C.; Papandreou, G.; Schroff, F.; Adam, H. Rethinking atrous convolution for semantic image segmentation. Computer Vision and Pattern Recognition. *arXiv* **2017**, arXiv:1706.05587.
29. Chen, L.C.; Zhu, Y.; Papandreou, G.; Schroff, F.; Adam, H. Encoder-decoder with atrous separable convolution for semantic image segmentation. In Proceedings of the European Conference on Computer Vision (ECCV), Munich, Germany, 8–14 September 2018; pp. 801–818.
30. Simonyan, K.; Zisserman, A. Very deep convolutional networks for large-scale image recognition. Computer Vision and Pattern Recognition (CVPR). *arXiv Preprint* **2014**, arXiv:1409.1556.
31. He, K.; Zhang, X.; Ren, S.; Sun, J. Deep residual learning for image recognition. In Proceedings of the IEEE Conference on Computer Vision and Pattern Recognition (CVPR), Las Vegas, NV, USA, 27–30 June 2016; pp. 770–778.
32. Su, H.; Maji, S.; Kalogerakis, E.; Learned-Miller, E. Multi-view Convolutional Neural Networks for 3D Shape Recognition. In Proceedings of the IEEE International Conference on Computer Vision (ICCV), Santiago, Chile, 7–13 December 2015; pp. 945–953.
33. Maturana, D.; Scherer, S. VoxNet: A 3D Convolutional Neural Network for real-time object recognition. In Proceedings of the IEEE/RSJ International Conference on Intelligent Robots and Systems (IROS), Hamburg, Germany, 28 September–2 October 2015.
34. Zhou, Y.; Tuzel, O. Voxelnet: End-to-end learning for point cloud based 3d object detection. In Proceedings of the IEEE Conference on Computer Vision and Pattern Recognition, Salt Lake City, UT, USA, 18–23 June 2018; pp. 4490–4499.
35. Yan, X.; Zheng, C.; Li, Z.; Wang, S.; Cui, S. PointASNL: Robust point clouds processing using nonlocal neural networks with adaptive sampling. In Proceedings of the IEEE/CVF Conference on Computer Vision and Pattern Recognition, Seattle, WA, USA, 13–19 June 2020; pp. 5589–5598.
36. Li, J.; Chen, B.M.; Lee, G.H. So-net: Self-organizing network for point cloud analysis. In Proceedings of the IEEE Conference on Computer Vision and Pattern Recognition, Salt Lake City, UT, USA, 18–23 June 2018; pp. 9397–9406.
37. Boulch, A. ConvPoint: Continuous convolutions for point cloud processing. *Comput. Graph.* **2020**, *88*, 24–34. [CrossRef]
38. Wang, Y.; Sun, Y.; Liu, Z.; Sarma, S.E.; Bronstein, M.M.; Solomon, J. Dynamic Graph CNN for Learning on Point Clouds. *ACM Trans. Graph.* **2019**, *38*, 1–12. [CrossRef]
39. Li, Y.; Ma, L.; Zhong, Z.; Cao, D.; Li, J. TGNet: Geometric Graph CNN on 3-D Point Cloud Segmentation. *IEEE Trans. Geosci. Remote Sens.* **2019**, *58*, 3588–3600. [CrossRef]
40. Wu, Z.; Song, S.; Khosla, A.; Yu, F.; Zhang, L.; Tang, X.; Xiao, J. 3D ShapeNets: A Deep Representation for Volumetric Shapes. In Proceedings of the 28th IEEE Conference on Computer Vision and Pattern Recognition (CVPR), Boston, MA, USA, 7–12 June 2015.
41. Niemeyer, J.; Rottensteiner, F.; Soergel, U. Contextual classification of lidar data and building object detection in urban areas. *ISPRS J. Photogramm. Remote Sens.* **2014**, *87*, 152–165. [CrossRef]
42. Kölle, M.; Laupheimer, D.; Schmohl, S.; Haala, N.; Rottensteiner, F.; Wegner, J.D.; Ledoux, H. The Hessigheim 3D (H3D) benchmark on semantic segmentation of high-resolution 3D point clouds and textured meshes from UAV LiDAR and Multi-View-Stereo. *ISPRS Open J. Photogramm. Remote Sens.* **2021**, *1*, 100001. [CrossRef]
43. Lian, Y.; Feng, T.; Zhou, J.; Jia, M.; Li, A.; Wu, Z.; Jiao, L.; Brown, M.; Hager, G.; Yokoya, N.; et al. Large-Scale Semantic 3-D Reconstruction: Outcome of the 2019 IEEE GRSS Data Fusion Contest-Part B. *IEEE Journal of Selected Topics in Applied Observations and Remote Sensing* **2021**, *14*, 1158–1170. [CrossRef]
44. Current Height File Netherlands 3 (AHN3). Available online: http://data.europa.eu/88u/dataset/41daef8b-155e-4608-b49c-c87ea45d931c (accessed on 8 April 2022).

45. Wichmann, A.; Agoub, A.; Kada, M. RoofN3D: Deep Learning Training Data for 3D Building Reconstruction. *ISPRS-Int. Arch. Photogramm. Remote Sens. Spat. Inf. Sci.* **2018**, *XLII-2*, 1191–1198. [CrossRef]
46. Behley, J.; Garbade, M.; Milioto, A.; Quenzel, J.; Behnke, S.; Stachniss, C.; Gall, J. SemanticKITTI: A Dataset for Semantic Scene Understanding of LiDAR Sequences. In Proceedings of the IEEE International Conference on Computer Vision, Seoul, Korea, 27–28 October 2019; pp. 9297–9307.
47. Thomas, H.; Goulette, F.; Deschaud, J.-E.; Marcotegui, B.; LeGall, Y. Semantic Classification of 3D Point Clouds with Multiscale Spherical Neighborhoods. In Proceedings of the International Conference on 3D Vision (3DV), Verona, Italy, 5–8 September 2018; pp. 390–398.
48. Roynard, X.; Deschaud, J.-E.; Goulette, F. Paris-Lille-3D: A large and high-quality ground-truth urban point cloud dataset for automatic segmentation and classification. *Int. J. Robot. Res.* **2018**, *37*, 545–557. [CrossRef]
49. Tan, W.; Qin, N.; Ma, L.; Li, Y.; Du, J.; Cai, G.; Li, J. Toronto-3D: A large-scale mobile lidar dataset for semantic segmentation of urban roadways. In Proceedings of the IEEE/CVF Conference on Computer Vision and Pattern Recognition Workshops, Seattle, WA, USA, 14–19 June 2020; pp. 202–203.
50. Matrone, F.; Lingua, A.; Pierdicca, R.; Malinverni, E.S.; Paolanti, M.; Grilli, E.; Remondino, F.; Murtiyoso, A.; Landes, T. A Benchmark For Large-Scale Heritage Point Cloud Semantic Segmentation. *ISPRS-Int. Arch. Photogramm. Remote Sens. Spat. Inf. Sci.* **2020**, *XLIII-B2-2*, 1419–1426. [CrossRef]
51. Hackel, T.; Savinov, N.; Ladicky, L.; Wegner, J.D.; Schindler, K.; Pollefeys, M. Schindler and M. Pollefeys. Semantic3d. net: A new large-scale point cloud classification benchmark. *ISPRS Ann. Photogramm. Remote Sens. Spat. Inf. Sci.* **2017**, *IV-1-W1*, 91–98. [CrossRef]
52. Trochta, J.; Krůček, M.; Vrška, T.; Král, K. 3D Forest: An application for descriptions of three-dimensional forest structures using terrestrial LiDAR. *PLoS ONE* **2017**, *12*, e0176871. [CrossRef]
53. Li, Y.; Ma, L.; Zhong, Z.; Liu, F.; Chapman, M.A.; Cao, D.; Li, J. Deep Learning for LiDAR Point Clouds in Autonomous Driving: A Review. *IEEE Trans. Neural Networks Learn. Syst.* **2020**, *32*, 3412–3432. [CrossRef] [PubMed]
54. Boulch, A.; Puy, G.; Marlet, R. FKAConv: Feature-kernel alignment for point cloud convolution. In Proceedings of the Asian Conference on Computer Vision, Kyoto, Japan, 30 November–4 December 2020.
55. Geng, X.; Ji, S.; Lu, M.; Zhao, L. Multi-Scale Attentive Aggregation for LiDAR Point Cloud Segmentation. *Remote Sens.* **2021**, *13*, 691. [CrossRef]
56. Han, X.; Dong, Z.; Yang, B. A point-based deep learning network for semantic segmentation of MLS point clouds. *ISPRS J. Photogramm. Remote Sens.* **2021**, *175*, 199–214. [CrossRef]
57. Özdemir, E.; Remondino, F.; Golkar, A. Aerial Point Cloud Classification with Deep Learning and Machine Learning Algorithms. *ISPRS-Int. Arch. Photogramm. Remote. Sens. Spat. Inf. Sci.* **2019**, *XLII-4/W18*, 843–849. [CrossRef]
58. Shajahan, D.A.; Nayel, V.; Muthuganapathy, R. Roof Classification From 3-D LiDAR Point Clouds Using Multiview CNN with Self-Attention. *IEEE Geosci. Remote Sens. Lett.* **2019**, *17*, 1465–1469. [CrossRef]
59. Zhang, Z.; Sun, L.; Zhong, R.; Chen, D.; Zhang, L.; Li, X.; Wang, Q.; Chen, S. Hierarchical Aggregated Deep Features for ALS Point Cloud Classification. *IEEE Trans. Geosci. Remote Sens.* **2020**, *59*, 1686–1699. [CrossRef]
60. Lei, X.; Wang, H.; Wang, C.; Zhao, Z.; Miao, J.; Tian, P. ALS Point Cloud Classification by Integrating an Improved Fully Convolutional Network into Transfer Learning with Multi-Scale and Multi-View Deep Features. *Sensors* **2020**, *20*, 6969. [CrossRef] [PubMed]
61. Huang, R.; Xu, Y.; Hong, D.; Yao, W.; Ghamisi, P.; Stilla, U. Deep point embedding for urban classification using ALS point clouds: A new perspective from local to global. *ISPRS J. Photogramm. Remote Sens.* **2020**, *163*, 62–81. [CrossRef]
62. Krisanski, S.; Taskhiri, M.; Aracil, S.G.; Herries, D.; Turner, P. Sensor Agnostic Semantic Segmentation of Structurally Diverse and Complex Forest Point Clouds Using Deep Learning. *Remote Sens.* **2021**, *13*, 1413. [CrossRef]
63. Shinohara, T.; Xiu, H.; Matsuoka, M. FWNet: Semantic Segmentation for Full-Waveform LiDAR Data Using Deep Learning. *Sensors* **2020**, *20*, 3568. [CrossRef]
64. Wen, C.; Yang, L.; Li, X.; Peng, L.; Chi, T. Directionally constrained fully convolutional neural network for airborne LiDAR point cloud classification. *ISPRS J. Photogramm. Remote Sens.* **2020**, *162*, 50–62. [CrossRef]
65. Turgeon-Pelchat, M.; Foucher, S.; Bouroubi, Y. Deep Learning-Based Classification of Large-Scale Airborne LiDAR Point Cloud. *Can. J. Remote Sens.* **2021**, *47*, 381–395. [CrossRef]
66. Zhang, L. Deep Learning-Based Classification and Reconstruction of Residential Scenes from Large-Scale Point Clouds. *IEEE Trans. Geosci. Remote Sens.* **2017**, *56*, 1887–1897. [CrossRef]
67. Wen, C.; Li, X.; Yao, X.; Peng, L.; Chi, T. Airborne LiDAR point cloud classification with global-local graph attention convolution neural network. *ISPRS J. Photogramm. Remote Sens.* **2021**, *173*, 181–194. [CrossRef]
68. Widyaningrum, E.; Bai, Q.; Fajari, M.; Lindenbergh, R. Airborne Laser Scanning Point Cloud Classification Using the DGCNN Deep Learning Method. *Remote Sens.* **2021**, *13*, 859. [CrossRef]
69. Ghasemieh, A.; Kashef, R. 3D object detection for autonomous driving: Methods, models, sensors, data, and challenges. *Transportation Engineering* **2022**, *8*, 100115. [CrossRef]
70. Guo, Y.; Wang, H.; Hu, Q.; Liu, H.; Liu, L.; Bennamoun, M. Deep Learning for 3D Point Clouds: A Survey. *IEEE Trans. Pattern Anal. Mach. Intell.* **2020**, *43*, 4338–4364. [CrossRef]

71. Jebamikyous, H.H.; Kashef, R. Autonomous Vehicles Perception (AVP) Using Deep Learning: Modeling, Assessment, and Challenges. *IEEE Access* **2022**, *10*, 10523–10535. [CrossRef]
72. Jebamikyous, H.H.; Kashef, R. (2021, December). Deep Learning-Based Semantic Segmentation in Autonomous Driving. In Proceedings of the 2021 IEEE 23rd Int Conf on High Performance Computing & Communications; 7th Int Conf on Data Science & Systems; 19th Int Conf on Smart City; 7th Int Conf on Dependability in Sensor, Cloud & Big Data Systems & Application (HPCC/DSS/SmartCity/DependSys), Haikou, Hainan, China, 20–22 December 2021.

MDPI
St. Alban-Anlage 66
4052 Basel
Switzerland
www.mdpi.com

Sensors Editorial Office
E-mail: sensors@mdpi.com
www.mdpi.com/journal/sensors

www.ingramcontent.com/pod-product-compliance
Lightning Source LLC
LaVergne TN
LVHW070501100526
838202LV00014B/1766
* 9 7 8 3 0 3 6 5 8 4 2 8 7 *